# SECOND EDITION
# ACUPUNCTURE
## an anatomical approach

## SECOND EDITION
# ACUPUNCTURE
## an anatomical approach

**HOUCHI DUNG**

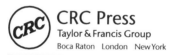

CRC Press
Taylor & Francis Group
Boca Raton London New York

CRC Press is an imprint of the
Taylor & Francis Group, an **informa** business

CRC Press
Taylor & Francis Group
6000 Broken Sound Parkway NW, Suite 300
Boca Raton, FL 33487-2742

© 2014 by Taylor & Francis Group, LLC
CRC Press is an imprint of Taylor & Francis Group, an Informa business

No claim to original U.S. Government works

Printed on acid-free paper
Version Date: 20130925

International Standard Book Number-13: 978-1-4665-8192-0 (Hardback)

This book contains information obtained from authentic and highly regarded sources. While all reasonable efforts have been made to publish reliable data and information, neither the author[s] nor the publisher can accept any legal responsibility or liability for any errors or omissions that may be made. The publishers wish to make clear that any views or opinions expressed in this book by individual editors, authors or contributors are personal to them and do not necessarily reflect the views/opinions of the publishers. The information or guidance contained in this book is intended for use by medical, scientific or health-care professionals and is provided strictly as a supplement to the medical or other professional's own judgement, their knowledge of the patient's medical history, relevant manufacturer's instructions and the appropriate best practice guidelines. Because of the rapid advances in medical science, any information or advice on dosages, procedures or diagnoses should be independently verified. The reader is strongly urged to consult the drug companies' printed instructions, and their websites, before administering any of the drugs recommended in this book. This book does not indicate whether a particular treatment is appropriate or suitable for a particular individual. Ultimately it is the sole responsibility of the medical professional to make his or her own professional judgements, so as to advise and treat patients appropriately. The authors and publishers have also attempted to trace the copyright holders of all material reproduced in this publication and apologize to copyright holders if permission to publish in this form has not been obtained. If any copyright material has not been acknowledged please write and let us know so we may rectify in any future reprint.

Except as permitted under U.S. Copyright Law, no part of this book may be reprinted, reproduced, transmitted, or utilized in any form by any electronic, mechanical, or other means, now known or hereafter invented, including photocopying, microfilming, and recording, or in any information storage or retrieval system, without written permission from the publishers.

For permission to photocopy or use material electronically from this work, please access www.copyright.com (http://www.copyright.com/) or contact the Copyright Clearance Center, Inc. (CCC), 222 Rosewood Drive, Danvers, MA 01923, 978-750-8400. CCC is a not-for-profit organization that provides licenses and registration for a variety of users. For organizations that have been granted a photocopy license by the CCC, a separate system of payment has been arranged.

**Trademark Notice:** Product or corporate names may be trademarks or registered trademarks, and are used only for identification and explanation without intent to infringe.

**Library of Congress Cataloging-in-Publication Data**

Dung, H. C., author.
   Acupuncture : an anatomical approach / Houchi Dung. -- Second edition.
   p. ; cm.
   Includes bibliographical references and index.
   ISBN 978-1-4665-8192-0 (hardcover : alk. paper)
   I. Title.
   [DNLM: 1.  Acupuncture. 2.  Neuroanatomy.  WB 369]
   RM184
   615.8'92--dc23
                                              2013038109

**Visit the Taylor & Francis Web site at**
http://www.taylorandfrancis.com

**and the CRC Press Web site at**
http://www.crcpress.com

# Dedication

*To my wife, Elizabeth Izu Dunn.*

# Contents

Preface to Second English Edition ........................................................................... xv
Preface to First English Edition .............................................................................. xxi
Preface to *Anatomical Acupuncture* ..................................................................... xxiii
Author ....................................................................................................................... xxv

**Chapter 1** Introduction ......................................................................................... 1

References ............................................................................................... 10

**Chapter 2** Anatomy in Acupuncture ................................................................... 11

2.1 General Consideration ............................................................... 11
2.2 Identity of Acupoints ................................................................. 11
2.3 All in the Sensory Nerves .......................................................... 12
    2.3.1 Organization of the Nervous System ............................ 12
    2.3.2 The Peripheral Nervous System ..................................... 13
    2.3.3 The Neuron ....................................................................... 13
    2.3.4 Histology of Nerves ......................................................... 14
    2.3.5 Divisions of the Nerves ................................................... 16
2.4 Efferent Fibers ............................................................................. 16
    2.4.1 Efferent Fibers to Skeletal Muscles ............................... 16
    2.4.2 Autonomic Nervous System ........................................... 16
2.5 Afferent Fibers ............................................................................ 16
    2.5.1 For Special Senses ........................................................... 17
    2.5.2 For General Senses .......................................................... 17
2.6 Muscular Nerve Branches ......................................................... 18
2.7 Cutaneous Nerve Branches ....................................................... 19
2.8 Anatomical Features Contributing to the Formation of Acupoints ................. 19
    2.8.1 Size ..................................................................................... 19
    2.8.2 Depth .................................................................................. 19
    2.8.3 Penetration of the Deep Fascia ...................................... 19
    2.8.4 Passage through Bone Foramina ................................... 20
    2.8.5 Motor Point ....................................................................... 20
    2.8.6 Concomitant Blood Vessels ............................................ 20
    2.8.7 Nerve Fiber Compositions .............................................. 21
    2.8.8 Points of Bifurcation ........................................................ 21
    2.8.9 Sensitive Points on Tendons and Ligaments ............... 21
    2.8.10 Suture Lines on the Skull ............................................... 22
2.9 Discussion and Conclusion ....................................................... 22
References ............................................................................................... 23

**Chapter 3** Acupoints of the Cranial Nerves ....................................................... 25

3.1 Cranial Nerves without Acupoints ........................................... 25
    3.1.1 Afferent Fibers Only ........................................................ 25
        3.1.1.1 Olfactory Nerve .............................................. 25
        3.1.1.2 Optic Nerve ..................................................... 25

|  |  | 3.1.1.3 | Statoacoustic Nerve | 25 |
|---|---|---|---|---|
|  | 3.1.2 | Efferent Fibers Only | | 26 |
|  |  | 3.1.2.1 | Oculomotor Nerve | 26 |
|  |  | 3.1.2.2 | Trochlear Nerve | 26 |
|  |  | 3.1.2.3 | Abducens Nerve | 26 |
|  |  | 3.1.2.4 | Hypoglossal Nerve | 26 |
| 3.2 | Cranial Nerves with Acupoints | | | 26 |
| 3.3 | Trigeminal Nerve | | | 26 |
|  | 3.3.1 | Acupoints of Cutaneous Branches | | 28 |
|  |  | 3.3.1.1 | Supraorbital | 28 |
|  |  | 3.3.1.2 | Supratrochlear and Infratrochlear | 28 |
|  |  | 3.3.1.3 | Lacrimal | 29 |
|  |  | 3.3.1.4 | Infraorbital | 29 |
|  |  | 3.3.1.5 | Zygomaticotemporal and Zygomaticofacial | 29 |
|  |  | 3.3.1.6 | Mental | 29 |
|  |  | 3.3.1.7 | Auriculotemporal | 29 |
|  |  | 3.3.1.8 | Paranasal | 30 |
|  | 3.3.2 | Acupoints of Connective Tissue | | 30 |
|  |  | 3.3.2.1 | Bregma | 32 |
|  |  | 3.3.2.2 | Pterion | 32 |
|  |  | 3.3.2.3 | Nasion | 32 |
|  |  | 3.3.2.4 | Coronal Suture | 32 |
|  |  | 3.3.2.5 | Temporomandibular | 32 |
|  | 3.3.3 | Acupoints of Muscular Branches | | 33 |
|  |  | 3.3.3.1 | Masseter | 33 |
|  |  | 3.3.3.2 | Temporalis | 34 |
|  |  | 3.3.3.3 | Anterior Auricular and Superior Auricular | 34 |
| 3.4 | Facial Nerve | | | 34 |
| 3.5 | Glossopharyngeal Nerve | | | 35 |
| 3.6 | Vagus Nerve | | | 35 |
| 3.7 | Spinal Accessory Nerve | | | 36 |
| References | | | | 37 |

**Chapter 4** Acupoints in the Neck Region ... 39

| 4.1 | Boundaries of the Neck | | 39 |
|---|---|---|---|
| 4.2 | Formation of the Cervical Plexus | | 39 |
| 4.3 | Acupoints of the Cutaneous Branches | | 40 |
|  | 4.3.1 | Greater Auricular | 40 |
|  | 4.3.2 | Lesser Occipital | 40 |
|  | 4.3.3 | Transverse Cervical | 41 |
|  | 4.3.4 | Supraclavicular | 42 |
| 4.4 | Acupoints of Muscular Branches | | 42 |
| References | | | 42 |

**Chapter 5** Acupoints in the Upper Limb ... 43

| 5.1 | Topography of the Upper Limb | | 43 |
|---|---|---|---|
| 5.2 | Organization of the Brachial Plexus | | 43 |
| 5.3 | Acupoints on the Pectoral Region | | 44 |
| 5.4 | Acupoints over the Scapular Region | | 45 |
|  | 5.4.1 | Dorsal Scapular | 45 |

|  |  |  |  |
|---|---|---|---|
| | 5.4.2 | Supraspinatus or Suprascapular II | 46 |
| | 5.4.3 | Infraspinatus or Suprascapular I | 46 |
| 5.5 | Arm and Forearm | | 47 |
| | 5.5.1 | The Muscular Branches | 47 |
| | | 5.5.1.1 Musculocutaneous or Biceps Brachii | 47 |
| | | 5.5.1.2 Median | 47 |
| | | 5.5.1.3 Axillary | 47 |
| | | 5.5.1.4 Teres Minor | 48 |
| | | 5.5.1.5 Deltoid | 49 |
| | | 5.5.1.6 Radial | 49 |
| | | 5.5.1.7 Deep Radial | 50 |
| | | 5.5.1.8 Posterior Interosseus | 50 |
| | 5.5.2 | Cutaneous Branches | 50 |
| | | 5.5.2.1 Posterior Brachial Cutaneous | 50 |
| | | 5.5.2.2 Lateral Brachial Cutaneous | 50 |
| | | 5.5.2.3 Medial Brachial Cutaneous | 51 |
| | | 5.5.2.4 Lateral Antebrachial Cutaneous | 51 |
| | | 5.5.2.5 Medial Antebrachial Cutaneous | 51 |
| | | 5.5.2.6 Posterior Antebrachial Cutaneous | 51 |
| | 5.5.3 | Acupoints over Tendons and Ligaments | 51 |
| | | 5.5.3.1 Tendon of the Biceps Brachii | 52 |
| | | 5.5.3.2 Lateral Epicondyle of the Elbow | 52 |
| | | 5.5.3.3 Flexor Retinaculum over the Wrist | 52 |
| 5.6 | Wrist and Hand | | 52 |
| | 5.6.1 | Muscular Branches | 53 |
| | | 5.6.1.1 Recurrent of Median | 53 |
| | | 5.6.1.2 Ulnar | 54 |
| | 5.6.2 | Cutaneous Branches | 54 |
| | | 5.6.2.1 Superficial Radial | 54 |
| | | 5.6.2.2 Interphalangeal Points | 54 |
| References | | | 54 |

**Chapter 6** Acupoints in the Body Trunk .................................................................. 55

| | | | |
|---|---|---|---|
| 6.1 | Defining a Typical Spinal Nerve | | 55 |
| | 6.1.1 | Two Roots with One Ganglion | 55 |
| | 6.1.2 | Two Primary Rami | 55 |
| | 6.1.3 | Muscular Branches without Anatomical Names | 55 |
| | 6.1.4 | Three Cutaneous Nerves with Six Terminal Branches | 55 |
| 6.2 | Composition of Fibers in the Typical Spinal Nerves | | 57 |
| | 6.2.1 | Efferent Fibers to Skeletal Muscles | 57 |
| | 6.2.2 | Autonomic Nervous System | 57 |
| | | 6.2.2.1 Sympathetic Nerves | 57 |
| | | 6.2.2.2 Parasympathetic Nerves | 58 |
| | 6.2.3 | Afferent Fibers for General Senses | 58 |
| 6.3 | Distributions of Acupoints | | 59 |
| | 6.3.1 | Back of the Body Trunk | 59 |
| | 6.3.2 | Front of the Body | 59 |
| | 6.3.3 | Lateral Side | 59 |
| 6.4 | Acupoints on Back of the Neck | | 60 |
| | 6.4.1 | Greater Occipital | 60 |

|  |  | 6.4.2 | Third Occipital .................................................................. 61 |
|---|---|---|---|

- 6.5 Acupoints on the Dorsal Surface of the Chest .................................................. 61
  - 6.5.1 Posterior Cutaneous Points ........................................................... 61
  - 6.5.2 Acupoints of the Thoracic Spinal Process ................................. 63
- 6.6 Acupoints on the Lumbar and Sacrum ............................................................. 63
  - 6.6.1 Posterior Cutaneous of the Lumbar Spinal Nerves ..................... 64
  - 6.6.2 On the Lumbar Spinous Processes ............................................. 65
  - 6.6.3 Posterior Cutaneous of the Sacral Spinal Nerves ....................... 65
  - 6.6.4 Superior Cluneal ......................................................................... 65
- 6.7 Acupoints in the Front .................................................................................... 65
  - 6.7.1 Anterior Cutaneous .................................................................... 65
  - 6.7.2 Xiphoid Point ............................................................................. 66
  - 6.7.3 Angle of the Chest Cage Point .................................................. 66
  - 6.7.4 Umbilical Point ......................................................................... 66
- 6.8 Lateral Side of the Chest Cage ....................................................................... 66
  - 6.8.1 Lateral Cutaneous ...................................................................... 66
  - 6.8.2 Intercostobrachial ...................................................................... 67
- References ................................................................................................................. 67

**Chapter 7** Acupoints in the Lower Limb ................................................................... 69

- 7.1 Regional Anatomy ......................................................................................... 69
- 7.2 Lumbar Plexus ............................................................................................... 69
- 7.3 Sacral Plexus .................................................................................................. 69
- 7.4 Acupoints of the Lumbar Plexus .................................................................... 71
  - 7.4.1 Cutaneous Branches .................................................................. 71
    - 7.4.1.1 Iliohypogastric ........................................................... 71
    - 7.4.1.2 Ilioinguinal ................................................................. 72
    - 7.4.1.3 Genitofemoral ............................................................ 73
    - 7.4.1.4 Cutaneous of Obturator ............................................. 73
    - 7.4.1.5 Lateral Femoral Cutaneous ....................................... 74
    - 7.4.1.6 Anterior Femoral Cutaneous ..................................... 74
    - 7.4.1.7 Parapatellar ................................................................ 75
    - 7.4.1.8 Saphenous .................................................................. 75
  - 7.4.2 Muscular Branches .................................................................... 75
    - 7.4.2.1 Obturator ................................................................... 75
    - 7.4.2.2 Rectus Femoris .......................................................... 75
    - 7.4.2.3 Vastus Lateralis ......................................................... 75
    - 7.4.2.4 Vastus Medialis ......................................................... 76
    - 7.4.2.5 Sartorius .................................................................... 76
    - 7.4.2.6 Femoral ...................................................................... 76
- 7.5 Acupoints of the Sacral Plexus ...................................................................... 76
- 7.6 Distributions to the Thigh .............................................................................. 76
  - 7.6.1 In the Posterior Compartment ................................................... 76
    - 7.6.1.1 Gluteal Fold Point ..................................................... 76
    - 7.6.1.2 Posterior Femoral Cutaneous .................................... 77
    - 7.6.1.3 Inferior Gluteal ......................................................... 77
  - 7.6.2 In the Lateral Compartment ...................................................... 77
    - 7.6.2.1 Greater Trochanter Point ........................................... 78
    - 7.6.2.2 Iliotibial Tract Point .................................................. 78
    - 7.6.2.3 Biceps Femoris Point ................................................ 79

Contents

- 7.7 Distributions in the Popliteal Fossa .................................................. 79
  - 7.7.1 Sciatic Point ........................................................................ 79
  - 7.7.2 Lateral Popliteal Point ........................................................ 79
  - 7.7.3 Medial Popliteal Point ........................................................ 79
- 7.8 Acupoints on the Posterior Compartment of the Leg and Ankle ..... 79
  - 7.8.1 Medial Sural ....................................................................... 80
  - 7.8.2 Sural ................................................................................... 80
  - 7.8.3 Medial Achilles ................................................................... 80
  - 7.8.4 Lateral Achilles .................................................................. 80
- 7.9 Acupoints on the Lateral Compartment of the Leg .......................... 80
  - 7.9.1 Peroneus Longus ................................................................ 80
  - 7.9.2 Peroneus Brevis .................................................................. 81
  - 7.9.3 Peroneus Tertius ................................................................. 81
- 7.10 Acupoints on the Anterior Compartment of the Leg ........................ 81
- 7.11 Acupoints on the Foot ...................................................................... 82
  - 7.11.1 Dorsal Surface of the Foot ................................................. 82
    - 7.11.1.1 Superficial Peroneal ......................................... 83
    - 7.11.1.2 Deep Peroneal .................................................. 83
    - 7.11.1.3 Metatarsal ......................................................... 83
    - 7.11.1.4 Talus .................................................................. 83
    - 7.11.1.5 Cuneiforms ....................................................... 83
    - 7.11.1.6 Dorsal Digital ................................................... 83
    - 7.11.1.7 Lateroinferior Malleolar ................................... 83
    - 7.11.1.8 Lateroanterior Malleolar .................................. 83
    - 7.11.1.9 Lateral Calcaneous ........................................... 83
    - 7.11.1.10 Cuboid .............................................................. 84
  - 7.11.2 Plantar Surface of the Foot ................................................ 84
    - 7.11.2.1 Tibial Point ....................................................... 84
    - 7.11.2.2 Medioanterior Malleolar .................................. 84
    - 7.11.2.3 Medioinferior Malleolar ................................... 84
    - 7.11.2.4 Medioposterior Malleolar ................................. 84
    - 7.11.2.5 Medial Calcaneous ........................................... 84
    - 7.11.2.6 Navicular Point ................................................. 85
    - 7.11.2.7 First Metatarsal Point ....................................... 85
    - 7.11.2.8 Flexor Digitorum Longus ................................. 85
    - 7.11.2.9 Plantar Point ..................................................... 85
    - 7.11.2.10 Medial Plantar Point ........................................ 85
    - 7.11.2.11 Lateral Plantar Point ........................................ 85
    - 7.11.2.12 Calcaneus ......................................................... 85
- References ................................................................................................. 85

**Chapter 8** Physiology in Acupuncture ........................................................... 87
- 8.1 Electrical Phenomena of the Body ................................................... 87
  - 8.1.1 Excitability ......................................................................... 87
  - 8.1.2 Polarization and Action Potential ...................................... 87
  - 8.1.3 Threshold ............................................................................ 88
  - 8.1.4 Conductivity ....................................................................... 88
  - 8.1.5 Fatigue ................................................................................ 88
- 8.2 Electrical Activity in Acupoints ....................................................... 88
- 8.3 Dynamic Nature of Acupoints .......................................................... 89

8.4 Three Phases of Acupoints ................................................................... 90
    8.4.1 Latent Phase .......................................................................... 90
    8.4.2 Passive Phase ........................................................................ 90
    8.4.3 Active Phase ......................................................................... 91
8.5 Physical Properties of Acupoints .......................................................... 92
    8.5.1 Sensitivity ............................................................................. 92
    8.5.2 Sequence ............................................................................... 93
    8.5.3 Specificity ............................................................................. 93
References ........................................................................................................ 94

**Chapter 9** Biochemistry in Acupuncture ................................................................. 95

9.1 Biochemistry in Relation to Acupuncture ............................................. 95
9.2 Terminologies in Neurotransmitters ...................................................... 95
    9.2.1 Neuroreceptor ....................................................................... 95
    9.2.2 Agonist and Antagonist ........................................................ 95
    9.2.3 Synapses ................................................................................ 96
    9.2.4 Granules ................................................................................ 96
    9.2.5 Neuromuscular Junction ...................................................... 96
9.3 Relevance of Neurotransmitters ............................................................ 96
9.4 Importance of Endorphin ....................................................................... 97
9.5 Other Neurotransmitters ........................................................................ 98
    9.5.1 Catecholamines .................................................................... 98
    9.5.2 Serotonin ............................................................................... 99
    9.5.3 Histamine .............................................................................. 99
    9.5.4 Neuroactive Peptides ......................................................... 100
    9.5.5 Amino Acids as Neurotransmitters ................................... 100
    9.5.6 Adenosine ........................................................................... 101
9.6 Immediate Acupuncture Reactions ..................................................... 101
    9.6.1 Atopic Erythroid Skin Change ........................................... 102
    9.6.2 Sweating ............................................................................. 102
    9.6.3 Syncope .............................................................................. 103
9.7 Reactions after Acupuncture ............................................................... 103
    9.7.1 Flare-Up of Pain ................................................................. 104
    9.7.2 Drowsiness and Sleeplessness ........................................... 104
    9.7.3 Parasympathetic Enhancement .......................................... 106
References ...................................................................................................... 106

**Chapter 10** Pathology in Acupuncture ................................................................ 107

10.1 Conventional Wisdom in Pathology .................................................. 107
10.2 Pathological Origins ........................................................................... 107
10.3 Endogenous Origins ............................................................................ 107
    10.3.1 Hormonal Imbalances ...................................................... 108
    10.3.2 Poor Blood Circulation .................................................... 109
    10.3.3 Degeneration .................................................................... 109
    10.3.4 Infections .......................................................................... 110
10.4 Exogenous Origins .............................................................................. 110
10.5 Modes for Trigger Points to Appear .................................................. 111
    10.5.1 Systemic ........................................................................... 112
    10.5.2 Regional ........................................................................... 114

Contents         xiii

       10.6     Combination of Systemic and Regional Appearances .................................. 115
       10.7     A Special Case.............................................................................................. 118
       10.8     A Few Conclusions ...................................................................................... 118
       References .................................................................................................................. 119

## Chapter 11   Psychology in Acupuncture........................................................................................ 121

       11.1     Psychology of Pain ...................................................................................... 121
       11.2     True or False................................................................................................ 123
       11.3     Historical Prospect of Pain Perception......................................................... 124
       11.4     Mental Attitude toward Pain ....................................................................... 125
       11.5     The Vicious Cycle of Pain ........................................................................... 127
       11.6     Rebutting Acupuncture as Placebo.............................................................. 128
       References .................................................................................................................. 128

## Chapter 12   Pain and Measurement .............................................................................................. 129

       12.1     A Challenge and a Puzzle............................................................................ 129
       12.2     Measurements of Pain ................................................................................. 129
       12.3     Subjective Pain versus Objective Pain......................................................... 130
       12.4     Ranking the Trigger Points ......................................................................... 131
       12.5     Trigger Points in Four Groups..................................................................... 132
                12.5.1    Primary Points.............................................................................. 133
                12.5.2    Secondary Points.......................................................................... 133
                12.5.3    Tertiary Points.............................................................................. 135
                12.5.4    Nonspecific Points........................................................................ 136
       12.6     Trigger Points on the Spinous Processes..................................................... 136
       12.7     Results of Pain Measurement...................................................................... 139
                12.7.1    Pain Measurement by Counting Trigger Points in the Thoracic
                             Vertebrae ..................................................................................... 141
                12.7.2    Pain Measurement by Counting Trigger Points in the Body........... 143
       12.8     Acute versus Chronic Pain .......................................................................... 146
       References .................................................................................................................. 147

## Chapter 13   Good to Excellent Applications ................................................................................ 149

       13.1     General Guidelines...................................................................................... 149
       13.2     Samples of Pain for Demonstration............................................................. 150
       13.3     Defining Good to Excellent Results............................................................ 152
       13.4     Pain in the Face and Head ........................................................................... 152
       13.5     Pain in the Neck and Shoulders................................................................... 155
       13.6     Pain in the Upper Limbs.............................................................................. 158
       13.7     Pain in the Body Trunk ............................................................................... 159
       13.8     Pain in the Lower Limbs ............................................................................. 163
                13.8.1    Meralgia Paraesthetica or Bernhardt Disease............................... 164
                13.8.2    Pain in the Region of the Knee Joint............................................ 164
                13.8.3    Pain in Other Locations of the Lower Limb ................................ 166
       References .................................................................................................................. 166

## Chapter 14   Applications with Mixed and Limited Results ......................................................... 167

       14.1     Defining Mixed and Limited....................................................................... 167

|  | 14.1.1 | In Terms of Patient Profiles | 167 |
|---|---|---|---|

        14.1.1  In Terms of Patient Profiles ......................................................... 167
        14.1.2  In Terms of Number of Treatments ............................................ 168
        14.1.3  In Terms of Pain Relief and Relapse ......................................... 168
  14.2  Irrelevant to Pain ....................................................................................... 168
        14.2.1  Weight Reduction ...................................................................... 168
        14.2.2  Infertile Pregnancy .................................................................... 170
  14.3  Subjective Pain Perceived ......................................................................... 172
  14.4  Pain in the Face and Head ........................................................................ 174
        14.4.1  Migraine ..................................................................................... 174
        14.4.2  Trigeminal Neuralgia or Tic Douloureux ................................. 177
        14.4.3  Postherpetic Neuralgia in the Face and Head ........................... 179
  14.5  Pain in the Neck and Shoulder ................................................................. 182
        14.5.1  Whiplash .................................................................................... 182
        14.5.2  Arthritic Neck ............................................................................ 183
  14.6  Pain in the Upper Limb ............................................................................ 184
        14.6.1  Biceps Tendinitis ....................................................................... 185
        14.6.2  Carpal Tunnel Syndrome .......................................................... 186
  14.7  Pain in the Body Trunk ............................................................................ 188
        14.7.1  Postherpetic Neuralgia .............................................................. 188
        14.7.2  Lower Back Pain ....................................................................... 190
  14.8  Pain in the Lower Limb ............................................................................ 193
        14.8.1  Knee Pain ................................................................................... 196
        14.8.2  Pain in the Foot ......................................................................... 197
  14.9  Diffuse Pain .............................................................................................. 198
  References ........................................................................................................... 199

**Chapter 15**  Difficult Patients with Poor Results ........................................................... 201
  15.1  Connecting Difficult and Poor .................................................................. 201
  15.2  Profiles of Difficult Patients ..................................................................... 201
  15.3  Pain in the Face and Head ........................................................................ 203
        15.3.1  Migraine ..................................................................................... 203
        15.3.2  Postherpetic Neuralgia .............................................................. 203
  15.4  Difficult Pain from the Neck to the Fingers ............................................. 206
        15.4.1  Torticollis in Perpetual Motion ................................................. 206
        15.4.2  Severe Arthritis inside the Shoulder Joint ................................ 207
        15.4.3  Carpal Tunnel Syndrome .......................................................... 207
        15.4.4  Deformities and Pain ................................................................ 208
  15.5  Pain after Surgery ..................................................................................... 209
        15.5.1  Lower Back Pain after Surgery ................................................ 210
        15.5.2  Pain after Hip Replacement ...................................................... 212
  15.6  Phantom Limb Pain .................................................................................. 213
  15.7  Spondylitic Abnormalities ........................................................................ 214
  15.8  Reflex Sympathetic Dystrophy ................................................................. 217
  15.9  Tailbone Fracture ...................................................................................... 217
  15.10  Difficult Patients with Different Results ................................................ 218
  15.11  A Few Afterthoughts ............................................................................... 218
  15.12  Editor's Afterword .................................................................................. 220
  References ........................................................................................................... 220

**Index** ............................................................................................................................. 223

# Preface to Second English Edition

In 1970, I was offered a tenure track faculty position in the Department of Anatomy, University of Texas Medical School at San Antonio, and arrived in July of that year to accept that position. By October of 1972, I began to receive inquiries from medical students about learning acupuncture. The timing was not coincidental; after nearly 30 years of Cold War era tension between China and the United States, President Richard Nixon had reopened the diplomatic doors to China.

Many Americans of myriad professions, physicians included, began to arrive in China, discovering new methods and practices almost completely unknown in the western world. When the travelers returned to the United States, they shared what they observed with their fellow countrymen. One astonishing technique that came back with a few physicians was acupuncture anesthesia. Patients received operations on surgical tables while totally awake. To doctors trained in the tradition of sedatives, acupuncture anesthesia appeared to be magic, sparking a quick and sudden soaring of interest in acupuncture, to which my medical students were no exception.

At the time, there were very few faculty members at the school who were ethnically Chinese. Although I was born in Taiwan and have absolutely no relationship with China in any sense, I do possess a certain degree of sophistication in relation to China's cultural heritage (including acupuncture). I did not hesitate to share the knowledge I have of acupuncture, and thus, I ultimately became infamous throughout campus as "the acupuncturist." So when *San Antonio Express/News* reporter D. Dreier was looking for someone who would know something about acupuncture, my name was suggested to him. He came to interview me and wrote a lengthy article that was published in the local newspaper on Sunday, February 27, 1972. The next morning, when I arrived at my office at the school, there were more than a dozen telephone calls awaiting me. All of the callers wanted to know if I could use acupuncture to relieve their pain. For the next few days, the phone rang off the hook with people asking the same thing. At that moment, I came to realize that acupuncture had marketing potential as a therapeutic modality for pain management, although I didn't yet know if acupuncture would indeed be effective to stop any pain.

Eventually, I agreed to offer an elective called theoretical acupuncture for students who were curious about the ancient Chinese practice. The registrar form shows that on October 25, 1972, Jeffery W. Jordan was the first student to enroll in the course. However, the elective didn't last long; after teaching theoretical acupuncture to a few students for just 2 years, I canceled the class. There were four reasons for making such a decision. First, I was a junior faculty member without tenure in the department. I had a family, and I needed the job security that only tenure offered. To better my position, I needed to devote all my time to research activities. Second, teaching an elective such as theoretical acupuncture doesn't help one advance, in terms of either promotion or salary. Why waste my valuable time doing something for nothing in return? Third, like many events or phenomena in medicine, there was always the looming possibility of acupuncture becoming another passing fad, destined to disappear in time from people's memory. If, indeed, acupuncture turned out to be another temporary trend, my effort would become an unattainable dream. Fourth, because the class focused on only the theoretical, the elective consisted only of oral presentation, without any practical applications. There was not a single patient available for bedside clinical training. Without a sensible purpose, the words I preached about acupuncture were useless. It took many more years before the teaching of anatomical acupuncture would be meaningful, with real patients to treat.

To my surprise, 10 years later, I still regularly received regular inquiries from medical students across the country who wanted to learn acupuncture. Such a fact drew me to conclude that interest in acupuncture among medical students in the United States was more pervasive than I had previously realized. By then, I was a tenured associate professor with a secure position, and I didn't have to worry about my livelihood.

There was another reason that I had to offer acupuncture. In the intervening years between 1978 and 1982, one freshman student, Shari Thomas, suffered from acute and severe neck pain because of an automobile accident. After different medical procedures failed to eradicate her pain, she approached me for help. One acupuncture session stopped her neck pain completely. She was so impressed and inspired that she begged me to teach her acupuncture. I promised that I would teach her during her senior year. Three years later, Shari came to knock on the door of my office and immediately asked, "Dr. Dung, do you remember me?" Without excuses and obligated to keep my promise to Shari, I indicated to my Chairman, Edward G. Rennels, PhD, that I had decided to give up my endeavors in scientific research and would like to devote my time to the study and practice acupuncture. He was not only sympathetic to my decision, but fully supportive of it. My elective was renamed "anatomical acupuncture."

That year, I ended up teaching anatomical acupuncture to eight medical students. The following year, in 1983, the number increased to 12. Soon, anatomical acupuncture, without exaggeration, became the most popular elective on campus. At that time, it came to my mind that I needed a suitable textbook to teach my elective. That was when I conceived the idea of writing a book on anatomical acupuncture.

Student evaluation forms from the end of the course always had inspiring comments. Here are just a few examples:

"Wonderful opportunity. Please, continue this elective. Great for anatomy and physical examination." (Joyce Mauk, May 1983.)

"If the medical school or MCH had an acupuncture clinic, students could practice acupuncture skills and would probably learn more." (Gail Scott Hovorka, April 20, 1983.)

"This may be one of the most useful courses I've taken in all the 4 years. Good review of anatomy." (Susan Joerns, February 14, 1983.)

"Based on what I observed, acupuncture can be very useful and should be researched much more extensively." (Mark Johnson, May 9, 1983.)

"After taking this elective, I find that there are certain cases when acupuncture is very beneficial. I was surprised at the level of pain relief, for example, some patients with chronic pain received. My suggestion is that the pain clinic at our hospital should use this mode of treatment in patients who are refractory to medicines or for some reason or another can't tolerate pain medications. I feel that acupuncture needs to be fully researched in a scientific manner in order to give it an objective evaluation as to its 'real' value for the treatment of pain. Our school has the opportunity and the acupuncturist to do this work." (Josue Montanoz, May 24, 1983.)

"Excellent course, good didactic and clinical instruction. Look forward to completion and publication of Dr. Dung's book, which will be an invaluable aid in the course." (Chris Wahlberg, May 5, 1983.)

"Dr. Dung was one of the most concerned teachers I have had at this medical school. Well-organized. Continue having students practice on one another." (Anna C. Miller, March 23, 1983.)

Unfortunately, the school hierarchy had a different opinion toward acupuncture than my students and I. One day in April of 1987, Erle K. Adrian, Jr., MD, PhD, Professor and Deputy Chairman of my department, handed me a memo addressed to him from Peter O. Kohler, MD, Dean of the Medical School. The memo stated: "We finally had a meeting of the Executive Committee. This was the first since you and I discussed acupuncture. As you may have anticipated, we decided that we do not want an acupuncture elective in the medical school. I will inform Doctor Grant and the Dean's Office so that no further elective forms are signed." And that was officially the end of my

## Preface to Second English Edition

elective. I often wonder what acupuncture would be today if I had been allowed to teach anatomical acupuncture in the medical school through the years.

Although anatomical acupuncture as an elective for medical students was officially killed and dead, the teaching and writing of acupuncture stayed alive and thrived because no one, not even a school bureaucracy, could terminate the desire to learn something that someone wants to know. Students who didn't care if the acupuncture course came with academic credits kept coming to take the class. I have no idea how many students ended up taking the course, as it was difficult to take a precise tally. Some of my students are listed on the pages of acknowledgments in the first edition of *Acupuncture: An Anatomical Approach.*

Apprentices of anatomical acupuncture were not limited to students in our medical school. There were medical doctors from several other countries, including Edwin Falconi (Philippines), Teruko Tashiro (Japan), Andreas Lee (Argentina), Jorge Villalobose (Venezuela), Stanley Chang (Taiwan), D. Embey-Isztin (Hungary), Dumele Andreea (Hungary), Abudul Chen (United Arab Emirates), and several others. Through my personal effort in teaching and in writing for publications in acupuncture journals, it seems that anatomical acupuncture has gradually become known inside and outside the United States. Still, denial, rejection, and refusal to acknowledge acupuncture as a legitimate pain treatment persisted in the medical mainstream, and medical publishing companies refused to print my research and findings.

I completed writing the first edition of *Anatomical Acupuncture*, the predecessor to *Acupuncture: An Anatomical Approach*, in 1996. I spent almost a year attempting to find an established printing company to publish the book, without avail. They all replied to my inquiries with a uniform answer: that the book had no potential market. Finally, in 1997, I financed the publication of *Anatomical Acupuncture* myself. Antarctic Press, a publishing company based in San Antonio, Texas and owned and operated (even to this day) by my sons, printed the book. Two thousand copies were printed; approximately 20 copies are in my inventory to this day. All others were either sold directly to the readers or given away as complementary gifts.

It is hard to say if what happened next to *Anatomical Acupuncture* was sheer luck or preordained destiny. On April 9, 2001, I received a copy of an e-mail sent to Mike Morse by Steve Zollo, both of whom were strangers to me. Steve asked Mike for my name and e-mail address so he could contact me.

Contact indeed occurred. After brief discussion during the spring of 2001, we decided to form a team of three coauthors to rewrite the book. Dr. Curtis Clogston began his career as a reporter for the *Houston Chronicle* before attending and graduating from the medical school where I taught. Not only did he possess a firm comprehension of the medical information in the book, his early years as a reporter guaranteed a proficiency in English that I lacked, so I left the writing to him. My son, Joeming Dunn, completed our team. By 2001, he'd already had a few years of acupuncture practice on his own. He proofread the book to make sure that there would be no mistakes like there were in the first edition, in which the writing was all my own.

*Acupuncture: An Anatomical Approach* was published in 2004. Despite the use of a different title, in my own mind, it is still the second edition of *Anatomical Acupuncture*. I have no idea how well the book has sold. All I know is that every so often, I receive a small royalty check for it. However, money was never my motivation for writing the book; what pleased me was the knowing that somewhere, someone was reading our book, and thus the knowledge of anatomical acupuncture was propagating.

In addition to two English editions, the book had one Chinese edition. Yun-tao Ma, PhD was doing his postgraduate work at the Department of Pharmacology and Experimental Therapeutics at the University of Maryland at Baltimore. He had had some acupuncture training in China. During the Thanksgiving holiday of 1997, he accidentally had a chance to read the first edition of the book. After reading it, he sent me a three-page letter in which he said that I have "revolutionized the traditional acupuncture modality, both its theoretical concepts and clinical practice," that I "have reached a depth in understanding acupuncture that no one has ever reached so far." He further said that my book is "an epoch-making milestone in acupuncture history…" He urged me to translate the book into Chinese.

It turned out that he ended up doing the translation himself, and he did a superb job. The first edition of *Anatomical Acupuncture* was translated to *Scientific Acupuncture for Health Professionals*, and in January of 2000, it was published in Beijing by the company known literally as the Chinese Medical and Pharmacological Technology Publication Company.

How the Chinese edition has been received in China is impossible to know, because since the Beijing publisher sent me four complementary copies of the book, I have not heard a word from them. I did have two readers write me, at least reassuring me that the book had indeed been published. One of them was a student in a traditional Chinese medical school from Anhue Province. This student expressed bewilderment after reading the book, as he was not quite sure if he could fully believe what it said. One question puzzling him was why no one in the last two thousand years since acupuncture began had come out and said what was described in the book. I wrote to provide my answer and explanation, but I never heard from him again.

I was used to the disappointment and frustration of waiting for letters. Only five of my many students have bothered to get in touch with me, so I have no idea whether the majority of my students still believe that acupuncture is a valid therapeutic modality. My faith in acupuncture, however, hasn't diminished an iota so far. I became a globe-trotter, traveling to many different countries to find out as much as I could about using and teaching acupuncture. Whenever I have time, I write about acupuncture and its relation to pain, leading to the publication of two more books in the past few years.

The first is *The Bipolar Nature of Pain*, coauthored with Shen-Kai Chen, MD, Chairman, Faculty of Sports Medicine, Kaohsiung Medical University, Taiwan. Yi Hsien Publishing Company in Taipei, Taiwan published our book in 2008. Only 600 copies were printed. Two hundred of them stayed in Taiwan, and the other 400 were shipped to America. All of them were sold.

The second book was written in Chinese, with a title which translates into English as *Pain Quantification*. It was coauthored with Yun-tao Ma, Tan Yuansen, and Fu Chuanghua. *Pain quantification*, which I will address later on in this book, is a new concept found to be used extensively in acupuncture. *Pain Quantification* was published in 2006 by Chemical Industrial Publication, based in Beijing, China. As usual, the outcome of any book published in China is unknown to me.

Previously, I mentioned that I cross the globe to learn about acupuncture. In traveling, I have had opportunities to meet health care professionals of different types in different ranks, and to understand their views toward acupuncture applications and educations. The newest person I've met as of this writing was just a week ago (June 15, 2012). His name is Orlando Alberto Escamilla, MD. His title is Medico Acupuncturist at U. Nacional Clinica del Dolor, located at Calle 22 B No.66-46, Bogota D.C. Clinica Universitaria, Colombia. He showed me his master's degree in acupuncture, which he'd received from Universidad Nacional de Colombia School of Medicine. I asked him what kind of acupuncture he learned, and in response, he pulled out a syllabus from a drawer. The syllabus contained traditional acupuncture indoctrination. This convinced me that an acupuncture textbook based on medical sciences, like *Anatomical Acupuncture*, is needed for medical communities throughout the world.

With the need evident and the hope that someday *Anatomical Acupuncture* might be used as a textbook in the teaching of acupuncture as part of a medical curriculum, the idea of a third edition was never far from my mind.

Eight years after the publication of the second edition, I began contemplating revising and publishing a third edition. Soon after, Barbara Ellen Norwitz, Executive Editor with Taylor & Francis Group/CRC Press, e-mailed me, asking if she could interest me in revising the second edition.

*Acupuncture: An Anatomical Approach* is needed because acupuncture practices have undergone substantial changes in the decade since the previous edition. The use of acupuncture has grown in the United States and around the world. This growth can be attributed to the demographic shift to longevity. As populations live longer, the number of people suffering from chronic pain can be

## Preface to Second English Edition

expected to increase. Many of them will turn to acupuncture for help, and consequently, there will be a demand for more acupuncturists. Thus, more medical professionals will want to learn acupuncture, and a book such as *Acupuncture: An Anatomical Approach,* based on medical sciences, will be increasingly useful.

The revised edition has some new information added, especially in the area of quantifying pain. Pain is an enigma to health care providers, partially because there is no reliable method to measure or quantify it. This edition offers a proposal for the quantification of pain. If the method is verified, it could be a major step for a better understanding of pain, increasing our ability to predict the outcome in pain management.

Another difficult issue facing pain management is the lack of a meaningful way to differentiate acute pain from chronic pain. Most define whether pain is acute or chronic based solely on time duration, which can be misleading. In this third edition, I will explain a revolutionary way to enable practitioners to determine if pain encountered is already in a chronic stage or is still in an acute phase.

It is my hope that reading this book will help you understand the scientific nature and basis of acupuncture. If you want to learn more, I will gladly address any questions or inquiries you have about the book or about acupuncture in general.

**H.C. Dung, PhD**
*San Antonio, Texas*

# Preface to First English Edition

I think it was probably 1999 when Houchi Dung first called to say he wanted to teach me acupuncture. I had known Dr. Dung for nearly 30 years; he was one of my interviewers when I applied to medical school, and once I was accepted and matriculated, he was one of my teachers of gross anatomy (a subject in which I did not excel). When he called those many years later, he said he was preparing to retire from the university and he wanted to teach me acupuncture. Why me? He did not say at the time, but later he admitted it was because of my journalistic background. He felt a communicator was necessary to convey what he had learned over his 30-year career of sticking some five million needles into some 16,000 patients. In fact, he said that the reason he pushed for my acceptance into medical school was because the medical profession needed to be able to communicate better.

I was skeptical. My (uninformed) opinion of acupuncture was that it was placebo, pure and simple. Furthermore, to my thinking, it was based on metaphysical concepts that are incongruent with the principles of medicine. I put Dr. Dung off for nearly a year before he wore me down. For one thing, I had a lot of respect for him, and I owed him a debt for his supporting my medical career at an important time. In retrospect, his persistence was uncanny. He wanted me to spend a week or two at his clinic—he said that would be enough time to learn all I needed to know. I could not spare the time as a block. Reluctantly, he agreed to let me come on Saturday mornings, although he feared that would not give me the needed perspective to learn how to manage patients. I went to his clinic every Saturday morning for over a year, observing his patients and then incorporating what I had learned in the treatment of my own patients.

As I said, I was skeptical. I was hoping to spend a few Saturdays at his clinic and then quietly fade away back to my more pressing duties. Little did I know of what was in store for me. First, I had to admit almost immediately that acupuncture was not a placebo; it was obvious that Dr. Dung's patients were helped! Second, there was nothing metaphysical about his teaching. He was the same scientist I had known as a student, and he disdained nonscientific concepts of acupuncture. Dr. Dung had taken classical acupuncture and reinvented it as a medical science. His meticulous observations of his patients (and some 2,000 cadavers) over his career had led to some important discoveries, which he was generously willing to share with any practitioner willing to take the time to learn them.

Dr. Dung has an overriding desire to see acupuncture understood as science and taught, along with gross anatomy, in medical schools throughout the world. He published his first book, *Anatomical Acupuncture*, in 1997; it contains a wealth of knowledge but is somewhat difficult to read. He wanted me to help him write a revised edition of that text, but we ultimately settled on the entirely new text here before you. This current text borrows heavily from the earlier one, with the authors' thanks to its publisher, Antarctic Press, for allowing us to do so. Dr. Dung has traveled throughout the United States and the world to promote the use of acupuncture in medical education, and his earlier book has been translated or is being translated into several languages. Its first printing in Chinese sold out in China, indicating its relevance in a country in which acupuncture is an accepted practice.

Almost immediately after beginning my studies with Dr. Dung, I began incorporating acupuncture into my practice. It was so easy and patients responded so well! It is gratifying in clinical practice to obtain such dramatic results, even in refractory cases, and with so little effort. Dr. Dung is an anatomist as well as an acupuncturist, but not a physician, so his career has been limited in that he cannot diagnose disease and has often been deprived of the benefit of knowing a patient's complete medical history. Some of the case histories in this text reflect that deficit. His son, coauthor Joeming

Dunn, MD, is a physician who limits his practice to acupuncture and has taken over his father's practice since his retirement.

I have a more comprehensive practice, seeing acute occupational injuries and offering a variety of therapeutic options other than acupuncture: medication, education, and physical therapy. Many of my patients are blue collar workers with little sophistication, and it has been difficult to introduce some of them to acupuncture. I rarely do at first, preferring to wait until it has become obvious that they are not progressing with other therapies and may require surgical intervention (I have had patients waiting interminably for insurance approval for epidural steroid injections by a pain medicine specialist. After I administered acupuncture in the interim to provide symptomatic relief, they refused the epidural injections once approval was finally obtained because by then they were asymptomatic).

I have had to overcome quite a bit of initial patient resistance, especially in males, because of a fear of needles. Employers are also resistant, often feeling, as I once did, that acupuncture is bogus. Although, the former are gradually finding acupuncture more palatable than other available options (and are gratified to find that the pain of an acupuncture needle is not at all like that of an injection). The latter are beginning to see that the judicious use of acupuncture saves them money because their employees' recoveries from painful conditions are accelerated without more extensive and expensive interventions. Gradually, I have begun to use acupuncture for sinus allergy and asthma with gratifying results, and I look forward to trying it in a number of other conditions, especially infertility.

I am grateful to Dr. Dung for his helping me to understand more about the subject of pain. This is a greatly overlooked topic in medical education, and he has added new knowledge to the understanding of pain throughout an individual's lifetime. This is one of the most important themes of this text—possibly more important than the description of the practice of acupuncture. I am also grateful for his giving me a tool to help so many patients so easily, and giving me the opportunity to assist in the production of this text. His selflessness and integrity as a person and as a scientist have propelled this project forward, hopefully to the benefit of millions of our readers' patients.

**Curtis P. Clogston, MD**

# Preface to *Anatomical Acupuncture*

Most knowledge is learned from reading. All skills have to be acquired by practice. These two axioms can be applied to my becoming an acupuncturist.

Right from the beginning in the process of learning and doing acupuncture, I quickly realized that everything available for reading on the subject was fictitious—totally lacking in scientific truth. So it remains today. Nevertheless, through years of clinical practice, I cannot help but accept the therapeutic validity of this healing antiquity. In my eyes, what should be a treasured medical heritage is substantially undervalued, for no other reason than a deficiency in its proper scientific aspects. Such a deficiency not only repels mainstream medical professionals from any affinity toward acupuncture, but also, far worse, foments hostility toward this benevolent and useful healing modality. As a result, a great heritage of human civilization has been neglected until it has reached a state of waste and decay. *Anatomical Acupuncture* is undertaken with a wish to change the minds of the medical communities, as well as of society in general. The possibility of such a change arises because acupuncture, for the first time in history, has been described and discussed in the well-established language of the basic and clinical sciences, with which we in the United States are so very familiar.

This book presents no data of hard scientific research to theorize about the mechanism of acupuncture. Rather, it contains a great deal of valuable information obtained from firsthand observations through years of personal practice. The information may be of interest to both laymen and professional people. It can be said with confidence that individuals who have an interest in knowing the medical art of acupuncture healing will find this book useful. The book is written in very much the same framework following the lecture series for anatomy and chronic pain, a senior elective offered to medical students in the University of Texas Health Science Center at San Antonio. Judging from the critiques and evaluations given by the students who have selected the course, the information seems to be well received.

The book consists of five parts. Part one has two chapters: One chapter describes the history of acupuncture in China, and the other in the United States. Part two also has two chapters: One chapter is used to discuss the absurd concepts and heretical suppositions of Chinese medicine, and the other is devoted specifically to nonscientific theories of traditional acupuncture. These four chapters should be comprehensible to all readers, with or without a sophisticated medical background. Such sophistication may be required to fully understand the rest of the book, however.

There are five chapters in part three. Their purposes are to provide established knowledge in the basic sciences of medicine, including anatomy, physiology, and biochemistry, for interpreting acupuncture. After a thorough understanding of the basic sciences in acupuncture, it will be possible to realize how acupuncture can be used in the clinical applications that are discussed in part four. Acupuncture can have good to excellent results for certain patients diagnosed with a clinical condition, and yet, other patients with the same condition may not benefit from such treatments. Thus, patients are categorized into different groups, each of which will have a chapter devoted to explaining why acupuncture will work and why it will not. Four chapters discuss different therapeutic results in acupuncture treatments. Part five is intended for scientific research. One chapter offers suggestions for clinical investigations using acupuncture as a vehicle in designing research protocols. The last chapter speculates on the possibility of using the information described in this book for studies of pain in terms of basic medical sciences.

Not much is known scientifically with respect to how acupuncture works. There are many reasons for this poor understanding of acupuncture's mechanism. One of the important reasons is the ambiguity of pain. With so much research carried out to study the nature of pain, the medical profession is still not quite sure of its true identity. Unless pain is better understood, it will be rather remote to explain how acupuncture can manage it. Acupuncture and chronic pain are two-way streets. Currently, the traffic on the streets is going in the wrong direction for increased knowledge. Such an increase can only be possible if acupuncture becomes an interesting subject for basic and clinical studies. It would be nice if this book can serve as a catalyst to stimulate some excitement among medical investigators to look into acupuncture more intensively and seriously.

**H.C. Dung, PhD**

# Author

The author graduated from the University of Louisville in 1970 with a Ph.D. in anatomy. Soon after, he accepted a faculty position in the Department of Anatomy, School of Medicine, at the University of Texas Health Science Center at San Antonio, which he held until his retirement in 2002. His main responsibilities were teaching gross human anatomy to medical and dental students and conducting research on a number of neurological mutations in mice.

During his 31-year academic career, he published a total of 77 papers. Twenty-six of these were in abstract form, while the rest were in full-paper form. Twenty-four of the full papers were on the field of acupuncture. These were the product of clinical experiences in acupuncture practice, obtained owing to the demands of medical students who wanted to learn acupuncture.

The first edition of *Anatomical Acupuncture* was published in 1977 and *Acupuncture: An Anatomical Approach* in 2003. This publication will be the Second Edition by that title. The author has published an additional six books on acupuncture and pain, three in English and three in Chinese.

New Editions of Previously Published Works:

*Anatomical Acupuncture, First Edition*, was published by the author himself, via Antarctic Press, San Antonio, TX (publisher: Ben Y. Dunn).

*Anatomical Acupuncture* was translated into Chinese by H.C. Dung, Ph.D., and Yun-tao Ma, Ph.D., and was published in 2000 in Beijing, China, under the title *Scientific Acupuncture for Health Professionals*.

*Acupuncture: An Anatomical Approach*, was coauthored by H.C. Dung, Ph.D., Curtis P. Clogston, and Joeming W. Dunn, M.D. It was published in 2004 by CRC Press.

# 1 Introduction

As explained in the preface, this book was written and prepared with the intent that it be used as the text for teaching Anatomical Acupuncture as a senior elective for medical students. School officials canceled the elective. Then, I retired. My wish to teach acupuncture based on medical sciences vanished, and I thought that the destiny of the book would be obliterated thereafter. Fortunately, in 2004 (2 years after my retirement), CRC Press agreed to publish a second, revised edition, and the book has survived to this date. With the advent of the third edition, it should be possible to expect its existence to last a few more years.

Acupuncture has been in use and practiced for more than 2 thousand years [1,2]. It would be difficult to make an accurate estimate of how many books have been written in its name during this long period of history. One book more or less about the topic will not make much difference to the reality of acupuncture. It will stay useful and remain in practice for the foreseeable future, despite the small, limited effect of this particular book on its usage and practice. There are several reasons for making the effort to publish this book that may be worth knowing if you want to learn to use acupuncture in your medical practice. It is a matter of professional respect and prestige. One does not want to be criticized as not knowing what he or she is doing, particularly in the field of medicine. Medicine is considered a branch of the sciences. Thus, we want to simply ask, "What is the scientific nature of acupuncture? Is it possible to use scientific terminology known in medical communities to explain what we do in acupuncture?"

Before I started writing this book, I had to collect data. From the beginning, it became a frustrating task to find acupuncture publications that were scientifically oriented. There is no basic medical science to speak of for acupuncture. To acupuncturists, even in this modern age of scientific medicine, human anatomy appears like what we see in Figure 1.1. This figure was taken from a publication intended to be a textbook of Chinese medicine. The book was printed sometime in 1946. The drawing displays an example of human anatomy, with many visceral organs shown in the thoracic and abdominal cavities. However, the division between these two cavities, the diaphragm, is not shown. Anatomically, there are many more obvious errors and gross mistakes. These cannot be unintended negligence because they are grotesque in scope. Even people without anatomical training will be able to detect errors in the drawing. So, why hasn't a single acupuncturist ever stood up to correct these mistakes? Why have they been perpetuated up to this date?

Anatomy in the medical curriculum consists of gross anatomy, microanatomy (histology), and neuroanatomy. No trace of microanatomy or neuroanatomy was found in my search of the literature for acupuncture. No known acupuncture book describes how nerve cells and fibers look histologically. Yet, the combination of nerve cell and fiber, known as a neuron, is the only anatomical entity that matters in acupuncture.

In addition to their dubious depictions of visceral organs in gross anatomy, many acupuncture books printed before 1960 were rather confusing in their presentation of locations or loci of most acupuncture points. The points' diameters were too large in proportion to the body surface. It was often difficult to determine their exact anatomical sites because the texts gave no precise anatomical features as landmarks to demarcate the points' locations. Taking into account these factors and several others, it was natural for individuals of scientific mind to begin questioning the merit of acupuncture's veracity. The willingness to accept acupuncture as something real in terms of medical practice began to subside, and skepticism about its use began to creep into our thoughts. Years later, we found that there were other medical professionals who had spent time learning acupuncture, then decided to forsake its practice for precisely the reasons given above. By then, we had changed our

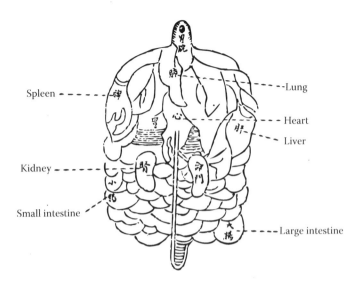

**FIGURE 1.1** Human anatomy as viewed by many acupuncturists.

view toward acupuncture because we had proved on our own that acupuncture works and is useful in managing pain of both an acute and chronic nature. This book is offered to share the experience we have gained from acupuncture practice. Don't give up on acupuncture because of what you have heard or read. Try it on your own, and in time, its advantages and benefits will become clear.

In 1976, I received an invitation from the Chinese government to visit China. During my stay in Beijing, I had enough spare time to visit a bookstore. On the shelves of the store was one particular book [3], the Chinese title of which can be translated as *Essentials of Chinese Acupuncture*. The name of the publisher can be translated from Chinese as "People's Hygienic Publishing Company."

I bought a copy and brought it back to Texas, where I thoroughly perused the book from beginning to end. What impressed me the most were the anatomical illustrations printed in the book. I had no doubt that the drawings and pictures seen in the book had been prepared and produced by people with good anatomical training. The anatomical positions of all acupuncture points were well defined. In fact, the book led me to realize that there was good anatomical identity for each point described. I began formulating my understanding of acupuncture as essentially anatomical in nature. Good anatomical knowledge, specifically of gross anatomy, would be the key to unlocking and revealing acupuncture's medical nature.

Coincidentally, on a visit to San Francisco in 1984, I discovered another book in a Chinatown bookstore. The book was titled *Essentials of Chinese Acupuncture* and was written in English [4]. It had been compiled by three colleges—from Beijing, Shanghai, and Nanjing—and the Acupuncture Institute of the Academy of Traditional Chinese Medicine. The drawings and photos used in both this book and the one I'd found in 1976 were basically the same. However, the written content was somewhat different. It was obvious to me that the Chinese edition was written for those who read Chinese, and the English edition was for non-Chinese foreigners. The differences were not entirely due to the separation of linguistic backgrounds. The need to introduce acupuncture to different audiences with different cultural backgrounds also played a factor. The Chinese version sounds more mystic and mythological to me than the English edition does. Editorial maneuvers of this nature could lead to the suspicion that one can interpret acupuncture any way to fit one's own ideas and thoughts. It raised the possibility for acupuncture to be pure fiction, making it harder for the medical mainstream, with its hardened views of science in medicine, to accept that the modality is real.

The maxim, "It is easier to change dynasties than to change minds," applies well for most people in the medical mainstream. Once they think that acupuncture has no scientific reasoning behind it,

# Introduction

it will be difficult for them to accept acupuncture. We know of incidences in which physicians spent time learning acupuncture, either abroad or in their own country. And yet, in the end, they decided to give up the chance to practice it, confessing that they still don't understand the medical explanation for acupuncture despite making efforts to study it. Here is an example:

I met Dr. Gonzalo Parra Flores (Figure 1.2) in 1998. From June 9 to June 18 of that year, I joined a Christian Medical Mission to go to Chilcapamba, Imbabura, Ecuador. The mission was organized by the Central Christian Church of San Antonio, Texas, and was led by Dr. Douglas Deuell, Senior Minister. The evening of our arrival, a couple of reporters came to interview members of the mission, and they found out that I was an acupuncturist. The next morning, a local newspaper reported that free acupuncture service would be available at Hospital Ibarra. Thereafter, every morning, more than 100 people were lined up to wait for my services. Soon, I realized that not all of them were patients. A few of them, in fact, were medical staff of the hospital. A couple of them even

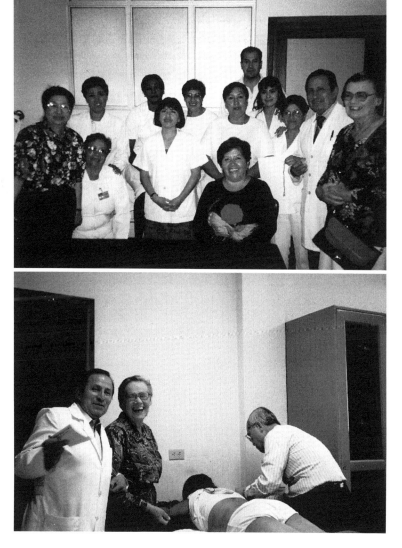

**FIGURE 1.2** Two photos taken on two different days at the Ibarra Hospital. Dr. Flores, wearing the white coat, is in both of them.

indicated that they wanted to learn to practice acupuncture. One of them, Dr. Parra, told me that he'd gone to Ukraine, then still a part of the Soviet Union, to learn acupuncture. He confessed that after his return, he had no courage to practice acupuncture because he still didn't understand what it was all about. What troubled him the most was not being able to remember the terminology of acupuncture points. I pointed my right index finger at the medial end of my right eyebrow, and asked him, "What is that point?" Naturally, he didn't remember that the point is known in acupuncture as *zanzhu*. Nor did he remember the terms *sibai* and *yifeng*. Then, I told him that *zanzhu* represents the supraorbital nerve, *sibai* the infraorbital, and *yifeng* the greater auricular. Naturally, he had no problem knowing what these three nerves were. What bothered him the most was why his acupuncture instructors in Ukraine didn't tell him so. I knew such puzzlement all too well because none of the students who took Anatomical Acupuncture as their elective were capable of mastering acupuncture points in Chinese, with the exception of a few commonly known points such as *heku*, which is the point representing the superficial radial nerve. Therefore, the main mission of this book is to name acupuncture points using terms learned from gross anatomy. These terms are familiar to every medical student. A big portion of this book—five chapters—is devoted to describing acupuncture points based on human gross anatomy.

Dr. Parra was not the only example of a disgruntled acupuncturist that we knew; the same thing had happened in the United States. We knew of students who had graduated from medical school, then gone to California to take an acupuncture training program for a week or so. After spending substantial sums of money, they returned to say that they still didn't know much about acupuncture. The difference between Dr. Parra and the physicians in the United States was that Dr. Parra's expenses were paid for by the government of the Soviet Union, whereas the American doctors had to pay for their own expenses. The difference occurred because it was during the Cold War, and the Soviet Union used acupuncture as a tool to lure intelligentsia in the Third World to support its political agenda. The same thing happened with Chinese acupuncture during that time.

Hurdles and obstacles that create inconvenience and hesitance in learning acupuncture can turn up in any direction. Some of them are self-inflicted, coming from within acupuncture communities themselves. Some are imposed from external environments. Examples of internally generated ambivalence will be discussed subsequently in this chapter to show why concepts, theories, or views presented by traditional acupuncture practitioners will be difficult for the medical mainstream to accept. Here, I offer three more examples to illustrate how and why external environments as educational systems in medicine can often hinder or obstruct the incorporation of acupuncture teaching into the medical curriculum.

The first example occurred in Cuba in June of 1999. Ralph Alan Dale, from a publication called *AfroCubaWeb* at acupunk.com, e-mailed me a 10-page printout message. The first line of the message was, "East and West Meet in the Caribbean: Is Cuba Developing the World's Best Health Care Model?" Dr. Dale had EdD, PhD, CA, and Dipl. Ac. degrees. He made three trips to Cuba in 1990, 1991, and 1992. His e-mail was a report about the observations made during the trips. One wonders why it took so long, almost 10 years after the first trip, to give such a report. Nevertheless, I took his report seriously and read it carefully. What attracted my attention most in the report was that the Cuban Ministry of Health appointed a National Commission of Acupuncture to facilitate the development of acupuncture throughout the country. The commission would develop acupuncture curricula in the medical colleges. According to Dr. Dale, "there are eight or nine medical colleges in Cuba, all of which will soon incorporate acupuncture as an important part of their curricula. All medical colleges have a 6-year program. In addition, there is a 3- to 4-year internship requirement. Acupuncture will become an integral part of every level of this program. Acupuncture has already been incorporated into the curriculum at many medical colleges, specifically, Giron and Julio Trigo Colleges in Havana, and the medical colleges in Holguin, Oriente (Santiago de Cuba), Villa Clara and Cienfuegos." In the same e-mail, he mentioned a few names: Leoncio Padron, Orlando Sanchez, Marta Perez, and Rita Beretervide. Dr. Sanchez, "a doctor just 2 years out of the University of Havana Medical School, recalled that his interest in a medical career began during his army service.

He was befriended by a medical school dropout who taught him the traditional Chinese health practice of *tai chi* and *quigong*."

After reading this information, I decided to go to Cuba, which was not that simple a matter at that time. One had to have a license from the U.S. Department of the Treasury to go. After acquiring license #CU-60406, I reached Cuba on June 1, 2000, and stayed there for 11 days. During that period, through rather complicated channels, I was able to meet Francisco Jose Moron Rodriguez, MD, PhD. Dr. Moron was a graduate of the Medical University of Havana, which was the oldest medical school established in the New World after the arrival of Christopher Columbus. At the time we met, he was Professor and Chairman of the Department of Pharmacology at his alma mater. He also had a title as Head of the Central Research Department of Pharmacology, Faculty of Medicine "Dr. Salvador Allende," Vice Minister for Research and Education, Ministry of Public Health. His numerous titles and credentials were so extensive that to write all of them down would take up an entire page. The most important part for me, however, would be whether he was in charge of incorporating acupuncture into their medical curriculum. I asked him if he already did so, and he answered "no," because he didn't know how to do it. I offered my free and voluntary service to help him set up an acupuncture teaching program for his medical students and the physicians in his country. He was most delighted to have such an opportunity come to him. We ended up meeting five times and took a few pictures, one of which is shown in Figure 1.3. I told him all I needed was a letter of invitation from either the dean of his medical school or, even better, from the president of the Medical University of Havana. The letter of invitation never arrived, and my hopes to set up a teaching program for scientific acupuncture never had the chance to be realized. Cuba was a tough country and a difficult place, both at that time and even now. I could tell after visiting that country that it would not be easy for Dr. Moron to arrange a feasible trip to his university. There were just too many logistical handicaps he needed to face and overcome to prepare for my stay.

It was obvious to me that Cuba was not a place where you could speak your mind freely. I didn't ask Dr. Moron why they decided to incorporate acupuncture into their curriculum. They ultimately didn't do it anyway, after almost 10 years of talking about it. He didn't voluntarily explain to me why they decided not to do so. One thing that puzzles me to this date is that Dr. Moron didn't know any of the names of the doctors mentioned in Dr. Dale's e-mail. One wonders how Dr. Dale came up with these people, who were supposedly in charge of incorporating acupuncture into medical

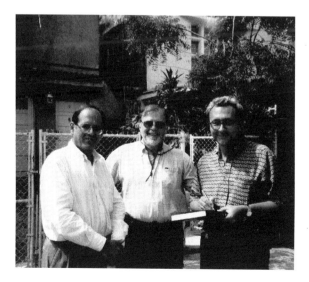

**FIGURE 1.3** Dr. Moron on the right. At center is Dr. Larry Hufford, professor of political sciences at St. Mary's University, San Antonio, Texas, the leader of the travel seminar group to Cuba. On the left is the Vice President of the Medical University of Havana, whose name the author has unfortunately forgotten.

curricula in Cuba. It is doubtful whether Cuba was ever able to incorporate acupuncture into their medical curricula. This example clearly indicated that doing so would not be as easy as expected, even if the intention had sanction from a government official and was clearly approved and supported, in this case for Cuban medical schools, by the highest authority in the country.

The second example took place locally in my neighborhood. My home is within walking distance from South Texas Medical Center, where the University of Texas Health Science Center and Audie L. Murphy Memorial Veterans Hospital are located. I taught at the Health Science Center for 31 years before my retirement, and volunteered to instruct tai chi exercise at the Bob Ross Senior Multi-Service Health and Resource Center, which is one street across from the VA hospital. I made quite a few new friends among enthusiastic tai chi practitioners. In time, a few of them became close friends. One of them was Mary Francis Uptain, who was also one of the acupuncture patients who obtained excellent results from my treatments. We frequently talked about acupuncture. She indicated that my altruistic conviction to share what I knew from practicing it was certainly admirable. One day in February of 2009, she brought me a newspaper clipping printed in the January 31, 2009 edition of the *San Antonio Express/News*. The headline article therein was "Military Expanding Acupuncture Treatments for Pain," written by Kamala Lane, an Associated Press reporter. Lane reported that Col. Richard Niemtzow, an Air Force physician, used auricular acupuncture to reduce pain at Walter Reed Army Medical Center in Washington for Chief Warrant Officer James Brand Smith, who had broken five ribs, punctured a lung, and shattered bones in his hand and thigh after falling more than 20 feet from a Black Hawk helicopter in Baghdad a month before. The results were positive, with an improvement level of perhaps 50%. Lane further said that the Air Force, which runs the military's only acupuncture clinic, was training doctors to take acupuncture to the war zones of Iraq and Afghanistan. At the end of the article, Lane quoted Niemtzow as saying that U.S. troops should start to learn acupuncture so they can treat each other while out on missions. For now, the Air Force program was limited to training physicians. Lane also said it was "remarkable" for the military, a "conservative institution," to incorporate acupuncture. I told Mary that I was curious to confirm the veracity of the report. Mary replied that she worked at VA hospital as a volunteer and had connections within hospital administration. She promised to arrange for me to talk with the proper personnel about offering to teach acupuncture to doctors in the VA hospital. The person she found was David Dooley, MD, Chief of Education Services in the hospital.

I had three meetings with Dr. Dooley, and we e-mailed each other on several occasions. In the first e-mail I received, he said that he "heard good things" about me. Basically, what I offered was very simple: I would provide free instruction in acupuncture to any physicians in his jurisdiction at any time and place of his choosing. A copy of an e-mail sent by Sandra Sanchez-Reilly to Dr. Dooley indicated that "All our fellows (PC and geriatrics) are interested. Some faculty (including myself and Dr. Chiodo, the geri program director) are very interested in learning acupuncture as well. We have three geri fellows and eight PC interprofessional fellows, in addition to about 10 other staff physicians, who could potentially attend these sessions once we organize this. I think we have a quorum. I will let Scotte know via this e-mail as well." The last time I saw Dr. Dooley was in March of 2009, when I gave him the Application for Physicians, Dentists, Podiatrists, and Optometrists, a four-page, double-sided form from the Department of Veterans Affairs. I have not heard a word from either Dr. Dooley or the Department of Veterans Affairs since. The incident made me wonder how substantially the acupuncture program promoted by Col. Richard Niemtzow has been advanced, or even whether the program is real or just one reporter's imagination. If military establishments really had the intention of training their medical staff to use acupuncture, who would have the qualifications or become qualified to teach the course, and where would these instructors be found? Are these not the obstacles that medical professionals will face in the teaching of acupuncture?

One more factor to mention regarding this example—Lane's report describes a case of acute pain. Using acupuncture to manage acute pain like that will be discussed in a later chapter of this book. Acute pain of that nature is very rarely seen in an ordinary acupuncture clinic. Patients who sustain traumatic injuries of that nature always end up in the emergency room of major hospitals.

Most acute pain will subside on its own in time without requiring auricular acupuncture treatment. It is chronic pain, most of which is intractable, for which acupuncture can be useful.

The third example demonstrates how feeble the connection between physicians and acupuncture can be. The slightest disturbance can disrupt it. Trust in acupuncture can vanish when claims made for the treatment fail to materialize. This was what happened to acupuncture anesthesia in a story told by a Hungarian doctor, Dr. Embey-Isztin. I met Dr. Embey-Isztin when I attended a meeting of the Hungarian Pain Society on October 21, 2005. The meeting was held in a fancy hotel near Balatan Lake, not too far from Budapest. His card indicated that he was a consultant anesthetist and head of a pain clinic, the National Institute of Oncology, Hungary, in Budapest. Soon, I learned that he was a well-known medical figure in his country and a leader of some kind in the establishment of Hungarian medicine. My presentation in the meeting was "Using Trigger Points to Differentiate Acute and Chronic Pain." After the meeting, Dr. Embey-Isztin approached me to talk about acupuncture. At that time, I was a chair professor at Meiho Institute of Technology in Neipu, Pingtung, Taiwan. I promised him that if he cared to come visit me there, I would be very glad to show him how acupuncture worked. Indeed, he showed up the next year, in 2006 (Figure 1.4), and brought with him one of his colleagues, neurologist Dumele Andreea, MD. They stayed with me for almost 2 weeks. During that time, we were together almost 24 hours a day. We spent a lot of time talking about almost everything in life and in the world. One thing we talked about was acupuncture anesthesia, discussions which I will not forget for the rest of my life.

Dr. Embey-Isztin said that he first heard about acupuncture anesthesia when he went to work at a hospital in Paris after graduating from medical school in Hungary. He'd previously known nothing about acupuncture and had never had a chance to observe how it was able to induce anesthesia for surgical purposes. At that time, there were also physicians from China working in the same hospital. Two of them were invited and agreed to demonstrate to the hospital's medical staff how acupuncture anesthesia worked. Dr. Embey-Isztin indicated that he was very excited and had great expectations to see for himself what the acupuncture anesthesia was really like. When the time arrived, he went to the surgical ward with a rather large group of hospital personnel. The two Chinese physicians entered the room and went to prepare acupuncture anesthesia by inserting a number of needles into various locations of the body, including loci in the ears, forearms, hands, legs, and feet. The needles then were twirled, pushed down, and pulled up now and then. The hand manipulation obviously

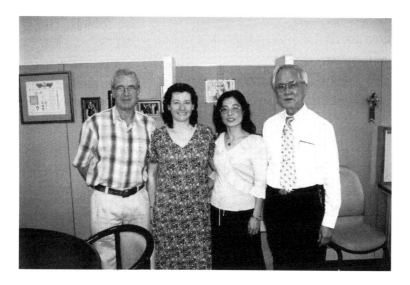

**FIGURE 1.4** Dr. Embey-Isztin on the left, beside him is Dr. Andreea, and then Faye Zu Wu, my secretary at the Meiho Institute of Technology.

generated certain discomfort, as could be seen from the patient's facial expressions. Such discomfort can be obvious even in some patients coming for regular acupuncture treatments that don't require much needle twisting. After approximately 10 to 15 minutes of needle manipulation, the patient was declared to be ready for surgery via scalpel. All the onlookers were astonished when, as the knife cut into the flesh, the patient almost jumped off the surgical table, weeping. That was the moment Dr. Embey-Isztin came to believe that miraculous acupuncture anesthesia was nothing but a folly, and began to doubt whether acupuncture could be accepted as a scientific entity in medical practice. It was impossible for me to tell whether his visit to the Meiho Institute changed his views on acupuncture. All I knew for sure was that acupuncture anesthesia in China had totally disappeared. In 2002, I stayed in China for 6 months, during which time I went to two medical schools as a visiting professor. During those visits, I kept asking if I could observe surgical operations under acupuncture anesthesia. No one could take me to see a single performance of such a treatment. Even today, we can definitively state that many physicians and medical doctors will use the failure of acupuncture anesthesia as an excuse to deny, discredit, or reject the real usefulness of acupuncture. More will be said about acupuncture anesthesia in a later chapter. All that needs to be said here is that it is not humbug. Acupuncturists need to learn how to screen out which patients are unsuitable for having acupuncture anesthesia. This book may provide a way to achieving that.

As pointed out above, there are elements of factual anatomy in acupuncture, although it is difficult to judge whether the presence of the said elements is sheer coincidence or luck. Because all we know at this time about acupuncture is limited to anatomy, anatomical sciences will occupy a major portion of this book. The next six chapters will be all about anatomy. Chapter 2 provides a general orientation to the nervous system, indicating which parts of it will be relevant for studying acupuncture. Our body can be divided into five regions: head, neck, upper limbs, body trunk, and lower limbs. Each of these regions will have a chapter devoted to covering a description of the acupuncture points located there. Chapter 3 describes acupuncture points located in the head and face, all of which are formed by the cranial nerves. Chapter 4 covers the cervical plexus, which forms acupuncture points in the neck region. Acupuncture points are similarly formed by the brachial plexus in the upper limbs (Chapter 5), the typical spinal nerves in the body trunk (Chapter 6), and the lumbar–sacral plexuses in the lower limbs (Chapter 7).

We know for sure that acupuncture began as a medical practice at the time the basic medical sciences were unknown in our civilization. The basic medical sciences started to evolve and develop from the time of the Renaissance in Europe, and although they have advanced continuously, acupuncture remains unchanged with respect to its scientific prospects. Besides anatomy, the basic medical sciences also include physiology and biochemistry. There is very little physiology to speak of in acupuncture. One commonly cited and widely known tenet that is insisted upon and promulgated by acupuncturists could be described as the theory of *qi* (pronounced "chi"). This qi is said to flow and circulate throughout the entire body within a number of channels, which are termed "meridians" in acupuncture. The flow of qi in the meridians is said to be controlled by two opposite forces, known as *yin* and *yang*. When yin and yang are out of balance, the flow of qi can become stagnated, or even blocked, resulting in sickness or pain. The fine needles used in acupuncture are inserted into the prescribed loci, spots, or points on the body that can adjust the flow of qi, or to reopen the meridians to allow the circulation of the qi. Thus, health can be restored and pain eradicated. The acceptability of such an explanation or theory is up to individual readers of this text. Opinions on this view of acupuncture can be found in many publications. The following quotation from the *Wall Street Journal* (March 23, 2010, p. 5) could be considered a typical example: "Acupuncture has long baffled medical experts, and no wonder: It holds that an invisible life force called qi (pronounced *chee*) travels up and down the body in 14 meridians. Illness and pain are due to blockages and imbalances in qi. Inserting thin needles into the body at precise points can unblock the meridians, practitioners believe, and treat everything from arthritis and asthma to anxiety, acne, and infertility." To us, this is just pure hogwash, without any scientific truth to it. Yet, the majority of acupuncturists keep repeating this worthless, nonsensical language to the world. We consider such behavior to be self-inflicted damage to the believability of the scientific nature of acupuncture. To deny this theory is easy: give us an investigator who has been able to identify the existence of meridians. No such meridians have ever been found in the body. However, there are many physiological activities, functions, and phenomena that can be described in the course of acupuncture reactions and usages. Thus, we need Chapter 8 to discuss physiology in acupuncture. There are known attempts to interpret acupuncture following the teachings of modern concepts in physiology. Two books on the topic [5,6] are cited for reference, if any readers are interested in studying this aspect of acupuncture.

Chapter 9, Biochemistry in Acupuncture, concludes the coverage of the basic medical sciences for acupuncture. There is no biochemistry to speak of in acupuncture. Yet, research in biochemical studies will provide the final answer to the question of how acupuncture works. Acupuncture needs to have biochemical substances in the nervous system to produce anesthesia so that pain can be reduced or eliminated. The substances are most likely to be synthesized and secreted as hormones or neural transmitters in the physiological system. What these substances could possibly be will be discussed in this chapter.

The last five chapters can be viewed as the clinical aspect of acupuncture studies. Chapter 12 will discuss several aspects of pain: what is pain? Can pain be measured and quantified? If we cannot measure how much pain patients are suffering, it will be difficult to know whether their pain can be managed. Does it make good sense to differentiate acute and chronic pain with the methods currently available in clinical practice? Several aspects concerning pain will be discussed in this chapter.

Chapters 13, 14, and 15 are devoted to the applications of acupuncture in clinical practices. Chapter 13 provides examples of patients whose pain is easy to manage, and for whom applications of acupuncture will produce excellent results. Chapter 14 will show that, often, the use of acupuncture can have mixed or limited results (or both), with several appropriate cases provided to demonstrate these mixtures and limitations. The purpose of Chapter 15 is to help acupuncture students understand that acupuncture is not a panacea. It will not reduce or stop all sorts of pain. The chapter provides examples of pain that are difficult or impossible to manage, and explains these in terms that are understandable from a medical point of view.

The final chapter, Chapter 16, theorizes where the future of acupuncture may be headed. Much is still unknown in acupuncture. Finding the correct answers for the unknown will take more research and study, and this chapter discusses what kinds of research and studies these should be. Investigators in the field of acupuncture know that there are numerous reports available in the medical literature. Unfortunately, spending time to study these reports will not be of much use in understanding what acupuncture is all about. One example to prove the point: one study of acupuncture was made to determine whether using needles would be more effective than using so-called sham stimulation. Whether real needles are more or less effective is beside the point. As long as acupuncture can reduce or stop pain in a minority of patients, its use in clinical applications can be justified. To me, most research studies consist of merely finding some logical excuse to oppose the use of acupuncture. It is doubtful that most of the investigators who wrote the research reports ever had a chance to really practice acupuncture in their medical careers as health care providers. We are very certain that, in the end, acupuncture will turn out to be a very useful tool for medical investigators and scientific researchers to advance our understanding of the physiological nature of pain. This chapter discusses such a possibility and many other aspects relating to pain.

For anyone with adequate education and training in the basic medical sciences, this book should be easy to read. Reading this book should make it easy to understand what acupuncture is. Furthermore, this book will enable physicians and medical practitioners to perform acupuncture for their patients who are suffering from acute and chronic pain. It is the author's hope that the practice of acupuncture will gain momentum in the medical field after the publication of this book. There are many individuals in this world who are afflicted with pain, and acupuncture is sure to give them some relief. Let medical professionals who are qualified to practice acupuncture provide this therapeutic treatment to those who need its services.

## REFERENCES

1. Veith, I. *The Yellow Emperor's Classic of Internal Medicine.* University of California Press, Berkeley, CA, 1970.
2. Veith, I. Acupuncture in traditional Chinese medicine—an historical review. *California Medicine* 118:70, 1973.
3. *Essentials of Chinese Acupuncture*, 1st ed. (in Chinese). People's Hygienic Publishing Company, Beijing, 1964.
4. *Essentials of Chinese Acupuncture*, 1st ed. (in English). Foreign Languages Press, Beijing, 1980.
5. Baldry, P.E. *Acupuncture, Trigger Points and Musculoskeletal Pain.* Churchill Livingstone, New York, 1993.
6. Ulett, G.A. and S.P. Han. *The Biology of Acupuncture.* Warren H. Green, St. Louis, MO, 2002.

# 2 Anatomy in Acupuncture

## 2.1 GENERAL CONSIDERATION

Any person who is or has been a medical student knows that anatomy consists of gross human anatomy, microanatomy (also known as histology), neuroanatomy, and sometimes embryology as well. The total instruction time required for all of them can require as much as 390 h. Of that, the time required for each can be approximately divided into 180 h for gross anatomy, 120 h for microanatomy, 60 h for neuroanatomy, and 30 h for embryology. Equipping an adequate facility for teaching these courses is extremely expensive. As far as the author is aware, dental and medical schools are the only educational institutions where such an opportunity could possibly be available. Chiropractic schools might be included, but certainly not oriental and acupuncture colleges. If oriental and acupuncture colleges do teach gross anatomy and microanatomy, the said teaching is most likely limited to didactic oral presentation, without practical dissection of cadavers and microscopic examination of tissue mountings on slides.

For all the times mentioned above, how many hours do medical professionals need to review their anatomy to properly learn to practice acupuncture? A reasonable estimate would be 26 h for gross anatomy, 4 h for microanatomy, and none for neuroanatomy or embryology. Out of the time spent for gross anatomy, 18 h can best be put to use by returning to the gross anatomy laboratory for dissecting cadavers. Many obscure and insignificant peripheral nerves need to be dissected out and examined to observe their unique anatomical features, which will be described and discussed in the following five chapters. Four hours for microanatomy can be spent to review the histology of nerve tissues, including the microstructure of neurons, nerve cells, and their fibers. The most difficult requirement in the entire ordeal in learning to practice acupuncture is getting the opportunity to return to a gross anatomy laboratory to dissect a cadaver for a review of anatomy. Of course, skipping this step does not necessarily mean that one cannot learn acupuncture. As long as medical professionals are capable of understanding what is described in this book, they can still achieve that mission. It is just more convincing if one can verify real morphological entities in an actual human body.

## 2.2 IDENTITY OF ACUPOINTS

Acupuncture can be defined merely as inserting fine, sterilized needles into specific points on the body for therapeutic purposes. These certain points are designated as acupuncture points, abbreviated hereafter in this book as acupoints.

Acupoints are the primary essence of acupuncture. To learn acupuncture, we must know what acupoints are. Certain aspects of acupoints are well established, such as their anatomical locations. Other aspects are uncertain, such as their real identity. Do they represent definite anatomical structures? Are these structures identifiable in our body? The answers to both these and many other similar questions is "no." There is no anatomical structure that can be said to represent acupoints, and no such structure has ever been identified in the body. We do know that some anatomical features, alone or in combination, contribute to the formation of acupoints. Ten such features are mentioned in Section 2.5 of this chapter.

We advise readers with scientific curiosity to check out two reports to learn more about the identity of acupoints. The first is an experimental study using monkeys as a model. The results of the study were reported by Dr. H.C. Ha [1] in 1980. The report describes that under the skin of one acupoint studied, there are more nerve receptors of different categories than in areas that are not beneath acupoints. Dr. Ha and I were acquaintances for many years. He told me that the study was only focused on just a couple of acupoint loci. It was impossible to conclude if all acupoints are located in skin areas where an abundance of nerve receptors are found. Thus, it will not be entirely accurate to attribute nerve receptors as the only anatomical structure in forming all acupoints.

A second opinion reported by a number of scientific investigators is that acupoints are actually trigger points [2,3], or motor points [4]. Many of these individuals, such as Melzack, are well-known researchers in the study of pain. It would be unruly to recant their opinions. Yet, the trouble is whether or not we know the real identity of a trigger point. If our bodies indeed have trigger points, why are they not mentioned in any gross anatomy textbook? There are points of numerous different names, in addition to acupoint, trigger point, and motor point, known in medical literature. They include such descriptors as tender, sensitive, and dermal points. More about these points will be discussed in Section 2.6 of this chapter. For the time being, one fact known about all these points, which are under different names, needs to be pointed out: they can all manifest sensitivity as aching or pain under certain physical conditions in certain times of our life. This sensitivity is due to our having nerve tissue in our body, particularly the sensory nerves. Thus, it is clear to us that it will be useful to know the nervous system—more specifically, the sensory nervous system.

## 2.3 ALL IN THE SENSORY NERVES

Sensory nerves are key players in forming acupoints. They are the only anatomic structures that are capable of generating sensations, painful or otherwise, uncomfortable or comfortable. With a few exceptions, such as the hair, the fingernails, the outermost epidermoid layers of the skin, and the corneas of the eyeballs, sensory nerves can be said to be ubiquitous throughout the body. This is why hair can be cut, nails can be clipped, epidermal skin can be thinly shaved with a razor blade, and the cornea can be damaged by diseases with no pain perceived. Injuries to parts of the body with sensory nerve innervation will make us experience pain. We know that the density of nerve distribution varies greatly from one area of the body to another. How many nerve fibers are needed to constitute the formation of one acupoint is not known at this moment. Nevertheless, it is reasonable to assume that our body surface must have quite a number of acupoints. The most commonly mentioned acupoint total in acupuncture books is 361 points. This is obviously an arbitrary number. In our view, every few square millimeters of body surface can be a potential acupoint. There is no location where acupuncture needles cannot be placed. However, for practical purposes, approximately 100 points are useful to recognize and identify. The difference is that some points will be used therapeutically 100% of the time, whereas others will rarely be used at all. These will be clarified in later chapters of the book, when clinical applications of acupoints are mentioned. The focus for the book will be where the useful acupoints are located. They are distributed along the localities of the peripheral nerve branches. Thus, we will begin our anatomical review by establishing an organization of the nervous system that is convenient for our descriptions.

### 2.3.1 Organization of the Nervous System

The system is divided into the central and peripheral divisions. The central nervous system consists of the brain and the spinal cord, the study of which falls under neuroanatomy. There is not much of importance for us regarding the neuroanatomy of the brain and the spinal cord. Acupuncture will not be of much help to treat pain due to diseases or injuries in the central nervous system. Pain originating in the brain and the spinal cord is described as central pain. Central pain is rarely seen in acupuncture clinics. Most pain encountered is viewed as somatic in nature, perceived in the outer portions of the body, such as the head, neck, limbs, and lower back. Nerve fibers distributing to these areas of the body are categorized as the peripheral nerves, and they form the peripheral nervous system.

# Anatomy in Acupuncture

## 2.3.2 THE PERIPHERAL NERVOUS SYSTEM

The peripheral system consists of the cranial and spinal nerves. The cranial nerves originate from the brain. There are 12 pairs: olfactory, optic, oculomotor, trochlear, trigeminal, abducens, facial, vestibulocochlear or statoacoustic, glossopharyngeal, vagus, spinal accessory, and hypoglossal. What roles each of these nerves play, whether they are relevant in acupuncture, and which of them will have acupoints formed along their anatomical locations will be the topics for the next chapter.

Peripheral nerves come from the spinal cord in 33 pairs. They are divided into five groups: cervical plexus, brachial plexus, typical spinal nerves, lumbar plexus, and sacral–coccygeal plexus. The numbers of spinal nerves that participate in forming these five groups are four for the cervical plexus, five for the brachial plexus, 11 for the typical spinal plexus, four for the lumbar plexus, five for the sacral plexus, and four for the coccygeal plexus. The nerve branches of the cervical plexus are distributed in the neck region. The acupoints formed by these nerve branches are described in Chapter 4. Acupoints formed in the upper limbs along nerve branches of the brachial plexus can be found in Chapter 5. Chapter 6 is for the acupoints located in the body trunk, or thorax and abdomen, where terminal branches of the typical spinal nerves are located. Acupoints located in the lower limbs are formed by nerve branches of either the lumbar or sacral–coccygeal plexus, and can be found in Chapter 7.

## 2.3.3 THE NEURON

The term "nerve branch" is used frequently in anatomy, and so it will be within this book. We all know that nerve branches can be microscopic, invisible to the naked eye, or as large as a finger. Tiny twig nerve branches are anatomically ubiquitous. Nerve branches with anatomical nomenclatures are physically larger and limited in number. They are what we will speak about in this book. Regardless of their size, all nerve branches are made of nerve fibers. A nerve fiber is a portion of the nerve cell, which is known as a neuron. Neurons are structural units of the nervous system. As can be seen from Figures 2.1 and 2.2, there are different kinds of neurons, such as unipolar, bipolar, and multipolar. They are also named according to their locations, such as pyramidal, Purkinje,

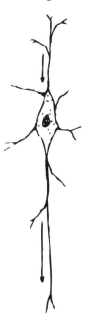

**FIGURE 2.1** A representative neuron. This particular type of neuron is known as multipolar. Arrows indicate the direction of nerve impulse transmission in the neuron.

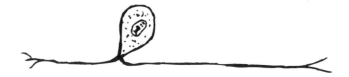

**FIGURE 2.2** Typical appearance of a bipolar neuron.

cerebellum, ventral horn, etc. Neurons can also be described by nomenclature according to physiological function. This can include motor, sensory, sympathetic, and parasympathetic. Sympathetic and parasympathetic neurons are subdivided into preganglionic and postganglionic neurons. Our main attention will be on the bipolar or sensory neurons.

All neurons have a cell body known as the perikarkyon, within which is the nucleus, and its extensions. The extensions of nerve cells are what we call nerve fibers, which are protoplasmic processes extending from the cell body. Neurons of the peripheral nervous system are all housed in a structure known as the ganglion. There are two types of nerve fibers, axons and dendrites, as shown in the two figures. The cells, dendrites, and axons are set in a framework of specialized and specific connective or interstitial tissues known as neuroglia. There is not much concern for knowing what the neuroglia is with regard to acupuncture. What needs to be known are the histologic or microscopic structures of the nerves or nerve fibers.

### 2.3.4 Histology of Nerves

Nerve fibers, often simply referred to as nerves, have a cord at their center, and this central cord is wrapped by a myelin sheath, as shown in Figure 2.3. There are six fibers seen in this figure. Five of them have only a single myelin sheath layer, and one has multiple sheath layers. The size of the central cord is very much the same for all nerves. However, the number of myelin sheath layers can vary from one to a hundred, as seen in Figure 2.4.

Thus, it is clear that the quantity of layers formed outside the central cord of the nerve determines the size of all nerve fibers. The fact that there are different nerve fibers of different sizes is important in explaining how and why acupuncture should and shouldn't work. More about the physiological aspects of acupuncture will be presented in Chapter 8.

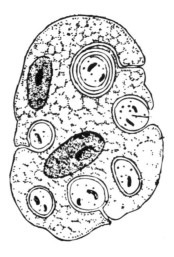

**FIGURE 2.3** A drawing depicting the formation of a myelin sheath around six axons or dendrites. One nerve has three layers of myelin sheath, whereas the other five nerves only have one layer. The two nuclei shown belong to neuroglia cells, which synthesize myelin. These particular neuroglia are known as Schwann cells.

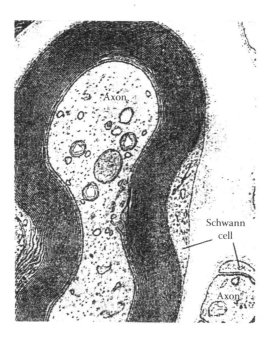

**FIGURE 2.4** An electron microscopic picture showing the detailed structures of a myelin sheath. There are two nerves shown; one is myelinated with more than 30 countable layers of sheath, and the other is unmyelinated and is often referred to as a naked nerve.

The myelin sheath is not only the microstructure that determines the size of the nerve, it also serves as the substance that insulates nerve fibers from shorting out each other. Figure 2.5 is a picture taken of a small nerve branch that was cut in a cross-section. From this picture, we can see nerves of different sizes. Not only is each nerve insulated by myelin but also the congregation of nerve fibers as a bundle is protected by a thick layer of connective tissue known as the perineurium. A number of small nerve bundles, such as those seen in Figure 2.5, can be collectively presented to form a larger bundle or branch, which will be wrapped in an even thicker layer called the epineurium. The myelin sheath outside a single nerve fiber is described as the endoneurium. It is obvious that neurons that become part of the nervous tissue are very well protected. This is the reason that, in the practice of acupuncture, needles properly inserted into the body are unlikely to produce substantial damage to nerve fibers. However, if the myelin is damaged or destroyed, pain will occur in

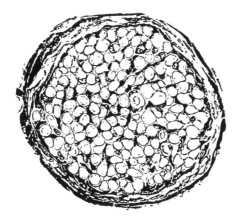

**FIGURE 2.5** A small nerve branch cut cross-sectionally to show nerve fibers of different diameters.

the body. It is very much like two uninsulated electric wires coming into contact, producing sparks and fire as a consequence.

### 2.3.5 Divisions of the Nerves

Anatomically, all nerve fibers are very much alike. They have a central cord wrapped in myelin sheath layers. Physiologically, however, they have different functions. These functions are motor and sensory. Motor functions are carried out by the efferent fibers, and sensory functions are performed by the afferent fibers. We need to categorize these two divisions in the instruction of acupuncture.

## 2.4 EFFERENT FIBERS

### 2.4.1 Efferent Fibers to Skeletal Muscles

Physiologically, "efferent" means move or run away from the cell bodies. What moves or runs away are impulses or messages generated or occurring in the neurons themselves. Efferent nerve fibers are also called motor nerve fibers. By this definition, we have efferent nerves to the skeletal muscles and in the autonomic nervous system. Efferent fibers to the skeletal muscles have two origins: one in the brain and the other in the spinal cord. The anatomy of efferent fibers—their origins, locations, and distributions—are described in the next five chapters. Here, we will briefly mention that skeletal muscles in the face and head are known as muscles of mastication and muscles of facial expression. Mastication muscles are controlled by the trigeminal nerve, and facial expression muscles are controlled by the facial nerves. Skeletal muscles in all other parts of the body are controlled by the spinal nerves. Nerves to the skeletal muscles originate from motor neurons in either the brain or the spinal cord. The signals to activate or move the muscles originate from these motor neurons to reach to the muscles. Therefore, the nerves are known as efferent fibers. The signals transmitted in the efferent fibers do not go from the muscles back to the neurons. This may explain why acupuncture does not have much effect on diseases involving efferent fibers, particularly efferent fibers to the skeletal muscles.

### 2.4.2 Autonomic Nervous System

Another kind of efferent fiber leads to cardiac and smooth muscles. Cardiac muscles are found in the heart. Smooth muscles are in the visceral organs, including—most importantly in the use of acupuncture—blood vessels in the arterial side. This group of efferent fibers is called the autonomic nerves. The autonomic nervous system has two subdivisions: sympathetic and parasympathetic nerves. Each division has two neuron stations, known as preganglionic and postganglionic cells. The system is far more complicated in organization and distribution. However, it is useful to be familiar with the anatomy of the autonomic nervous system because it plays a minor role in understanding the reactions created by acupuncture stimulation. More will be discussed about the nervous system in the next six chapters.

## 2.5 AFFERENT FIBERS

Afferent fibers carry nerve messages from the peripheral to the central nervous system. The messages are sensory in nature. Each nerve is believed to have a sensory receptor at the peripheral terminal end of the fiber. The receptor receives sensory messages generated along the afferent fibers. There are two types of sensory receptors: one for receiving the special senses, and the other for the general senses. Histologically, the receptor types are different in form and are distributed in different areas of the body. Special senses occur exclusively in the face and head, and general senses occur throughout the entire body.

## 2.5.1 FOR SPECIAL SENSES

We have five special senses. Their receptors and nerve fibers are located in the face and head regions of five special areas. These five special senses are smell sensation, located in the olfactory of the first cranial nerve; sight sensation, located in the optic of the secondary cranial nerve; taste sensation, located in the facial of the seventh cranial nerves; and hearing and equilibrium, located in the vestibulocochlear or statoacoustic of the eighth cranial nerve. The sensory receptors for smell are in the upper portion of the nasal cavity, known as the olfactory epithelium. The receptors for vision are located in the retina, which is inside the eyeball. The receptors known as taste buds, which make the discernment of sweet or sour possible, are located on the surface of the tongue. The receptors for hearing sound and balancing our body are located inside the inner ears, deep in the temporal bone in the structure known as the cochlea, which is a portion of the endolymphatic system. From these anatomical descriptions, it should be readily understood that functional deficits in all these special senses will not be easy to improve or correct by acupuncture treatments because none of the afferent nerve fibers that transmit special senses are accessible from the body surface. No known acupoints are formed by the olfactory, optic, or statoacoustic nerves. Acupuncture is useless if no acupoints are available to insert needles. More about facial nerves will be covered in the next chapter.

## 2.5.2 FOR GENERAL SENSES

"General senses" refers to sensations felt throughout the entire body. Physiologically, there are said to be five kinds of general senses: temperature, the sensation of hot or cold; tactile, the sensation of physical contact with the body; stereognostic, the sensation for detecting the form and nature of objects by palpation; proprioception; the awareness of body position and movements of the musculoskeletal system; and nociception, the ability to feel pain. Their respective peripheral receptors at the terminal end of the nerve fibers are the thermoreceptor, mechanoreceptor, stereognostic receptor, proprioceptor, and nociceptor.

There are quite a few histological terms used to describe different receptors in the general sensations. Known examples include Merkel's disk, Meissner's corpuscle, Paciniform ending, Vater–Pacini corpuscle, Ruffini's corpuscle, Krause's end bulb, neuromuscular spindle, neurotendinous organ, tactile corpuscle, free nerve ending, etc. We do not know for sure which of these structures represent what receptor. It is also not certain if any one of these receptors is responsible for one of the five senses we have, or more than one sense. Even though we have divided the sensory abilities into five categories, the reality of sensory functions may be much more complicated than we are able to comprehend. Take nociception, the sensation of pain, for example. Many different kinds of pain are known to us. It can be burning, excruciating, dull, numbing, prickling, tingling, and many more types. Do these terms describe the same phenomenon produced by the same sensory nerve, or is only one type of afferent sensory fiber responsible for our feeling each type of pain? Does each of these pain sensations have one specific receptor, or do multiple receptors act together to produce different kinds of nociception? We don't really know. Receptors for pain sensation are always described as free nerve endings, which have no or very little myelination. Because of their scanty myelin sheath, they are often considered to be naked nerves. A few free nerve endings are seen in Figure 2.6.

Thus, different sizes of afferent fibers, which are known to mediate different sensations, play an important role in our understanding of how acupuncture works. More will be said in the last few chapters about the relationship between the size of afferent fibers and how acupuncture can reduce or stop pain. In general, the different sizes of afferent nerve fibers are described as A, B, and C fibers. For our purposes, it is not necessary to know their exact diameters, only that A fibers are the largest in diameter, B fibers are second in size, and C fibers are the smallest. Using this distinction, we will be able to say that proprioceptors and mechanoreceptors have A fibers, thermoreceptors and stereognoceptors have B fibers, and nociceptors have C fibers. Within group C, numbing and

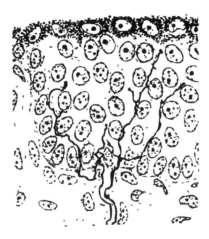

**FIGURE 2.6** A few free nerve endings are shown to run in the stratum spinosum and germinativum of the skin.

dull pain are transmitted by larger afferent fibers. Next to numbing and dull pain, the fibers to transmit sensation for pricking or tingling pain will be smaller in size. The smallest afferent fibers are the naked free nerve endings, which are nociceptors transmitting burning and excruciating pain. Knowing this is helpful for understanding why it is easier and quicker for acupuncture needles to stop burning and excruciating pain than dull, numbing, prickling or tingling pain. Different sizes for afferent nerves play an important role in the manageability of pain in acupuncture treatments.

By now, the anatomical differences between afferent fibers for the special senses and for the general senses should be clear. Each special sense is confined to the branches of only one cranial nerve. Within that cranial nerve, all afferent fibers perform one identical function for detecting one special sense. Afferent fibers for the five general senses are all mixed inside every peripheral nerve branch, meaning that all peripheral nerve branches contain afferent fibers of different sizes, from A to C groups. In the gross dissection of a cadaver, it is impossible to separate A, B, and C fibers. Thus, we must treat all afferent fibers for the general senses as one anatomical entity, and we will refer to them as afferent fibers for the general senses in this book.

In summary, we have stated that acupoints are the most important thing in acupuncture. From our observations, the identity of acupoints is in the nerve fibers. There are two kinds of fibers—efferent and afferent. Efferent fibers go to innervating skeletal muscles and structures that contain cardiac and smooth muscles. Efferent fibers that innervate cardiac and smooth muscles are known as autonomic nerves. Autonomic nerves are divided into sympathetic and parasympathetic, each of which consists of preganglionic and postganglionic segments. Afferent fibers are sensory nerves. There are afferent fibers for special senses, and afferent fibers for general senses. Combinations of a number of these nerve fibers exist in the body as nerve branches. Nerve branches are what are needed to locate acupoints.

There two types of nerve branches, muscular and cutaneous nerves, which takes us to our next topic.

## 2.6 MUSCULAR NERVE BRANCHES

The term *motor nerve* can be confused with *muscular nerve*. Innervation to skeletal muscle is not by motor nerves alone. Keep in mind that motor nerves are limited to the efferent fibers originating from motor neurons in the brain and spinal cord. Motor nerves are joined with afferent fibers for general sensations and with postganglionic sympathetic nerves to form a muscular nerve branch. This is why describing the locus where a muscular nerve enters a muscle as a "motor point" is not exactly accurate. However, it is such a commonly accepted term that we will adopt it in this book.

Muscular nerves or nerve branches, as used in our definition, are implied to contain three types of nerve fibers: efferent nerves to the skeletal muscles, postganglionic sympathetic nerves, and afferent fibers for the general senses.

## 2.7 CUTANEOUS NERVE BRANCHES

Another type of peripheral nerve branch is cutaneous. Cutaneous branches contain only two kinds of nerve fibers: afferent fibers for the general senses and postganglionic sympathetic nerves. Postganglionic sympathetic nerves control the activity of smooth muscles in blood vessels, secretory glands, and hair follicles.

In the end, what matters with respect to acupoints, are the muscular and cutaneous nerve branches. We can claim that all acupoints are a portion of either muscular or cutaneous nerves because, along these nerve branches, there are certain anatomical features that contribute to acupoints forming at those particular locations.

## 2.8 ANATOMICAL FEATURES CONTRIBUTING TO THE FORMATION OF ACUPOINTS

The distribution of acupoints in the body is not as random as it may seem to be. Every acupoint has a functional justification to be where it is located. A number of justifications turn out to be anatomical features that form acupoints. Therefore, it is reasonable to assume that acupoints are not formed by an identifiable structure as an anatomical entity, but rather by certain anatomical features that are observable upon gross dissection. How many of these anatomical features do we have? Here, we list 10 that have been previously reported [5].

### 2.8.1 Size

Acupoints are invariably distributed along either muscular or cutaneous nerve branches. The bigger the branches are, the higher the possibility for acupoints to be formed. Of course, size is not the sole feature to determine whether an acupoint will be located on a particular nerve branch. There are many fairly large nerves, such as the sciatic, femoral, medial, lateral, and posterior cords of the brachial plexus where no acupoints are found. The reason is that these nerve branches are deep in the body.

### 2.8.2 Depth

The sciatic nerve is buried deep inside three muscles: the gluteus maximus, gluteus medius, and gluteus minimus in the gluteal region. This region is a relatively large area, but only one acupoint is known to be in the gluteal region. After descending to the posterior compartment of the thigh, the sciatic divides into two branches, the tibial and common peroneal. Both are more superficially located in their courses of distribution. A few acupoints are formed along the distal portions of both branches. The same occurrence will be found for the femoral and other nerves mentioned. In general, it is true that muscular nerves are more deeply located than cutaneous branches.

### 2.8.3 Penetration of the Deep Fascia

This feature is appropriate for cutaneous nerves only. As covered in gross anatomy, structures in the body are arranged layer upon layer. Between layers, particularly of the musculature, there are fasciae of connective tissue. We have superficial and deep fasciae. All cutaneous nerves have to penetrate the deep fascia to go into the superficial fascia under the skin. The location where a cutaneous nerve branch identifiable in gross anatomy can be seen to penetrate the deep fascia will unmistakably form an acupoint. Many realistic examples will be provided in the next few chapters. No muscular nerve has a need to penetrate deep fascia.

### 2.8.4 Passage through Bone Foramina

Some cutaneous nerves pierce deep fascia to go superficially into skin. Others pass through bone foramina to distribute subcutaneously. This anatomical feature applies specifically to the trigeminal nerve. There are five foramina identifiable on the skull bone of the face: the supraorbital, infraorbital, mental, zygomaticotemporal, and zygomaticofacial. Each of these has a cutaneous nerve running through it, carrying the same anatomical name as its foramen. Of these five foramina, the difference in size is visible in gross anatomy. Thus, the size of the five cutaneous nerve branches can be expected to be different. The biggest of them is the infraorbital. Next is the supraorbital, followed by the mental, zygomaticotemporal, and zygomaticofacial. The clinical significance of these differences will become obvious when we discuss headaches in the latter chapters of the book relating to their applications in acupuncture.

### 2.8.5 Motor Point

The original term used for this anatomical feature was "neuromuscular attachment." Another, more appropriate, name to describe this feature would be "neuromuscular junction." However, neuromuscular junction is a well-established anatomical nomenclature, so using that here could cause confusion. We thus adopt the term "motor point" because it is well known in the medical community. According to *Dorland's Illustrated Medical Dictionary*, a motor point is "the point at which a motor nerve enters a muscle." As explained above, this definition is neither accurate nor true, unless "motor nerve" is intended to be "muscular nerve branch." There is no way for a motor nerve to enter a muscle alone. Nerves that enter a muscle will have to be in a muscular branch, which must contain efferent fibers to skeletal muscle, afferent fibers for general senses, and postganglionic sympathetic nerves. In gross anatomy dissections, it is not important for students to know the precise location where a muscular nerve branch enters the muscle. The site of the motor point is very constant from person to person. Most muscles have only one motor point, with the exception of a few long muscles, such as the biceps brachii. Many motor points are deep under the muscle mass. They do not have the potential to become acupoints.

### 2.8.6 Concomitant Blood Vessels

Nerve branches are often accompanied by vascular supplies, called concomitant arteries and veins. Nerves, arteries, and veins stay and run together as neurovascular bundles. We don't know whether blood vessels play an important role in the formation of acupoints. We do notice that there is a dense, rich blood supply in the vicinity of several important acupoints. The importance of what constitutes acupoints will be explained in Chapter 8 when their physiological activities and functions are discussed. The significance of concomitant blood vessels in the formation of acupoints is found in the fact that cutaneous nerves are frequently distributed anatomically without visible blood supply. A cutaneous nerve with a known acupoint, but without concomitant blood vessels, is more superficially located than a motor point formed by a muscular nerve of the same size that is situated deeper inside the muscle mass. The acupoint formed by this cutaneous nerve cannot be as useful as that formed by the muscular branch (what we mean here by "useful" will be discussed in later chapters). The deep radial nerve is a good example. It is a muscular nerve located deeply between the brachioradialis and extensor carpi radialis longus muscles. The muscles form a bulgy portion at the proximal region of the forearm over the lateral compartment. According to acupuncture books, there are four acupoints described in the area, as shown in Figure 2.7. These four acupoints can be considered as motor points formed by the deep radial nerve as it branches upon entering

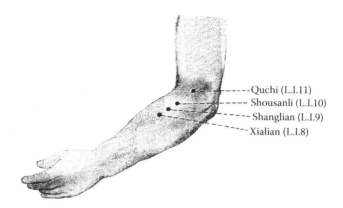

**FIGURE 2.7** Four acupoints shown over the proximal region of the forearm lying along the lateral compartment.

the extensor muscle group in the forearm. There are six extensor muscles lying superficially in this region. The motor points of these muscles have potential to become acupoints.

### 2.8.7 Nerve Fiber Compositions

Nerve fibers in both cutaneous and muscular branches are variable in size. The variability is considered to be greater and higher for muscular nerves than for cutaneous nerves because muscular branches have a greater variety of nerve fibers than cutaneous branches do. This difference could be a reason that acupoints formed by muscular branches often are more useful than those formed by cutaneous branches.

### 2.8.8 Points of Bifurcation

Several acupoints are located at the point where a relatively large nerve branch divides. The point formed by the superficial radial nerve on the dorsal surface of the hand between thumb and index finger is an example. All larger nerve branches will eventually divide to become smaller nerves. Most of the divisions are too minute to be seen gross-anatomically. They are microscopic in histological nature. Those which are visible under gross dissection are cutaneous nerves at the localities where they penetrate the deep fascia or go through bone foramina. These localities are where acupoints come to be. As the nerves divide into smaller branches, one possible consequence with respect to anatomy is that sensory fields become smaller. A sensory field is defined as a unit of area loaded with a number of sensory receptors. Sensory fields in the palm and plantar skin are more sensitive than skin in the dorsal surface of the body trunk. This difference is due to differences in the density of sensory fields. The skin on the palm is said to have a higher density of sensory fields than skin in other parts of the body. This explains why it is more painful to prick a needle into the palm than the buttock. The highest density of sensory fields, at the opening of a deep fascia where the penetration of a cutaneous nerve branch occurs, is a suitable location to have an acupoint. The same applies to cutaneous branches going through bone foramina on the face.

### 2.8.9 Sensitive Points on Tendons and Ligaments

Our body has muscle tendons, retinacula of various joints connecting separate pieces of bone, thick fascial sheets such as the iliotibial tract (which cover the lateral surface of the thigh deep under the skin), joint capsules, and collateral ligaments around the knee. These are formed by dense, fibrous connective tissue. These tissue structures are known to have rich proprioceptors, stereognostic

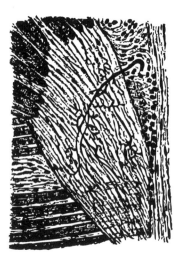

**FIGURE 2.8** A drawing to illustrate muscle and its tendon with afferent fibers and sensory receptors. (Adapted from Copenhaver, W.H. et al., *Bailey's Textbook of Histology*, 7th ed. Williams and Wilkins, Baltimore, 342, 1978.)

receptors, and nociceptors, as can be seen in Figure 2.8. Sensitive points detected along tendons and ligaments can be considered as acupoints and will be used as such. Two of the most frequently detectable acupoints are in the tendon of the long head of the biceps brachii. This segment of tendon is lodged in the intertubercular groove of the humerus head. The tendon will have anywhere from one to three tender points palpable in people who have pain in the shoulder joint. Another example is the acupoint located in the tendon of the long extensor muscles in the forearm. The tendon originates from and is attached to the lateral epicondyle of the humerus. People with "tennis elbow" will not have much difficulty in finding tender points over the surface of the lateral epicondyle. These tender points can surely be considered as acupoints.

### 2.8.10 SUTURE LINES ON THE SKULL

Our skull is constructed of a number of bone pieces. These bone pieces are cemented together by connective tissue that become suture lines as our body matures. These include the coronal suture, sagittal suture, lambdoidal suture, and so on. Some areas of suture lines have more connective tissue than others. The areas where there are more connective tissues in the embryonic stage are known as fontanelles. We have the anterior, posterior, anterolateral or sphenoidal, and the posterolateral or mastoid fontanelles. These fontanelles become the bregma, pterion, asterion, etc. The spots where fontanelles were previously located have more afferent nerve receptors remaining. Thus, there is a better possibility for acupoints to appear in such localities.

## 2.9 DISCUSSION AND CONCLUSION

Assuming what is portrayed above in this chapter to be correct and true, it will be no surprise that the real identity of acupoints is difficult or impossible to find. If a person has multiple shadows, which one of them is really his or hers could be hard to decide. What is more confounding is that there are other points, such as trigger points, which are very well known clinically. Yet, no one has been able to clearly dissect out the real anatomical identity of these intriguing points in the body. This is because trigger points and acupoints have identical anatomical features. They actually are the same in their anatomical localities. Under normal and healthy conditions, the localities are

# Anatomy in Acupuncture

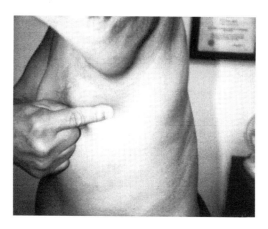

**FIGURE 2.9** The patient uses an index finger to point at an acupoint, which has become a trigger point with the pain this patient felt. This acupoint is called the intercostobrachial, and will be discussed in Chapter 6.

acupoints. When pain appears in the body, they become trigger points. More about the conversion between acupoints and trigger points will be discussed in later chapters.

Other names used in the medical literature that may have certain relevance to acupuncture include motor point, dermal point, sensitive point, and tender point, and there may be others of which we are not aware. None of them will be used in this book. We have previously explained what a motor point is. Dermal, sensitive, and tender points are simply the spots in the body where pain sometimes appears and can be perceivable. If the patients having one or more of these points are requested to identify where a sensitive or tender points is, the location they indicate will always turn out to be an acupoint or trigger point, as seen in Figure 2.9.

## REFERENCES

1. Ha, H.C. et al. Muscle sensory neurons in the spinal ganglia in the rat determined by retrograde transport of horseradish peroxidase. *Experimental Neurology* 70:438, 1980.
2. Vanderschodt, L. Trigger points vs. acupuncture points. *American Journal of Acupuncture* 4:233, 1976.
3. Melzack, R. Myofascial trigger points: Relation to acupuncture and mechanisms of pain. *Archives of Physical Medicine and Rehabilitation* 62:114, 1981.
4. Liu, Y.K. et al. Correspondence between some motor points in acupuncture loci. *American Journal of Chinese Medicine* 3:347, 1975.
5. Dung, H.C. Anatomical features contributing to the formation of acupuncture points. *American Journal of Acupuncture* 12:139, 1984.

# 3 Acupoints of the Cranial Nerves

Acupoints formed by the cranial nerves were first reported by the author in 1984 [1]. There are 12 pairs of cranial nerves, which can be divided into two groups. One group is composed of cranial nerves that have no known affiliated acupoints. Seven nerve pairs belong to this group. The other group is composed of cranial nerves that have anatomical features, which can be viewed as possible indicators for forming acupoints. Thus, for the sake of convenience, the contents of this chapter can be divided between cranial nerves with acupoints and cranial nerves without acupoints. The cranial nerves without acupoints will be discussed first.

## 3.1 CRANIAL NERVES WITHOUT ACUPOINTS

We have seven cranial nerve pairs without identifiable acupoints. Three of them contain afferent fibers only, whereas the other four carry only efferent fibers.

### 3.1.1 Afferent Fibers Only

As mentioned in the previous chapter, we have five special senses. The cranial nerves that are responsible for these five special senses are the olfactory, optic, facial, and statoacoustic nerves. Afferent fibers for these special senses run in unexposed routes and are distributed to localities that are not approachable from outside of the body.

#### 3.1.1.1 Olfactory Nerve

This originates from the olfactory epithelium, which is the lining of the roof and adjacent surface of the septum and of the superior nasal concha. Afferent fibers extend from olfactory cells in the epithelium to pass through the cribriform plate to enter the undersurface of the olfactory bulb of the brain. Loss of olfactory sensation due to any disease or damage along this nerve cannot be treated with acupuncture needles. Pain inside the nasal cavity is very rare. Afferent fibers for general senses in the nasal cavity are from cutaneous branches of the ophthalmic and maxillary divisions of the trigeminal nerves. The names of these nerves for pain sensation are nasociliary from the ophthalmic and nasopalatine from the maxillary.

#### 3.1.1.2 Optic Nerve

This nerve consists of the axon of the ganglion cells of the retina in the eye. It is not possible for acupoints to form along this cranial nerve.

#### 3.1.1.3 Statoacoustic Nerve

This nerve, also known as the vestibulocochlear, consists of two functionally distinct and incompletely united nerve fibers, the cochlear nerve and the vestibular nerve. No acupoints are known to be formed on either of the two nerves. However, conditions such as vertigo and tinnitus will respond to acupuncture by stimulating acupoints around the ears. Those acupoints are related to the trigeminal and facial nerves, which have a very close anatomical relationship with the statoacoustic nerve.

### 3.1.2 EFFERENT FIBERS ONLY

The four cranial nerves containing only efferent fibers are the oculomotor, trochlear, abducens, and hypoglossal nerves.

#### 3.1.2.1 Oculomotor Nerve

There is one key difference between the oculomotor nerve and the other three cranial nerves in this group. In addition to efferent fibers to the skeletal muscles, the oculomotor nerve is also composed of a parasympathetic portion of the autonomic nervous system. The preganglionic neurons of these parasympathetic nerves are located at the Edinger–Westphal nucleus inside the brain, and the postganglionic neurons in the ciliary ganglion are located behind the orbits. Short ciliary nerves carry the postganglionic parasympathetic fibers to the sphincter pupillae muscle of the iris and to the ciliary muscle of accommodation. Afferent fibers for the general sensations of the eye are from trigeminal nerves. Interneural communications between branches of the trigeminal and oculomotor nerves can produce reactions in the pupil when acupuncture needles are placed in the acupoints formed by the trigeminal nerve branches around the eyes.

#### 3.1.2.2 Trochlear Nerve

This is the smallest of the cranial nerves and supplies only one muscle. The human eye has seven muscles. Five of them are controlled by the oculomotor nerve. One, the superior oblique muscle, is controlled by the trochlear nerve.

#### 3.1.2.3 Abducens Nerve

This nerve controls the lateral rectus muscle. No acupoints are formed by the abducens nerve or the trochlear nerve.

#### 3.1.2.4 Hypoglossal Nerve

This is the motor nerve of the tongue. The tongue is composed of skeletal muscles. Its intrinsic muscles have no anatomical designations. The names of the extrinsic muscles are the styloglossus, hyoglossus, and genioglossus. Motor points formed by the hypoglossal nerve at these muscles are obscure and difficult, if not impossible, to dissect out in cadavers.

## 3.2 CRANIAL NERVES WITH ACUPOINTS

Five cranial nerves are qualified to be placed in this group: the trigeminal, facial, glossopharyngeal, vagus, and spinal accessory nerves. The most important of these, in terms of acupoints, is the trigeminal nerve, followed by the facial nerve, and then the spinal accessory nerve. The glossopharyngeal and vagus nerves are placed in this group for one practical reason: their anatomical complexity.

## 3.3 TRIGEMINAL NERVE

Where acupoints are concerned, the trigeminal nerve is the most important and most useful of the 12 cranial nerve pairs. There are several reasons for this nerve's importance. Anatomically, it is large in size, and possibly the biggest of the cranial nerves. It has more branches than any other cranial nerve, more than 50 with proper anatomical names. Many of them have communications with the neurons of other cranial nerves. Their anatomical relations are too complicated for all of them to be mentioned, but here are a couple of examples. The chorda tympani is a branch of the facial nerve carrying the special sense of taste from the tongue by way of the lingual branch of the mandibular division of the trigeminal. Then, there is the autonomic nerve controlling the secretion of mucus in the nose and saliva in the mouth. The sympathetic section of the autonomic nerve to the secretory glands in the head is from the cervical spinal nerves. The parasympathetic section is from the superior salivatory nucleus in the brain, where preganglionic neurons are found. Preganglionic nerves coming out of the brain in the facial nerve than synapse at the postganglionic neurons in the pterygopalatine, otic, and submandibular ganglia. Finally, postganglionic nerves from these ganglia reach their target glands in the nasal and oral cavities. Such a brief and simple description of interneural connections explains why acupuncture can be useful for relieving nasal congestion in people suffering from allergic ailments. However, the physiological mechanism by which acupuncture is beneficial for treating certain kinds of allergies is too complicated to thoroughly explain in this book.

Acupoints formed by the branches of the trigeminal are useful because they are necessary to treat patients suffering from headaches or pain in the head region. Headaches and pain in the head region are not necessarily the same. Varieties of headache include tension, cluster, migraine, and tic douloureux. These headaches are not the same as postherpetic neuralgia along the trigeminal nerve and atypical facial pain. Acupoints located along the branches of the trigeminal nerve are useful for managing both headaches and pain in the head and facial regions.

The anatomy of the trigeminal nerve is rather complex. Because of this complexity, we have a few ways to categorize the acupoints that are located along the branches of the nerve. Acupoints can be identified following the three divisions of the trigeminal: the ophthalmic, maxillary, and mandibular divisions. Each of these divisions has a number of branches that will eventually end up having acupoints. Inconveniently, not all of the terminal branches that form acupoints will come directly from one of the three divisions. The mental nerve is from the inferior alveolar branch, which branches from the mandibular division. The maxillary division has 10 identified branches, one of which is the infraorbital. The ophthalmic division has three terminal branches: the supraorbital, supratrochlear, and infratrochlear. They do not directly branch from the ophthalmic division but are from the frontal nerve which in turn is a direct branch of the division. We have decided that it will be easier to describe acupoints using the denominations of cutaneous and muscular nerve branches given in Chapter 2. However, Figure 3.1 is offered for reference as an overview of the cutaneous nerve supply in the face and scalp by the three divisions of the trigeminal nerve. For all acupoints formed by the cutaneous nerve branches, it should be fairly easy to recognize from which division the nerve comes. If the point is located in the region innervated by that particular division, then the nerve which forms that point must belong to that division.

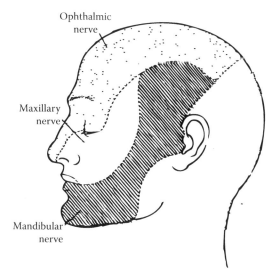

**FIGURE 3.1** A schematic drawing of cutaneous nerve supply by the three divisions of the trigeminal nerve.

### 3.3.1 ACUPOINTS OF CUTANEOUS BRANCHES

A total of 10 acupoints are considered to be formed by the cutaneous branches of the trigeminal nerve. Their locations are shown in Figure 3.2. Four different symbols are used to mark these acupoints: stars, squares, triangles, and circles. The acupoints designated by stars are considered as the primary acupoints in this book, squares as the secondary, triangles as the tertiary, and circles as the nonspecific points. Their meaning and significance in pain and acupuncture will be extensively explained in Chapters 8 and 10. For the time being, their implications can be ignored. We will frequently come back to figures showing acupoints in this chapter and in the subsequent four chapters when we talk about the clinical applications of acupuncture. These 10 acupoints are listed below with a brief description for each, and are provided to highlight their anatomical locations and significance.

#### 3.3.1.1 Supraorbital

This is located toward the medial end of the eyebrows. The nerve branch forming this point is the second biggest of the 10. With its concomitant blood vessels, the branch runs through the supraorbital foramen to distribute subcutaneously.

#### 3.3.1.2 Supratrochlear and Infratrochlear

The nerve branches that form these two points are too small to be identifiable for gross dissection. They are very rarely used in clinical applications for the practice of acupuncture. Acupoints that are categorized as nonspecific points are not often used in clinical practice.

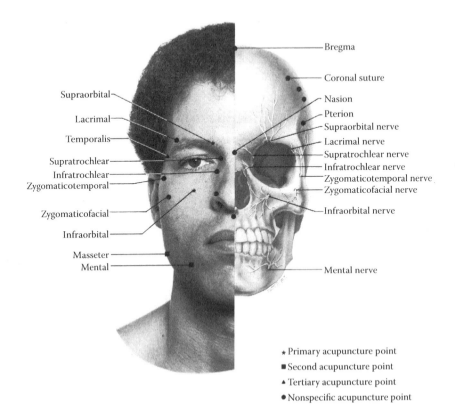

**FIGURE 3.2** The right half of the photo shows the cutaneous nerve branches of the trigeminal, which form the acupoints shown on the left half of the photo.

# Acupoints of the Cranial Nerves

### 3.3.1.3 Lacrimal

These points are located toward the lateral ends of the eyebrows but superior to them. The nerve becomes cutaneous after giving away innervation to the lacrimal glands. Stimulating the lacrimal points around the eye has the potential of increasing tear secretion. The nerves that form these four points are all branches of the ophthalmic division.

### 3.3.1.4 Infraorbital

This is formed by the biggest cutaneous nerve branch. It is accompanied by the infraorbital artery and vein to pass through the infraorbital foramen to reach the skin. This is the most important acupoint in the entire head and face area because it is the most frequently used point, which is why it is classified as a primary point. There are only two primary points among these 10 acupoints, the other being the supraorbital point.

### 3.3.1.5 Zygomaticotemporal and Zygomaticofacial

These can be considered as one point. The cutaneous nerves forming both of the acupoints are terminal branches of the maxillary division. Like the supratrochlear and infratrochlear nerves, it is very difficult to dissect out these two nerves in the gross laboratory. They are also nonspecific acupoints and can be located over the cheek bones in people who have been suffering from chronic and severe headaches for a long time.

### 3.3.1.6 Mental

This is one of the terminal branches of the mandibular division. If the supraorbital, infraorbital, and mental points were connected, it would form a straight line. Of these three points, the mental is formed by the smallest nerve. The concomitant vessels are also mental as well as the foramen they go through together. The mental is considered as a secondary point. It will not become tender as often as the supraorbital and infraorbital points, and it is used less frequently, although it ranks the third in usefulness among all the acupoints located in the head and face.

### 3.3.1.7 Auriculotemporal

This is the only point not seen in Figure 3.2 because of its location on the side of head. However, Figure 3.3 is a drawing of a right ear, in which the location of the acupoint formed by the auriculotemporal nerve can be found. The name of the foramen that the auriculotemporal nerve runs through under the base of the skull is the spinosum. Once it is outside the skull, the nerve then passes laterally behind the temporomandibular joint (TMJ). Because of their proximity, there is no question that the joint receives innervation from the auriculotemporal nerve. As indicated in Figure 3.3, the

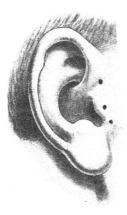

**FIGURE 3.3** Three acupoints in front of the right ear. They are the temporomandibular, auriculotemporal, and anterior auricular.

temporomandibular and auriculotemporal points are right next to each other vertically, although both are formed by the same auriculotemporal nerve. The temporomandibular point is relatively important because of pain in the TMJ. Pain from TMJ is rather frequently encountered in acupuncture clinics. In teaching gross anatomy for 31 years, the author has never had a chance to identify a branch of the auriculotemporal nerve to the TMJ. Because the temporomandibular point is formed in a joint, the point is grouped with tendinous acupoints following acupoints of muscular branches.

### 3.3.1.8 Paranasal

This extraordinary point is located right on top of the wings of the nose, as can be seen in Figures 3.2, 3.4, and 3.5, each of which has a circled, unnamed, nonspecific point. It is extraordinary because there is no cutaneous nerve to represent the point. The point obviously is inside the territory innervated by the nerve branches of the mandibular division. This point is very useful in dealing with problems involving the nasal airway, such as nasal congestion, coughing, and smoking cessation.

## 3.3.2 ACUPOINTS OF CONNECTIVE TISSUE

A number of acupoints are known to be located along the suture lines of the skull or on the fibrous capsules of joints—specifically, the TMJ. Sutures existing between bones of the skull and on the joint capsule are formed by connective tissue [2]. The areas where two suture lines cross each other are fontanelles during the embryonic stage. Figures 3.6 and 3.7 show where some of the fontanelles are located. Fontanelles will eventually become acupoints, as shown in Figure 3.2. Fontanelles, sutures, and joint capsules must contain sensory receptors of afferent fibers. Yet no cutaneous nerve branches can be found to come from any of the acupoints described in this section. Thus, they have to be assembled together as a separate group. Five of the acupoints in this group are listed in the

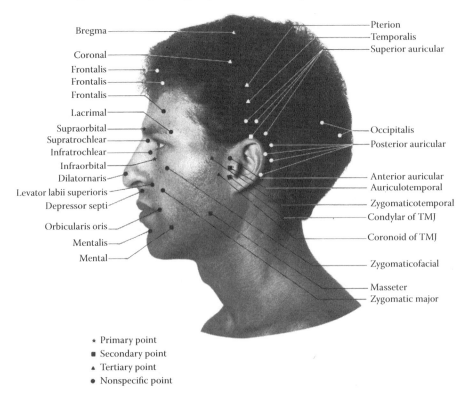

**FIGURE 3.4** A lateral view of the head and face. The nonspecific point marked on the side of the nose is the paranasal point.

# Acupoints of the Cranial Nerves

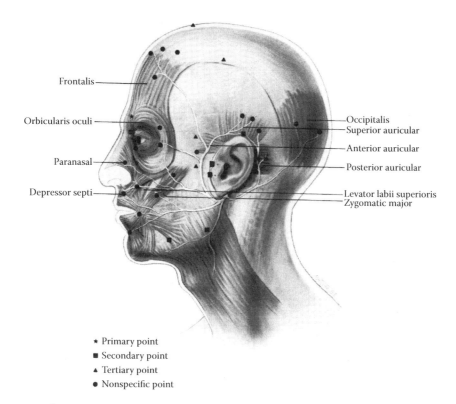

★ Primary point
■ Secondary point
▲ Tertiary point
● Nonspecific point

**FIGURE 3.5** Lateral view of the head showing a variety of acupoints.

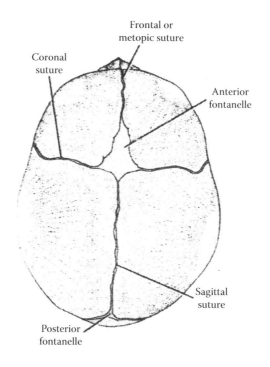

**FIGURE 3.6** Top view of the skull in a newborn.

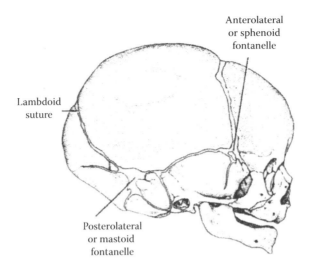

**FIGURE 3.7** Lateral view of the skull in a newborn.

following sections. The other acupoints in this group are not described, not only because they lack anatomical nomenclature but also because they lack importance as they are not used clinically at all.

### 3.3.2.1 Bregma

This point is at the meeting of the coronal and sagittal sutures. In the fetal skull, it is the site of the anterior fontanelle. This acupoint is not used very often because it is a tertiary point.

### 3.3.2.2 Pterion

This is the area where the frontal, sphenoid, and temporal bones closely adjoin one another. Surgically, it is an important landmark, but again, it is not an important acupoint.

### 3.3.2.3 Nasion

This is the point where the internasal and frontonasal sutures meet. Occasionally, this acupoint will be useful to ease headaches and severe nasal congestion.

### 3.3.2.4 Coronal Suture

This acupoint can appear along the coronal suture line between the bregma and the pterion, although such a case might never be encountered among all the patients seen in an acupuncture clinic.

### 3.3.2.5 Temporomandibular

This acupoint is formed by a branch that comes from the auriculotemporal nerve to the TMJ. It is a very useful point for managing pain in TMJ. As shown in Figures 3.3 and 3.5, there are three acupoints located immediately in front of the anterior line of the external ear: the temporomandibular (secondary point, as indicated by a square), auriculotemporal (tertiary point, as indicated by a triangle), and anterior auricular (nonspecific point, as indicated by a circle). These three points can be used as indicators to evaluate the severity of a TMJ condition. Tenderness in the temporomandibular point alone indicates that TMJ is in the early stages. The pain is often minor and very easy to eradicate. If both the temporomandibular and auriculotemporal points become tender, it indicates that TMJ is getting worse, and pain will bother the patient more frequently. It will be harder to manage, although it is still manageable. When all three points are tender, TMJ is sure to be in an advanced condition. Pain certainly is in the chronic stage, and will be present most of the time. Managing pain in TMJ at this stage is not easy; even the use of acupuncture will not guarantee success.

Each afferent fiber is supposed to have a sensory receptor at the peripheral end of the nerve. All afferent nerves travel to sensory neurons inside the semilunar ganglion. From this ganglion, axons of nerve

# Acupoints of the Cranial Nerves

fibers enter the midbrain to terminate in the mesencephalic nucleus and the spinal tract. The spinal tract of the trigeminal descends inferiorly in the spinal cord to as low as the segment of the fourth cervical spinal nerve, which contributes to the upper portion of the brachial plexus, making intercommunication possible between acupoints in the head and in the upper limbs. Some of this intercommunication will be dealt with in Chapter 5, where acupoints of the brachial plexus will be discussed in our study.

Intercommunications between the trigeminal and other cranial nerves belong to the study of neuroanatomy [3]. These communications involve superior and inferior salivatory nuclei. The superior salivatory is part of the facial nerve, and the inferior salivatory is part of the glossopharyngeal. Other nuclei that have nerve cells interconnected to axons of the trigeminal include the vestibulocochlear and vagus. The complexity of these neuro-relationships is beyond the reach of acupuncture. All we need to keep in mind is that stimulating acupoints in the head and face can have profound consequences for physiological activities and functions in these regions.

### 3.3.3 Acupoints of Muscular Branches

The muscles of the head and face can be divided into two functional groups [4,5]. One group is composed of muscles of mastication, the other group is composed of the muscles of facial expression. The muscles of mastication are the subject of this current description. The muscles of expression will be dealt with in Section 3.4 of this chapter.

All muscles of mastication are innervated by muscular branches coming from the mandibular division of the trigeminal. We know that at least six muscles receive nerve supplies from the mandibular division. A couple of these, the medial and lateral pterygoid muscles, are deep in the wing of the mandible. Their motor points will not be accessible, assuming that they indeed exist. The other four muscles are superficially located. The motor points of these four muscles form acupoints as follows.

#### 3.3.3.1 Masseter

This muscle overlies the angle of the mandible as shown in Figures 3.2, 3.4, and 3.8. The masseteric nerve passes laterally to go through the mandibular notch and enter the deep surface of the masseter muscle. The masseteric nerve also provides branches to the TMJ.

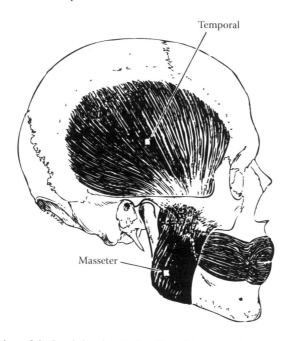

**FIGURE 3.8** Lateral view of the head showing the location of two acupoints.

### 3.3.3.2 Temporalis

This acupoint (Figures 3.2, 3.4, and 3.8) is formed by the deep temporal nerve. The nerve enters the temporalis muscle on its deep aspect. Both the masseter (secondary acupoint) and temporalis (tertiary) are frequently used for acupuncture therapy. Patients with tension headaches often have pain in the temporalis point.

### 3.3.3.3 Anterior Auricular and Superior Auricular

These two acupoints can be seen in Figures 3.4. and 3.5. There are three auricular muscles: the anterior, superior, and posterior muscles. Muscular branches to the first two muscles come from the motor nerves of the mandibular division. Nerves to the posterior auricular muscle are derived from the facial nerve, which will be covered subsequently.

## 3.4 FACIAL NERVE

This cranial nerve (VII) is second in importance only to the trigeminal. All acupoints formed by the facial nerve are motor points in nature. Each motor point can act as an acupoint. Thus, depending on how many muscles are innervated by the facial nerve, we will have that many acupoints in the head and face. According to our calculations, there are at least 21 muscles for which innervations come from the facial nerve. They are what we call the muscles of facial expression. Acupoints formed by the muscular branches from the mandibular division, in general, are not of much use in acupuncture. One disease involving facial nerves is facial paralysis, also known as Bell's palsy. Efferent fibers in the facial nerve going to the muscles of facial expression all originate from neurons of the motor nucleus of that cranial nerve. If the paralysis or palsy is due to a disease in the central nervous system, such as a brain tumor or cancer resulting in damage to or destruction of these motor neurons, acupuncture is absolutely useless. However, facial paralysis is almost always caused by injury to the facial nerve in the stylomastoid foramen, which is relatively far away from the brain. At that location, the facial nerve is already considered to be a portion of the peripheral nerves. Peripheral nerve fibers have the potential to regenerate, and acupuncture is capable of accelerating the regeneration process of nerve fibers. Under ordinary circumstances, Bell's palsy is a self-limiting disease. For most patients suffering from this type of illness, the paralysis will improve and diminish on its own without clinical treatment. From our own clinical experiences, acupuncture indeed has the potential to further improve the symptoms of paralysis by using motor points on the facial muscles. Which acupoints will be useful for treating Bell's palsy? The answer will be almost any of the acupoints that are located in the head and face regions. Example acupoints are depicted in Figures 3.4 and 3.5, and include the frontalis, dilatonaris, levator labii superioris, depressor septi, orbicularis oris, mentalis, occipitalis, posterior auricular, and orbicularis oculi.

Compared with muscles from the rest of body, the muscles of facial expression are relatively small in size and short in length. The nerves of these muscles are tiny. They can be difficult to visualize and impossible to dissect out grossly. Such anatomical conditions make the acupoints formed by the muscular branches of the facial nerve insignificant for use in acupuncture. They are considered as nonspecific acupoints, meaning that if an acupuncturist decides to use any of them in clinical applications, the locations where the needles need to be inserted don't have to be precisely where the motor points are supposed to be, but only in the general loci of the acupoints.

In addition to efferent fibers to skeletal muscles, the facial nerve also contains autonomic and afferent fibers. The autonomic portion is in the parasympathetic division. Its efferent fibers begin at preganglionic cells in the superior salivatory ganglion. The preganglionic nerves end in postganglionic neurons located inside the sphenopalatine and submandibular ganglia, from which the postganglionic nerves are distributed to their target organs by way of the trigeminal branches. The afferent fibers in the facial nerve transmit the special sense of taste generated in the tongue back to the geniculate ganglion. Afferent fibers for the general senses to the muscles of facial expression are entirely contributed by the trigeminal nerves. None of these autonomic and afferent nerves for the special senses separately form any acupoint on their own. Therefore, there is no need to describe their presence further.

## 3.5 GLOSSOPHARYNGEAL NERVE

This ninth cranial nerve is primarily related to the tongue and pharynx. The nerves have no practical relation to acupuncture because no acupoint could be considered to be formed by any branch of this cranial nerve. However, the nerve has a couple of anatomical features that are unique in contrast with the other 11 cranial nerves. The first feature is that it contains all kinds of nerve fibers known in our body. It has efferent fibers to a skeletal muscle, the stylopharyngeus. It has autonomic nerves, both sympathetic and parasympathetic. The inferior ganglion of the glossopharyngeal communicates with the superior cervical ganglion. Nerve fibers of this communication reach the otic ganglion, which contains postganglionic parasympathetic nerve cells. The postganglionic parasympathetic nerve fibers from the otic ganglion proceed to control the secretions of the parotid gland. The afferent fibers in the glossopharyngeal are both for special and general senses. The special sense is the taste sensation for the posterior one-third of tongue. The general sensations are delivered from the parotid gland, carotid sinus, mucous membrane of the pharynx, middle ear, posterior one-third of the tongue, and skin of external ear. The second feature is that the glossopharyngeal has connections with the facial and vagus nerves. This complicated network of communication can produce unexpected physiological responses during acupuncture sessions. Many of these reactions are understood only poorly, if at all, in medical science. The results of these reactions can often turn out to be positive for patients, particularly in cases of abnormalities with indications of hypersympathetic activities.

## 3.6 VAGUS NERVE

The glossopharyngeal and vagus nerves have both anatomical similarities and dissimilarities. The relationship between the similarities and differences are intertwined, so separating them for the purposes of description and discussion will not be that easy. For example, the vagus contains efferent fibers to skeletal muscles. These efferent fibers provide motor innervation to voluntary muscles of the larynx, pharynx, upper two-thirds of the esophagus, and palate (except the tensor veli palatini, which is innervated by a branch of the mandibular division of the trigeminal nerve). With respect to the autonomic nervous system, the vagus contains parasympathetic nerves, but no sympathetic nerves. Preganglionic nerves of the parasympathetic start from preganglionic neurons in the dorsal nucleus of the medulla oblongata. Their postganglionic nerves extend inferiorly to as low as the stomach and intestine. Thus, it is obvious that the vagus nerves have extensive course and distribution, actually more than any of the other 11 cranial nerves. This extensive course and distribution make the vagus more useful in acupuncture than the glossopharyngeal nerve.

Vagus nerves have many branches, two of which are of interest in acupuncture. These are the auricular branch and vagal trunks, which can be divided into anterior and posterior. Anterior refers to the anterior surface of the stomach, and posterior to the posterior surface. In reality, the anterior vagal trunk comes from the right vagus nerve, and the posterior from the left. The auricular branch first enters the temporal bone through the mastoid canaliculus in the lateral wall of the jugular fossa, then emerges through the tympanomastoid fissure to distribute to the back of the external ear, the floor of the external acoustic meatus, and the lower part of the tympanic membrane. The skin area in the external acoustic meatus, where nerve fibers from the auricular branch are known to distribute, is called the concha and is shown in Figure 3.3. Afferent fibers for general sensation from the concha are transmitted to the vagus nerve to the joint of the anterior and posterior vagal trunks. This communication makes it possible to suppress appetite, which is a general sensation and is generated in

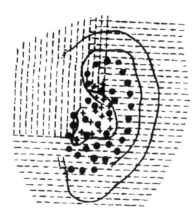

**FIGURE 3.9** Lateral view of an ear showing cutaneous innervation. The area with horizontal dotted lines is innervated by the cervical spinal nerves, the area with vertical broken lines is innervated by the trigeminal nerve, the area with crosses is innervated by the glossopharyngeal and vagus nerves, and the area with black circles is innervated by the facial nerve.

the stomach. Many acupuncture practitioners claim that body weight can be reduced by placing a few needles around the concha. This is known as auriculopuncture and involves acupoints in the ear.

Anatomically, innervation to the external ear has five sources [6,7], as shown in Figure 3.9. They are the trigeminal, facial, glossopharyngeal, vagus, and cervical spinal nerves. In addition to using acupoints in the ears for weight reduction, they are also used in helping smokers stop their cigarette smoking. Acupoints for this latter purpose are located in the area of the external ear marked as being innervated by the glossopharyngeal and cervical spinal nerves. From Figure 3.9, it seems that some areas of the skin that cover the external ear have dual sources of nerve innervations. The significance of two afferent fibers in two different nerves coming from the same skin area is unknown in acupuncture practice.

## 3.7 SPINAL ACCESSORY NERVE

This cranial nerve contains only two kinds of fibers, efferent fibers for skeletal muscles and afferent fibers for general sensation. Their nerve rootlets come from two separate regions, the brain and the cervical spinal cord. They join together to form a single nerve, then separate to go to another nerve branch, then again join to become another nerve branch. Familiarity with this complicated anatomical relation is not essential in learning to practice acupuncture. There is only one acupoint associated with the spinal accessory nerve that needs to be known. This acupoint is also designated the spinal accessory, and its location can be seen in Figure 4.2. In fact, there are five acupoints in Figure 4.2 that are labeled as spinal accessory. This is because the first point to appear and become tender at that spot is considered the primary point. Tenderness at this point is always detectable in patients who arrive at the clinic to seek acupuncture treatments. The tender sensation will expand outward of the vicinity as the duration of pain is prolonged. In time, more acupoints will appear in the area. Depending on the sequence of their appearance, each of these acupoints can be designated as secondary, tertiary, or nonspecific points. This is why there are multiple spinal accessory points indicated in Figure 4.2.

The spinal accessory nerve innervates two muscles, the sternocleidomastoid and trapezius. There is no acupoint formed in the sternocleidomastoid muscle. The motor point where the nerve branch enters the trapezius is right in the middle of the origin and insertion of the muscle. The muscle arises from the medial one-third of the superior nuchal line, the external occipital protuberance of the occipital bone, the ligmentum nuchae, the spine of the seventh cervical and all thoracic vertebrae, and from the intervening supraspinal ligament. The muscle inserts into the scapula, and forms a bridge across the shoulder. The acupoint formed by the motor point between the spinal accessory nerve and the trapezius muscle is located right at the center of this bridge.

Efferent fibers in the spinal accessory come from the cervical spinal cord. They enter the cranial cavity through the foramen magnum, then exit the cavity by way of the jugular foramen to go to the trapezius. Before entering the muscle, the efferent fibers are joined by afferent fibers for general sensations coming from the four upper cervical spinal nerves. This connection has physiological significance because it allows pain to be transmitted from the scapular area to the occipital region by way of the dorsal scapular nerve to the spinal accessory nerve to reach the greater occipital nerve behind the head. More about the pathways for the spread of pain from one anatomical region to another will be discussed in later chapters.

The spinal accessory point is tender not only for patients with headaches, neck stiffness, and shoulder pain but the point is also tender when adequately and appropriately palpated with a fingertip. This point is used 100% of the time for all patients seen in acupuncture clinics.

## REFERENCES

1. Dung, H.C. Acupuncture points of the cranial nerves. *American Journal of Chinese Medicine* 12:80, 1984.
2. Langman, J. *Medical Embryology*, 4th ed. Williams & Wilkins, Baltimore, 1981.
3. Truex, R.C. *Strong and Elwyn's Human Neuroanatomy*, 4th ed. Williams & Wilkins, Baltimore, 1959.
4. Woodburne, R.T. *Essentials of Human Anatomy*, 3rd ed. Oxford University Press, New York, 1965.
5. Warwick, R. and P.L. Williams. *Gray's Anatomy*, 35th British ed. W.B. Saunders Company, Philadelphia, 1973.
6. Cushing, H. The sensory distribution of the fifth cranial nerve. *Bulletin of the Johns Hopkins Hospital* 15:213, 1904.
7. Hollinshead, W.H. *Anatomy for Surgeons*, vol. 1: The Head and Neck, 3rd ed. Harper & Rowe, New York, 1969.

# 4 Acupoints in the Neck Region

## 4.1 BOUNDARIES OF THE NECK

Not much attention has been given to defining the boundaries of the neck in anatomy. Some anatomy textbooks [1] even describe the head and neck under one heading in the same topography. Clearly, we have separated the head and neck in this book. We have learned all the acupoints in the head, so in this chapter, the subject is acupoints in the neck. We are going to divide the neck into two territories, the anterior and posterior regions. The acupoints described in this chapter are all located in the anterior region. Acupoints found in the posterior region belong to another family, the back or dorsal side of the body, and will be covered in Chapter 6.

The anterior region of the neck is divided into two equal halves, right and left, by the median line connecting the center point of the lower margin of the mandible and the midsuperior border of the manubrium of the sternum. The upper boundary of each half is the lower margin of the mandible, and the lower boundary is the clavicle. The posterior boundary is the anterior border of the trapezius muscle. Each half is square in shape. The square is transected by two muscles, the omohyoid and sternocleidomastoid, resulting in the formation of four triangles. These are known as the muscular, carotid, posterior cervical, and omoclavicular triangles. Recognizing these triangles is clinically significant. There are many important structures underneath them, and any decision to insert needles into any of these triangles will require prudence.

The neck is a cylindrical structure that can be visualized as being wrapped in three layers of tissue. The outermost layer is the skin. Deep within the skin is subcutaneous tissue, which has one unique anatomical feature: the platysma muscle. The platysma is one of the two skeletal muscles in the body to be in the fascia of the subcutaneous tissue. The platysma is in the neck, but is not innervated by the cervical plexus. Rather, it is innervated by the cervical branch of the facial nerve. The muscles deep under the platysma form the third layer. Large blood vessels and nerve branches can be thought of the last internal portion. There are four infrahyoid muscles in the anterior region of the neck. Like other skeletal muscles, each of them has a motor point formed by a muscular branch of the cervical plexus. In addition to these muscular branches, the plexus also has cutaneous branches. All cutaneous branches reach the layer of subcutaneous tissue where most acupoints in the neck are formed. Both cutaneous and muscular branches in the neck are from the cervical plexus, the formation of which will be the next topic.

## 4.2 FORMATION OF THE CERVICAL PLEXUS

The cervical nerve plexus is formed by the interconnecting branches of the ventral primary rami of the first four cervical spinal nerves. Acupoints formed by the dorsal primary rami will be found on the back of the body, and are discussed in Chapter 6. As shown in Figure 4.1, the ventral primary rami of the first four cervical spinal nerves congregate at the midpoint along the posterior border of the sternocleidomastoid muscle. Nerve fibers at this location, which forms the cervical plexus acupoint, are fairly massive but relatively deep.

From the point of the cervical plexus, the nerves divide to become four cutaneous branches. There is one muscular branch, the ansa cervicalis, deep inside the muscle layer.

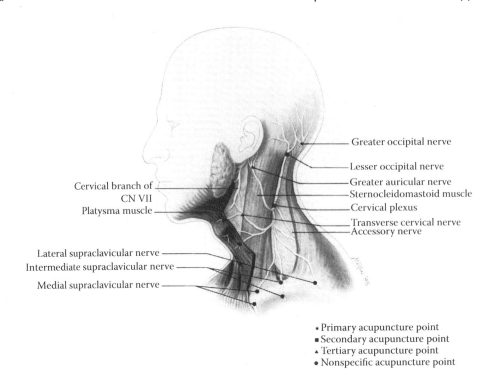

**FIGURE 4.1** A lateral view of the neck. Except for the cervical branch of the trigeminal nerve, all other branches belong to the cervical plexus. Circular black dots indicate the locations where the cutaneous nerves pierce the deep fascia to become subcutaneous. These are the places where acupoints are formed.

## 4.3 ACUPOINTS OF THE CUTANEOUS BRANCHES

The four cutaneous branches in the cervical plexus, which forms the acupoints, are the greater auricular, lesser occipital, transverse cervical, and supraclavicular nerves.

### 4.3.1 Greater Auricular

After separating from the point of the cervical plexus, this nerve branch runs upward to cross the sternocleidomastoid muscle obliquely. It reaches behind the earlobe at the angle of the mandible (Figure 4.2). The nerve pierces the deep fascia just below the ear. Most cutaneous branches stay as a single nerve bundle inside the deep fascia. It spreads outward to become many smaller fascicles, which will distribute to the subcutaneous layer in the area. The greater auricular point forms at the location where the nerve branch pierces the deep fascia. This nerve is important for acupuncture, and apparently shows tenderness in most patients who have pain in other parts of the body.

### 4.3.2 Lesser Occipital

This nerve characteristically ascends within the posterior cervical triangle along the posterior border of the sternocleidomastoid muscle. It pierces the deep cervical fascia near the intermuscular gap between the insertions of the sternocleidomastoid and the trapezius muscles on the occipital bone. This intermuscular gap is where the lesser occipital acupoint is formed. Both the greater auricular and lesser occipital are cutaneous and reside at the same depth. Their main difference is in their size; the greater auricular nerve is invariably larger than the lesser occipital. The greater auricular point invariably becomes tender sooner than the lesser occipital point does. Very often, the greater

Acupoints in the Neck Region

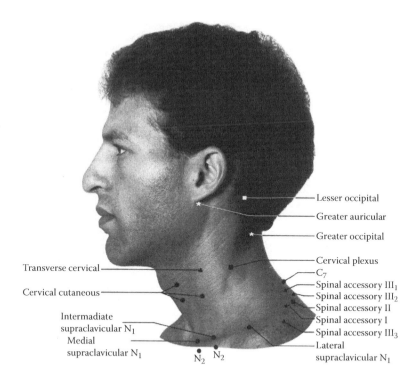

**FIGURE 4.2** A photograph showing acupoints in the neck and shoulder regions. Acupoints are indicated with different shapes to designate their different significances in clinical applications.

auricular will experience tenderness in patients whose lesser occipital turns out to have less sensitivity or none at all.

### 4.3.3 TRANSVERSE CERVICAL

As the name implies, this nerve branch literally traverses the neck by crossing over the sternocleidomastoid muscle, as shown in Figure 4.1. The single branch of the nerve divides into three smaller bundles. These smaller bundles are all recognized anatomically as the transverse cervical (with no additional individual anatomical nomenclatures). However, for acupuncture purposes, we can name the point at the highest location as the upper transverse cervical, the point at the lowest position as the lower transverse cervical, and the point in the center as the middle cervical. These points are formed as the nerve branches of the transverse cervical penetrate through the deep fascia, which covers the anterior surface of the sternohyoid muscle in the muscular triangle of the neck. All branches of the transverse cervical are visible during dissections of cadavers in gross laboratory. However, they are all too small to form acupoints to be important in the practice of acupuncture. By the time acupoints of the transverse cervical become detectably tender, pain in the neck will be too serious to manage easily with needles.

With respect to tender points in the neck with identical locations of acupoints, other investigators [2,3] have reported that they are trigger points or motor points formed on the scalene muscles. In our view, the scalene muscles are too deep inside the neck. It is almost impossible to palpate deep muscles, such as the scalene, from the skin's surface.

### 4.3.4 Supraclavicular

The branches that travel over the clavicle bone are anatomically known as the supraclavicular. There are three of them: the medial or anterior, the middle, and the lateral or posterior supraclavicular nerves, as shown in Figure 4.1. Each of these supraclavicular nerves has two small divisions. One runs superiorly through the deep fascia and another inferiorly to the clavicle, making a total of six acupoints along the length of the bone (Figure 4.2). Because of their small size, these six supraclavicular acupoints are functionally very similar to those of the transverse cervical nerves. They are all categorized as nonspecific acupoints and are not used much in the practice of acupuncture.

## 4.4 ACUPOINTS OF MUSCULAR BRANCHES

The cervical plexus is known to have one muscular branch, the ansa cervicalis, as mentioned in Section 4.2. The nerve innervates the infrahyoid muscles: the sternohyoid, omohyoid, sternothyroid, and thyrohyoid. Each of these has a motor point formed by the muscular nerves of the cervical plexus. The motor points are deep inside the muscle masses. They are never used as acupoints, and will not be mentioned further in the book.

## REFERENCES

1. Woodburne, R.T. *Essentials of Human Anatomy*, 3rd ed. Oxford University Press, New York, 1965.
2. Bonica, J.J. *The Management of Pain*, vol. 1, 2nd ed. Lea & Febiger, Philadelphia, 1990.
3. Travell, J.G. and D.G. Simons. *Myofascial Pain and Dysfunction: The Trigger Point Manual*. Williams & Wilkins, Baltimore, 1983.

# 5 Acupoints in the Upper Limb

## 5.1 TOPOGRAPHY OF THE UPPER LIMB

We view the topography of the upper limb as having four separate regions. These are the chest wall (pectoral region) in the anterior, shoulder (scapular region) in the posterior, arm (brachium) and forearm (antebrachium) dropping down laterally, and wrist (carpus) and hand (manus) at the distal end of the limb. The pectoral region is covered by two muscles, the pectoralis major and the pectoralis minor. The shoulder is bound by two bones, the clavicle and the scapula, and the muscles connecting these two bones, which are the deltoid and the trapezius. Besides the deltoid and trapezius, only a few other muscles attached to the scapula need to be remembered for our purposes. They are the levator scapulae and the rhomboideus minor and major, all of which insert along the medial border of the scapula. The supraspinatus and infraspinatus muscles lodge separately in the supraspinous and infraspinous fossa. Their tendons attach to the humeral head and conjoin with tendons of the subscapularis and teres minor muscles to build up the rotator cuff. Clinically, the rotator cuff is almost always blamed as the culprit for shoulder joint pain. More will be said about pain in the shoulder joint in a later chapter. Here, it is useful to keep in mind that such pain is invariably initiated at one acupoint, which sits right on the top of tendon of the long head of the biceps brachii muscle.

The arm and forearm are each divided into two muscle compartments: the anterior and posterior in the arm, and the lateral and medial in the forearm. Motor points formed by the muscular nerve branches in some of the muscles enclosed within different compartments will become acupoints. Cutaneous nerve branches in the arm and forearm are relatively large. Acupoints formed by a couple of the cutaneous branches are important in acupuncture, particularly when they are used in the quantification of pain. These points are easy to find and conveniently accessible.

The wrist and hand are different from other regions of the upper limb, as they are relatively flat. The flat surface has radial and ulnar sides or margins, between which are the palm and dorsum of the hand. The dorsal surface of the hand has no muscles but is rich in cutaneous nerve distribution. The palmar side of the hand is occupied by quite a number of muscles and is likewise rich in cutaneous nerves. Thus, acupoints formed by the muscular and cutaneous nerves can be expected to be found in both sides and surfaces of the wrist and hand.

## 5.2 ORGANIZATION OF THE BRACHIAL PLEXUS

The brachial plexus is a rather complicated structure; Figure 5.1 is presented for help in visualizing it. It is a diagrammatic sketch showing most of the nerve branches that participate in creating the plexus. Several nerve branches that don't contribute to the formation of acupoints are not labeled. These are the long thoracic nerve, phrenic nerve, upper subscapular nerve, middle subscapular or thoracodorsal nerve, lower subscapular nerve, nerve to the subclavius muscle, nerve to the longus colli, and scaleni. They are either hidden behind bones or are too deep to be accessible. Other nerves are not included because they are located far too peripherally to be in the diagram.

As can be seen from Figure 5.1, the brachial plexus is formed by the ventral rami of the fifth to eighth cervical spinal nerves and the greater part of the ramus of the first thoracic spinal nerve. A small portion of the fourth cervical and the second thoracic spinal nerves also contribute to the formation of the plexus. Such a contribution is important to know because the portion coming from

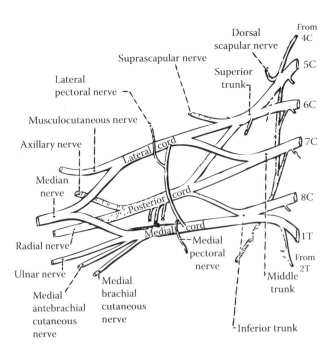

**FIGURE 5.1** A diagrammatic sketch of the brachial plexus.

the fourth cervical nerve makes communication possible between the cervical and brachial plexi. Thus, sensory impulses are capable of transmitting from the upper limb to the neck and the occipital region of the head, and vice versa.

The ventral rami of five spinal nerves join one another to form three trunks: the upper (superior), middle, and lower (inferior). Each trunk then splits into two divisions, the anterior and posterior. The union of the two anterior divisions from the upper and middle trunks becomes the lateral cord. The anterior division of the lower trunk stays alone to become the medial cord. All three posterior divisions join together to become the posterior cord. There is only one nerve branch from the ventral rami of the fourth and fifth cervical spinal nerves that is pertinent for acupuncture, and that is the dorsal scapular nerve. The other branches that are useful to know are derivations from the three cords and nerves distal to them.

In principle, nerve branches coming from the medial and lateral cords will go to the pectoral region, anterior compartment of the arm, medial compartment of the forearm, ulnar side of the wrist, and palmar surface of the hand. Nerve branches coming from the posterior cord supply the scapular region, posterior compartment of the arm, lateral compartment of the forearm, radial side of the wrist, and dorsal surface of the hand. Acupoints that can be found in the upper limb have been previously reported [1] and are described below.

## 5.3 ACUPOINTS ON THE PECTORAL REGION

There are two acupoints on the pectoral region (Figure 5.2). They are formed by the motor points of the lateral and medial pectoral nerves. Both of them are muscular branches. The lateral pectoral is a branch from the lateral cord, and the medial pectoral is from the medial cord. The lateral pectoral nerve is bigger than the medial pectoral because the lateral pectoral innervates the pectoralis major muscle, whereas the medial pectoral innervates the pectoralis minor. For this reason, the lateral pectoral point always becomes tender sooner than the medial pectoral point. The lateral pectoral is thus a primary point, and the medial pectoral a secondary point. The lateral pectoral is located 1.5 inches inferior to the midclavicular point. The medial pectoral is about 1.5 inches lateroinferior to the lateral pectoral point.

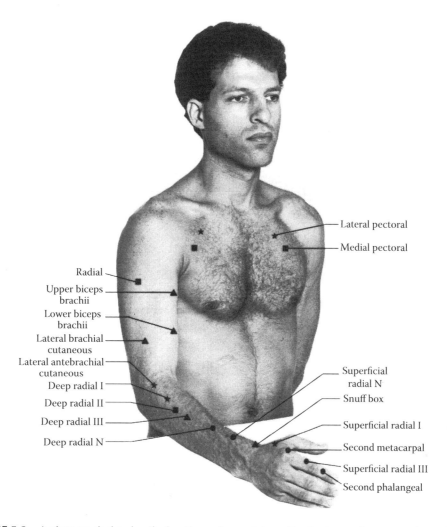

**FIGURE 5.2** A photograph showing the locations of acupoints on the chest, arm, forearm, wrist, and hand.

## 5.4 ACUPOINTS OVER THE SCAPULAR REGION

There are three acupoints over the scapular region: the dorsal scapular, the supraspinatus, and the infraspinatus. Their locations can be seen in Figure 5.3.

Dorsal scapular is the name for a nerve, whereas supraspinatus and infaspinatus are names for muscles. The nerve branches to these two muscles are the suprascapular. Thus, the acupoint formed by the motor point in the infraspinatus muscle can be called the primary suprascapular or suprascapular I to indicate that it is a primary acupoint, and the acupoint formed by the motor point in the suprascapular muscle can be named the secondary suprascapular or suprascapular II to indicate that it is a secondary acupoint. Both names for each of these two acupoints will be used interchangeably.

### 5.4.1 Dorsal Scapular

The dorsal scapular nerve innervates three muscles: the levator scapulae, the rhomboid major, and the rhomboid minor. The nerve arises from the ventral ramus of the fifth cervical spinal with a contribution from the fourth cervical spinal nerve, as mentioned above. It descends from the cervical region down to the medial border of the scapula. Along the medial border, the dorsal scapular nerve enters the rhomboid minor muscle at the base of the spine of the scapula to form an acupoint. This

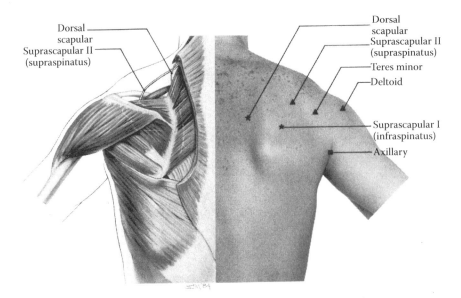

**FIGURE 5.3** Rearview anatomic illustration to show the dorsal scapular and suprascapular nerves on the left, and a human model with six acupoints on the right. Three of the six points—the teres minor, deltoid, and axillary—belong to acupoints in the arm.

acupoint is the dorsal scapular point (Figure 5.3), which has attracted the attention of some clinical scientists. Reports by Calabro [2], Campbell [3], Sheon et al. [4], and Travell and Simons [5] have indicated that pain can manifest at the dorsal scapular point in some patients with fibromyalgia. The opinions of where this motor point is located vary from rhomboid [3] to levator scapulae [4,5]. This disagreement can be easily resolved by dissecting a cadaver.

### 5.4.2 Supraspinatus or Suprascapular II

As shown in Figure 5.1, the suprascapular nerve arises from the superior trunk. The nerve passes laterally across the posterior cervical triangle along the anterior border of the trapezius muscle to reach the scapular notch. The notch forms a pathway by the transverse scapular ligament. Above the ligament, runs the suprascapular artery and vein, and below it, the nerve enters the supraspinous fossa within which it lodges in the supraspinatus muscle. A branch of the suprascapular nerve enters the muscle by running under it, and it is here that the acupoint of the supraspinatus or suprascapular II (Figure 5.3) is formed. The supraspinatus is a round, thick muscle. If the acupoint formed by this motor point deep inside the muscle becomes tender, the sensitivity will be relatively difficult to detect.

### 5.4.3 Infraspinatus or Suprascapular I

After splitting off the branch to the supraspinatus muscle in the supraspinous fossa, the suprascapular nerve then descends through the notch of the scapular neck to the infraspinous fossa to terminate at the motor point of the infraspinatus muscle. The infraspinatus is a broad, thin muscle, and the motor point is located right in its center. This motor point is the infraspinatus or suprascapular I acupoint (Figure 5.3). The suprascapular I in the infraspinatus muscle is a primary acupoint, and the suprascapular II in the supraspinatus muscle is a secondary point. The infraspinatus point always becomes tender sooner than the supraspinatus.

Regarding the suprascapular nerve, there is a condition known as suprascapular nerve entrapment, believed to stem from the nerve becoming entrapped inside the scapular notch by the transverse scapular ligament. The consequence is pain over the scapular region. Actually, it is impossible for this entrapment to occur because the transverse scapular ligament is a tough, tight structure, and will have difficulty bending to entrap anything above or below it.

## 5.5 ARM AND FOREARM

Acupoints found in the arm and forearm can be divided into three groups. They are acupoints formed by the muscular nerve branches, acupoints formed by the cutaneous nerve branches, and acupoints formed over the tendons and ligaments.

### 5.5.1 THE MUSCULAR BRANCHES

In the arm, there are three muscles in the anterior and four in the posterior compartment. In the forearm, the medial compartment has eight muscles and the lateral has 11 muscles. Among the nerve branches to these 26 muscles, it is possible to locate a total of eight acupoints.

#### 5.5.1.1 Musculocutaneous or Biceps Brachii

The most superficially placed muscle in the anterior compartment of the arm is the biceps brachii. It is a relatively thick and long muscle. The nerve innervating this muscle is the musculocutaneous, a branch of the lateral cord. Because of its length, although the nerve runs underneath deep to the muscle, it apparently needs to provide two muscular branches for innervation. The biceps brachii is one of only a few muscles with multiple nerve innervations, obviously due to its length. These two muscular branches form two acupoints in the biceps brachii muscle, known as the musculocutaneous points or upper and lower biceps brachii, as indicated in Figures 5.2 and 5.4. These two acupoints are situated along the midline on the biceps brachii muscle. The distance between the upper and lower biceps brachii points divides this midline into three equal segments. These two acupoints are seldom used and are categorized as tertiary points in acupuncture because of their deep locations.

#### 5.5.1.2 Median

This acupoint is called the median point because it is located right on the median nerve. The median nerve is formed by a branch from the lateral and another branch from the medial cord in the axillary area. It is one of the four relatively large nerve trunks enclosed inside the neurovascular compartment in the medial aspect of the arm. The other three are the ulnar, medial brachial, and medial antebrachial cutaneous nerves. There is no division or branching for these four nerve trunks inside the neurovascular compartment. Thus, there are no acupoints formed by these nerves in the arm. They all descend down to the forearm. In the forearm, the median nerve sends branches to innervate some long flexor muscles in the medial compartment. Motor points formed between branches of the median nerve and flexor muscles don't become acupoints because they are buried deep inside the muscle masses.

As the median nerve descends distally in the forearm, it gradually emerges to become more superficial. The course of the nerve is right along the center line of the forearm. Toward the distal end of the forearm, approximately 3 inches (40 mm) above the proximal skin crease on the wrist, the nerve runs right under the skin without any muscle coverage. This is the location where the median nerve will divide into small branches to contribute to the formation of the acupoint designated as the median point (Figure 5.4). It is a tertiary acupoint.

#### 5.5.1.3 Axillary

The next six acupoints, axillary included, are either located in the posterior compartment of the arm or lateral compartment of the forearm. The axillary point is not formed from the motor point of the nerve. As shown in Figure 5.5, the axillary nerve passes through the quadrangular space to reach

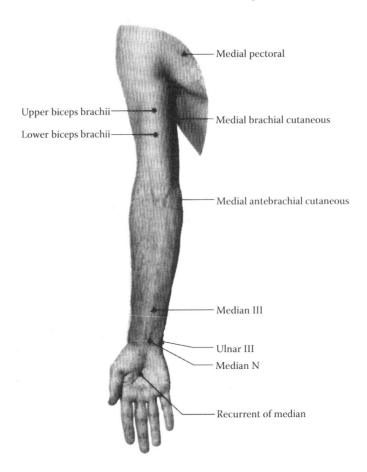

**FIGURE 5.4** Acupoints located on the anterior side of the upper limb.

the back of the shoulder joint region. As the nerve emerges out of the space, it divides into several small branches. The acupoint known as the axillary (Figure 5.3) is formed because of the division at this branch. As mentioned in Chapter 2, the spot where a larger nerve divides into smaller branches is an anatomical feature that contributes to the formation of acupoints. The median nerve, which is located toward the distal end of the forearm to become the median point, as mentioned in Section 5.5.1.2, is another example. The location of the axillary point is easy to determine, particularly when it becomes a trigger point. A trigger point always exhibits tenderness when adequate pressure is applied. In the case of the axillary point, use the thumb and index finger to squeeze the posterior axillary fold until a tender spot is found.

### 5.5.1.4 Teres Minor

The axillary nerve sends branches to other muscles, two examples being the teres minor and deltoid muscles. The teres minor is a narrow, elongated muscle that arises from the lateral border of the scapula in the upper two-thirds of its extent. Its tendon is directed obliquely upward and lateralward to insert into the lower facet of the greater tubercle of the humerus. This makes the muscle a portion of the posterior compartment of the arm. The axillary nerve lies just immediately below the teres minor muscle and sends a branch to the lateral margin of the muscle at the midpoint of its length. The motor point formed by this branch of the axillary nerve on the teres minor muscle is immediately underneath the skin. The acupoint formed by this motor point is called the teres minor (Figure 5.3).

# Acupoints in the Upper Limb

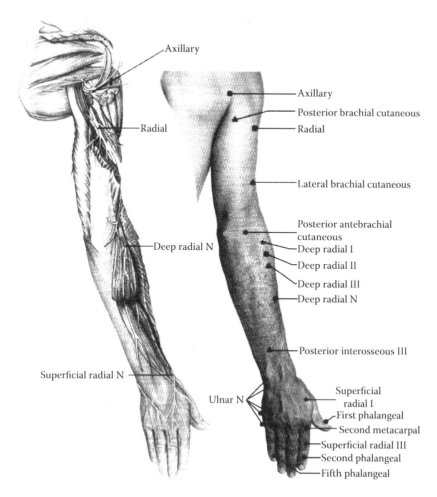

**FIGURE 5.5** The drawing on the left shows the locations of four nerves in the posterior compartment of the arm and the lateral compartment of the forearm. All five nerves are branches coming directly or indirectly from the posterior cord. The photograph on the right shows acupoints formed by the nerves rising from the posterior cord, except for the acupoints of the ulnar nerve, which is a branch of the medial cord.

### 5.5.1.5 Deltoid

Another muscle that receives innervation from a branch of the axillary nerve, the deltoid caps the point of the shoulder joint, as can be seen in Figure 5.3. The point at which a branch of the axillary enters the deltoideus is right on the deltoid tuberosity situated on the lateral surface of the middle acromion of the scapula, or the highest ground on the posterior surface of the shoulder joint. That is the motor point which forms the acupoint for the deltoid.

### 5.5.1.6 Radial

The posterior cord extends distally to become the radial nerve, one of the largest nerves in the upper limb. It supplies innervations to the extensor muscles in the posterior compartment of the arm. After leaving the axillary, the radial nerve runs downward, backward, and laterally between the long and medial heads of the triceps muscle to enter the radial groove of the humerus (Figure 5.5). The trunk of the radial nerve can be palpated at the location where it lies in the groove immediately below the insertion of the deltoid muscle. At this point, the radial nerve divides to create the posterior brachial cutaneous nerve. The posterior brachial nerve will be discussed later. The point of this division between the radial and the cutaneous nerves becomes an acupoint, which we call the radial point, as indicated in Figure 5.5. It is not an important point acupuncture-wise, simply because it is buried deep inside the muscle mass.

### 5.5.1.7 Deep Radial

The radial nerve penetrates the lateral intermuscular septum of the brachium to enter the lateral compartment of the antebrachium. In the forearm, the radial nerve bifurcates into two terminal branches, the deep and superficial radial nerves. The deep radial is a muscular branch, and the superficial is a cutaneous branch, which is the next topic for description.

Acupoints formed by the deep radial are the most important of all acupoints. More than 99% of all patients received in our acupuncture clinic have been tested to exhibit tenderness at the location of at least one of the acupoints along the deep radial nerve. The deep radial nerve supplies branches to all extensor muscles in the lateral compartment of the forearm. The nerve travels along the forearm in the intermuscular septum between the brachoradialis and the extensor carpi radialis longus muscles. This septum can be easily discerned in a person with a well-developed musculature. Ask the person to clench a fist tightly, and a linear groove will become visible, running between the brachioradialis and extensor radialis longus. The formation of the groove is due to the pulling of the intermuscular septum. Soon after entering the septum, the main trunk of the deep radial nerve begins to branch, and acupoints start to appear at these branching locations. The first point occurs approximately 4 cm distal to the lateral epicondyle of the humerus. Both the lateral and medial epicondyles are easy to palpate for their locations. As the nerve branches out, its size diminishes. This decrease in size is counted as a factor for the decrease in frequency of appearance for the subsequent acupoints. Up to four acupoints may occur along the course of the deep radial nerve. The location of these four acupoints is shown in Figures 5.2 and 5.5. Another reason there are so many acupoints in the region is that there is a rich vascular bed at this location. The vascular bed is contributed by the radial artery and vein, as well as their tributaries. The four acupoints of the deep radial, from the proximal to distal positions, are categorized as primary, secondary, tertiary, and nonspecific. Their respective designated names are deep radial I, deep radial II, deep radial III, and deep radial IV.

### 5.5.1.8 Posterior Interosseus

As the deep radial nerve reaches the distal one-third of the forearm, it divides, producing the posterior interosseus nerve, which descends on the posterior side of the interosseus membrane. The posterior interosseus nerve passes deep to the extensor pollicis longus muscle and ends at the wrist to supply the intercarpal joints. Where the posterior interosseus nerve splits from the deep radial nerve is the acupoint called the posterior interosseus (Figure 5.5). It is a tertiary point, but is used often in acupuncture because of its convenient position and ease of access.

## 5.5.2 CUTANEOUS BRANCHES

Posterior cutaneous branches to the arm and forearm are from the nerves of the posterior cord. The medial and lateral cutaneous branches to the arm and forearm are from the nerves of the medial and lateral cords. The cutaneous innervation can be defined as having six territories, three in the arm and three in the forearm.

### 5.5.2.1 Posterior Brachial Cutaneous

This cutaneous nerve is a branch of the radial. As shown in Figure 5.5, it pierces the deep fascia at the proximal end of the arm, where the posterior brachial cutaneous point is found. It is a small cutaneous nerve, and the acupoint it forms is not that important. We categorize this point in the tertiary group.

### 5.5.2.2 Lateral Brachial Cutaneous

There are two nerves innervating the skin on the lateral side of the arm, the axillary and the radial. The axillary nerve supplies the upper area of the lateral side, and the radial supplies the lower area.

The branch from the axillary is too small to form acupoints. The branch from the radial forms the lateral brachial cutaneous point, as can be seen in Figure 5.5. This is also a tertiary point.

### 5.5.2.3 Medial Brachial Cutaneous

This nerve is a direct branch of the medial cord in the brachial plexus. It pierces the deep fascia at the midpoint of the line connecting the armpit and the medial epicondyle of the humerus. The medial brachial cutaneous point (Figure 5.4) is also a tertiary point. Yet, it is a very useful point for rapidly quantifying pain when used in combination with the next two points.

### 5.5.2.4 Lateral Antebrachial Cutaneous

After giving away its muscular branches in the anterior compartment of the arm, the musculocutaneous nerve runs distally to penetrate the deep fascia at the lateral end of the cubital fossa to become the lateral antebrachial cutaneous nerve, which means that this nerve extends from the musculocutaneous nerve. The nerve innervates the skin covering the lateral compartment of the forearm. When the forearm is brought close to the arm, the cubital fossa will become a line. The lateral end of that line is where the acupoint of the lateral antebrachial cutaneous is located (Figure 5.2). This is a primary point; it is formed by the biggest cutaneous nerve in the entire upper limb.

### 5.5.2.5 Medial Antebrachial Cutaneous

This is the second biggest cutaneous branch in the upper limb. The nerve comes directly from the medial cord of the brachial plexus. It runs through the deep fascia right over the medial epicondyle of the humerus at the medial end of the line created by the folding of the cubital fossa to become subcutaneous over the skin of the medial compartment of the forearm. At that location, the acupoint of the medial antebrachial cutaneous (Figure 5.4) is formed.

These three acupoints formed by the three cutaneous nerve branches described above have a very useful relationship with respect to pain quantification. The nerve which forms the lateral antebrachial cutaneous point is the biggest of the three. The next biggest is that which forms the medial antebrachial cutaneous point, and the smallest forms the medial brachial cutaneous point. The difference in size for these three nerves is easy to discern by mere visual observation in cadaver dissections. The lateral antebrachial cutaneous is a primary point, the medial antebrachial cutaneous is a secondary point, and the medial brachial cutaneous is a tertiary point. A patient with tenderness detectable only at the primary point indicates that the quantity of pain in that patient is less than any patient whose secondary point is also tender. Patients having detectable tenderness in all three acupoints are bound to have the highest quantity of pain. More will be said and about pain quantification in Chapter 10.

### 5.5.2.6 Posterior Antebrachial Cutaneous

This nerve is a branch of the radial. It pierces the deep fascia between the lateral epicondyle of the humerus and the olecranon of the radius above the elbow joint. The acupoint of the posterior antebrachial cutaneous (Figure 5.5) is formed at the location where the nerve goes through the fascia. It is a nonspecific acupoint and is rarely used in acupuncture treatments.

### 5.5.3 Acupoints over Tendons and Ligaments

A few acupoints are found to form by sitting on a tendon, ligament, or retinaculum. There is no muscular or cutaneous nerve that can be traced to these structures. No doubt they must have innervation from nerve branches nearby. It will be inappropriate to name such acupoints using the names of nerves that are merely passing by. Instead, they will be named using nomenclatures of the muscular tendons, ligaments, retinacula, or bones of their attachments. Three examples are provided.

#### 5.5.3.1 Tendon of the Biceps Brachii

The biceps brachii muscle has two heads, long and short. The tendon of the long head is round, arising from the supraglenoid tubercle of the scapula. This tendon crosses the head of the humerus within the capsule of the shoulder joint and then, covered by a prolongation of the synovial membrane, it emerges from the joint beneath the transverse humeral ligament. It then descends in the intertubercular groove of the humerus. Inside this groove, the tendon must sustain a great deal of friction as the arm and the forearm are extended and flexed. It is quite conceivable that this friction can produce tissue damage or injury to the tendon, consequently forming tender points on the tendon. There can be anywhere from one to three tender points formed. The person in Figure 5.6 is shown to have two nonspecific acupoints on the biceps brachii tendon. People who experience pain in the shoulder joint will always exhibit tender sensation in one to three acupoints on the tendon. Locating these acupoints is not difficult. The biceps brachii tendon in the intertubercular groove can be palpated using a fingertip. One then applies adequate pressure with the fingertip while moving it along the tendon.

#### 5.5.3.2 Lateral Epicondyle of the Elbow

This epicondyle is covered by the tendons of the origin of the extensor carpi radialis longus and brevis muscles. Overuse of these two muscles, particularly by amateur tennis players, can result in pain in the elbow. The pain almost always manifests in the acupoints of the lateral epicondyle, shown in Figure 5.7. The number of acupoints in the region can range from one to as many as five.

#### 5.5.3.3 Flexor Retinaculum over the Wrist

This retinaculum stretches between the ends of the concavity of the carpal bones and converts their arch into a fibro-osseous tunnel, through which a considerable number of tendons and the median nerve pass into the hand. The nerve sends a cutaneous branch to this retinaculum, which may be the reason that an acupoint will appear on it. This acupoint is also described as the median N point (Figure 5.4), indicating it as a nonspecific point.

### 5.6 WRIST AND HAND

The number of acupoints in the wrist and hand is hard to estimate. Occurrences of acupoints vary greatly from individual to individual, disease to disease, and by how long a patient has had a disease.

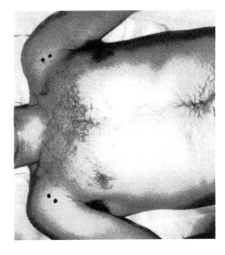

**FIGURE 5.6** Two circular black dots indicate the locations of acupoints formed on the biceps brachii tendon on each side of the anterior surface of the shoulder joint.

Acupoints in the Upper Limb

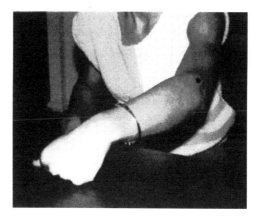

**FIGURE 5.7** An acupoint marked by a circular black point over the lateral epicondyle of the left forearm.

For example, identifiable acupoints in patients with carpal tunnel syndrome will be substantially different from those in patients who have suffered advanced rheumatoid arthritis for many years, as can be seen in Figure 5.8.

For illustrative purposes, only a couple of examples are given for the palmar and dorsal surfaces of the wrist and hand. In fact, the median N over the flexor retinaculum mentioned in Section 5.5.3.3 can be considered as an acupoint of the wrist region.

### 5.6.1 Muscular Branches

#### 5.6.1.1 Recurrent of Median

The median nerve passes through the carpal tunnel in the wrist under the flexor retinaculum to enter the palm. At the distal border of the flexor retinaculum, it gives off a stout branch to the muscles in the thenar compartment on the palm. This branch is known as the recurrent of median because it curves sharply from the median to the muscles in the thenar compartment. The motor point established by this recurrent branch on the thenar muscles is likewise known as the recurrent of median. This point always seems tender in patients diagnosed with carpal tunnel syndrome.

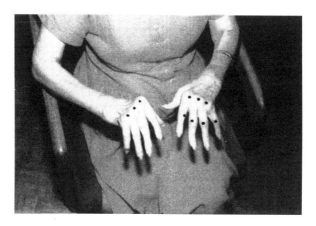

**FIGURE 5.8** The hands of a patient suffering for years from rheumatoid arthritis. The circular black points indicate only a fraction of the number of acupoints found on the patient.

### 5.6.1.2 Ulnar

Like the median nerve, the ulnar stays inside the deep fascia until it reaches the wrist region, specifically distal to the styloid process of the ulnar bone. Neurological pain is known to manifest on the ulnar side of the wrist and hand. When the pain occurs in the ulnar nerve, several acupoints can manifest along the ulnar side of the wrist and hand, as can be seen in Figures 5.4 and 5.5. Which muscular or cutaneous branches from the ulnar nerve contribute to the formation of acupoints is difficult to say because the ulnar nerve has both muscular and cutaneous branches in this area.

### 5.6.2 Cutaneous Branches

The wrist and hand have a rich distribution of afferent fibers for general senses, particular the palm side, because of its high sensory field due to the density of sensory receptors. Anatomically, the best known cutaneous branch in the wrist and hand is the superficial radial nerve.

### 5.6.2.1 Superficial Radial

The radial nerve bifurcates into two terminal branches, the deep and superficial radial. The superficial is the smaller of the two, which is the reason that the acupoint formed by the deep radial always becomes tender earlier than that of the superficial radial, even though the superficial radial is, by definition, closer to the surface of the body. As the superficial radial nerve descends to the lower one-third of the forearm, it runs right on the top of the outer border of the radius bone to pierce the deep antebrachial fascia, then enters the dorsum of the web of the hand between the thumb and index finger (Figure 5.5). At this location, the superficial radial nerve splits into branches. The point where the bifurcation occurs is an acupoint, the superficial radial. The superficial radial point or points can also appear on the lower one-third of the forearm, where the nerve almost adheres to the surface of the radius bone when the nerve is hit by a blunt force, producing a condition clinically known as superficial radial nerve neuropathy.

### 5.6.2.2 Interphalangeal Points

The cutaneous branches in the hand are called the common palmar digital or common dorsal digital nerves. They reach the margin of the web between two fingers, then split into two branches. Each of these runs along one side of a finger. All these cutaneous branches are known as proper digital nerves. Common digital and proper digital nerves have the potential to form acupoints. Some of them are shown in Figures 5.2, 5.5, and 5.8. These acupoints located between fingers can be called interphalangeal points. Their vast number makes it difficult for us to describe them individually with proper anatomical names, however.

Keep in mind that there are more acupoints than those we have mentioned. The reality is that acupoints can appear at almost any place in the body, depending on where damage to nerve tissue is sustained. However, for practical purposes, the number of acupoints introduced in this book will be sufficient for use in acupuncture.

## REFERENCES

1. Dung, H.C. Acupuncture points of the brachial plexus. *American Journal of Chinese Medicine* 13:49, 1985.
2. Calabro, J.J. Fibromyalgia: Chronic aches, diffuse pain. *Medical Student* March–April, 1982.
3. Campbell, S.M. Referred shoulder pain. *Postgraduate Medicine* 73:193, 1983.
4. Sheon, R.P. et al. *Soft Tissue Rheumatic Pain: Recognition, Management, Prevention.* Lea & Febiger, Philadelphia, 1982.
5. Travell, J.D. and D.G. Simons. *Myofascial Pain and Dysfunction: The Trigger Point Manual.* Williams & Wilkins, Baltimore, 1983.

# 6 Acupoints in the Body Trunk

## 6.1 DEFINING A TYPICAL SPINAL NERVE

We consider only 11 out of all spinal nerves as typical. All others, including the eight cervical, first thoracic, five lumbar, and five sacral spinal nerves are not typical because they participate in the formation of the cervical, brachial, lumbar, and sacral plexuses. Spinal nerves, which form a portion of any plexus, are different from one another in their divisions, connections, and terminal distributions. In contrast, all 11 typical spinal nerves are, with few exceptions, almost identical anatomically in their divisions and distributions. Typical spinal nerves have practically no interconnections, even though their tiny terminal branches do overlap to a certain extent. All acupoints that will be described in this chapter are formed by the typical spinal nerves. Thus, it is useful to define what a typical spinal nerve is. Figure 6.1 is a schematic illustration of a typical spinal nerve.

### 6.1.1 Two Roots with One Ganglion

A typical spinal nerve has two roots. They can be described as ventral (or anterior) and dorsal (or posterior) roots. The ventral root contains solely efferent fibers, whereas the dorsal root carries only afferent fibers for the general senses. Neurons for these afferent fibers reside in a ganglion attaching to its root, and this ganglion is known as the dorsal root or spinal ganglion. Efferent fibers in the ventral root are either efferent to the skeletal muscles or nerves of the autonomic system, specifically in the division of the sympathetic nerves. The ventral and dorsal roots join to become a spinal nerve, a short but relatively large nerve trunk. The trunk of the spinal nerves quickly divides into two primary rami.

### 6.1.2 Two Primary Rami

The two primary rami of a spinal nerve are the anterior (or ventral) and posterior (or dorsal). Each of the two rami has branches that we need to recognize. There are four branches useful to know from the anterior ramus: the gray and white rami communicantes, and the lateral and anterior cutaneous branches. Only one branch from the posterior ramus is of concern to us: the posterior cutaneous nerve. These branches are all shown in Figure 6.1.

### 6.1.3 Muscular Branches without Anatomical Names

Both primary rami of all typical spinal nerves have muscular branches to the thorax and abdomen. Muscular branches in the thorax and abdomen are not anatomically named, and there are no acupoints that can be attributed to these nerves. One can expect many motor points to be present in these areas. All of them are formed by small muscular nerve branches and are too small to be easily identifiable. In addition, they are very rarely used in acupuncture therapy.

### 6.1.4 Three Cutaneous Nerves with Six Terminal Branches

As mentioned above, each typical spinal nerve has three cutaneous branches. They are the anterior and lateral cutaneous from the ventral primary ramus, and the posterior cutaneous from the

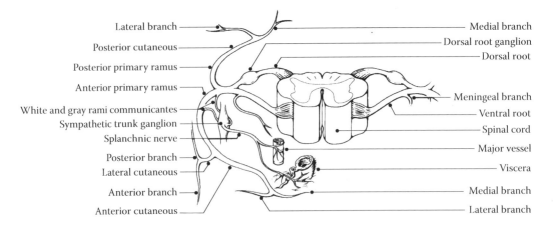

**FIGURE 6.1**  A schematic illustration of a typical spinal nerve.

dorsal primary ramus. Each of these three cutaneous nerves bifurcates into two terminal branches. Anatomically, these terminal branches all penetrate the deep fascia to become subcutaneously located. Their locations (Figure 6.2) are all identifiable in a careful dissection of the cadaver. Thus, a typical nerve will have six acupoints at the terminal ends of its three cutaneous branches. For practical purposes, only one acupoint is needed to represent each cutaneous branch on the body surface, as shown in Figure 6.3.

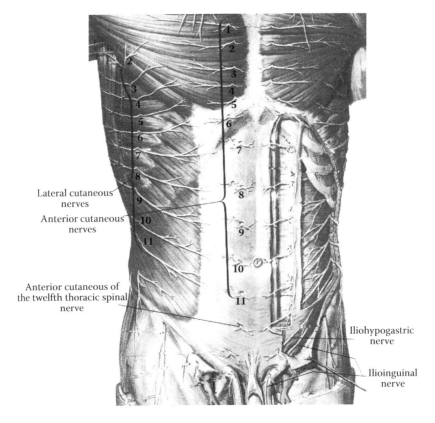

**FIGURE 6.2**  Distribution of the cutaneous nerves in the chest and abdominal walls.

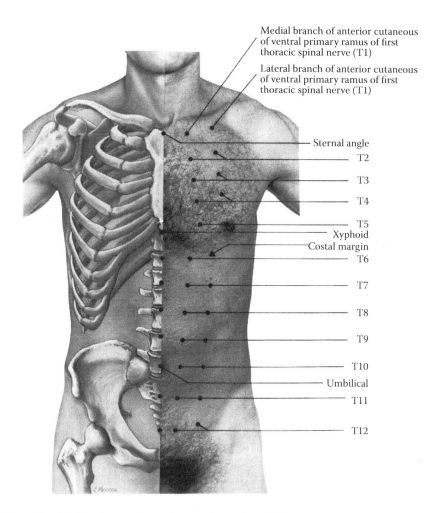

**FIGURE 6.3** Distribution of acupoints on the anterior surface of the body.

## 6.2 COMPOSITION OF FIBERS IN THE TYPICAL SPINAL NERVES

Here is a suitable point to review the different fibers that compose different nerve branches in the typical spinal nerves.

### 6.2.1 Efferent Fibers to Skeletal Muscles

The nerves originate from motor neurons in the ventral horn of the spinal cord. They are described as nerve fibers with single neurons. The nerves leave the spinal cord by way of the ventral root to become part of the spinal nerve. Because they are efferent fibers, impulses generated by the nerves will travel and will be transmitted outward to their target tissues and organs of the skeletal muscles. Abnormalities or malfunctions due to damage or injury along the efferent fibers to skeletal muscles are not of much use in acupuncture.

### 6.2.2 Autonomic Nervous System

#### 6.2.2.1 Sympathetic Nerves

Sympathetic nerves originate from preganglionic cells in the intermediate cell column of the spinal cord between the first thoracic and the second lumbar spinal nerves. The route through which the preganglionic sympathetic nerve travels is along the ventral root and white rami communicantes to end in the postganglionic neurons in the sympathetic chain. Postganglionic sympathetic nerves from the sympathetic chain are important to know because they are the efferent fibers to smooth muscles in the blood vessels and secretory glands in the skin. These efferent fibers of the sympathetic nerves will enter spinal nerves by the gray rami communicantes, and then follow both the anterior and posterior primary rami to reach acupoints by way of the cutaneous branches. This is the anatomical reason that sympathetic nerve reactions [1] are often observed in the course of acupuncture treatments. Patients with chronic pain tend to have hyperactivity in the sympathetic nerves. Consequently, their parasympathetic nerves can become hypoactive. Acupuncture seems to have the tendency to suppress sympathetic function, and in turn to enhance efficiency in the parasympathetic nerves. Another group of preganglionic sympathetic nerves will just bypass the sympathetic chain without synapses. The preganglionic fibers in this group go through a sympathetic chain to become splanchnic nerves. There are three splanchnic branches: the greater, lesser, and least. They are known as the visceral nerves. The greater splanchnic branch carries preganglionic sympathetic fibers from the first to ninth thoracic spinal nerves to reach postganglionic sympathetic neurons in the celiac ganglion. From this ganglion, postganglionic sympathetic nerves are supplied to organs developed from the embryonic foregut, including the esophagus to the proximal portion of the duodenum. The postganglionic nerves are supplied to these visceral organs by vascular branches of the celiac artery. The lesser splanchnic has a similar anatomical arrangement, from the tenth thoracic to the first lumbar spinal nerves ending in the superior mesentery ganglion, where another bunch of postganglionic sympathetic nerve cells are located. Postganglionic sympathetic nerves from these nerve cells link to the segment of the digestive tract between the duodenum and the end of the transverse colon. This segment of the digestive tract is derived from the embryonic midgut. Postganglionic nerve fibers to this part of the gut are supplied by vascular branches of the superior mesenteric artery. The same applies to the least splanchnic branch, which originates from the last two lumbar and the first sacral spinal nerves. Postganglionic neurons of this branch are in the inferior mesenteric ganglion from which the postganglionic fibers to the descending and sigmoid colons are distributed by the inferior mesenteric artery. Thus, it becomes obvious that there is a segmental and dermatomal relationship between the spinal cord and the cutaneous branches of the typical spinal nerves, making somato-visceral reflexes [2,3] possible in acupuncture stimulation. Examples of this relation will be provided in the rest of this chapter.

#### 6.2.2.2 Parasympathetic Nerves

Parasympathetic nerves in typical spinal nerves are not as relevant to us as sympathetic nerves, primarily because they have no way to reach to the skin's surface and thus become accessible by acupuncture needles. Parasympathetic fibers in the typical spinal nerves are from two sources, one from the hindbrain and the other from the lumbosacral segment of the spinal cord. The preganglionic parasympathetic fibers from the brain are carried to their target organs by the anterior and posterior vagal trunks. Inside the organs, this group of nerves synapses with postganglionic cells from which short postganglionic fibers spread out inside the organs. Similar arrangements are found for the parasympathetic nerves from the lumbosacral portion.

### 6.2.3 Afferent Fibers for General Senses

None of the branches from typical spinal nerves contain afferent fibers for the special senses. Afferent fibers for general senses, however, are ubiquitous. They can be found in every branch of the nerves. The existence of this anatomical reality is understandable. Sensory receptors exist all over the skin and inside all visceral organs. Afferent nerves extending from these receptors travel inward to their neurons in the spinal or dorsal root ganglia, eventually ending at the substantia gelatinosa in the spinal cord. Reference of pain from internal organs to the skin surface can be occasionally observed in patients with chronic illness inside the body cavity. Such pain on the body surface often reflects the number of typical spinal nerves to the visceral organs by way of the splanchnic branch and also to the skin by way of the cutaneous branch. Pain in a particular area of the digestive tract is most likely to have this type of reflective occurrence.

## 6.3 DISTRIBUTIONS OF ACUPOINTS

Using what is presented in the previous sections for typical spinal nerves, their branches, and what kinds of nerve fibers they contain, we will be able to identify acupoints formed by nerve branches of all the typical spinal nerves. These acupoints are distributed following the locations of their cutaneous branches: the anterior, lateral, and posterior cutaneous nerves. All acupoints described in this chapter have been previously reported [4].

### 6.3.1 BACK OF THE BODY TRUNK

We will divide the human back into three regions. First, is the upper region, defined as the back of the neck. Second, is the middle region, which begins from the spinal process of the first thoracic vertebra. Third, is the lower region, which includes the five lumbar vertebrae and sacrum. Acupoints in each of these regions will be described in Sections 6.4, 6.5, and 6.6 of this chapter.

### 6.3.2 FRONT OF THE BODY

Acupoints on the anterior surface of the body are all formed by the anterior cutaneous nerve branches. As explained above, typical spinal nerves have muscular branches. The intercostal muscles they innervate are small, and acupoints formed by their motor points are inconspicuous. Very occasionally, pain does occur in the chest cage when ribs are broken. Under these circumstances, acupoints are used nonspecifically, depending on where the tender points appear.

### 6.3.3 LATERAL SIDE

Both the anterior and lateral cutaneous nerves are branches of the ventral primary ramus of typical spinal nerves. We have only a few clinical examples of perceivable pain in the lateral side of the body. One of them is a herpes infection, as shown in Figure 6.4. There is only one acupoint that will be described for acupoints on the lateral side of the body trunk.

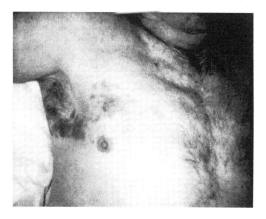

**FIGURE 6.4** A patient with herpes infection, showing the scars left by skin lesions on the right thoracic wall along the lateral cutaneous branches of the ventral primary rami of the third and fourth thoracic spinal nerves.

## 6.4 ACUPOINTS ON BACK OF THE NECK

Only the first three cervical spinal nerves have the posterior primary ramus run to the back of the neck. The remaining five cervical spinal nerves go to become mostly the ventral primary rami, with only a very small portion each becoming a posterior primary ramus. Their big ventral primary rami are going to become either the cervical or brachial plexus. The posterior primary ramus of the first cervical spinal nerve is known as the suboccipital branch. This suboccipital nerve innervates four muscles: the rectus capitis posterior major, rectus capitis posterior minor, obliquus capitis inferior, and obliquus capitis superior. These four muscles occupy a space deep in the occipital and posterior cervical regions, known as the suboccipital triangle. Because of their depth, motor points of these muscles do not become acupoints. Because the posterior primary ramus of the first cervical spinal is needed to take the nerves of the muscles of the suboccipital triangle, it doesn't spare any of itself for being the cutaneous branch. Thus, it is possible only for two remaining cervical spinal nerves to have posterior cutaneous branches.

### 6.4.1 Greater Occipital

The greater occipital nerve is the final extension of the posterior primary ramus of the second cervical spinal nerve. Remember, there is a lesser occipital nerve, a branch coming from the cervical plexus. The greater occipital emerges between the posterior arch of the atlas and the lamina of the axis, below the obliquus capitis inferior muscle. The branch becomes superficial dorsal to the suboccipital triangle to supply the skin of the occipital region, as indicated in Figure 6.5. The suboccipital

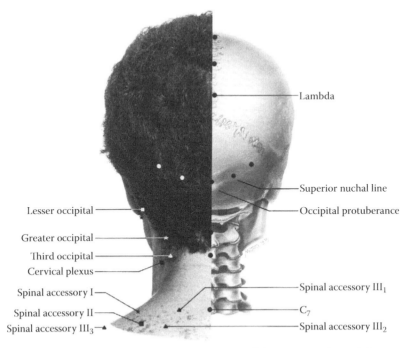

**FIGURE 6.5** Acupoints on the back of the head and neck. Some of the acupoints shown are formed by the cranial nerve of the spinal accessory and the lesser occipital of the cervical plexus.

triangle lies deep in the concavity between the trapezius and sternocleidomastoid muscles at the base of the occipital region. Because it is big in size and superficially located, acupoints formed by the greater occipital nerve are primary points and thus important in acupuncture. Examining the presence of the greater occipital point is relatively easy by palpating the hairline on the back of the head.

### 6.4.2 Third Occipital

The third occipital nerve is the extension of the posterior primary ramus of the third cervical spinal nerve. The nerve penetrates the deep fascia of the neck to become superficial approximately two or three centimeters medio-inferiorly to the greater occipital point (Figure 6.5). The third occipital nerve is smaller than the greater occipital. Therefore, even though they are located at the same depth, because both of them are cutaneous, acupoints of the greater occipital always become tender earlier than those of the third occipital. The third occipital is thus categorized as a secondary point.

Posterior cutaneous branches of the fourth to eighth cervical and first thoracic spinal nerves are gross-anatomically invisible, because their posterior primary rami are drafted to join ventral primary rami to contribute for the formation of the cervical and brachial plexus. There is not one acupoint found on the back of the neck between the spinal process of the fifth cervical to first thoracic vertebra. Very occasionally, an acupoint appears next to the spinal process of the fourth cervical vertebra in patients with a long history of chronic pain.

## 6.5 ACUPOINTS ON THE DORSAL SURFACE OF THE CHEST

The area referred to is shown in Figure 6.6. Acupoints in this area can be described as being in two groups: one is on the posterior cutaneous point of the thoracic spinal nerve and the other is on the thoracic spinal process.

### 6.5.1 Posterior Cutaneous Points

The skin on the dorsal surface of the chest is innervated by the posterior cutaneous branches derived from the posterior primary rami of the thoracic spinal nerves. Each posterior cutaneous nerve is divided into two terminal branches: the medial and lateral branches of the posterior cutaneous nerve of the posterior primary ramus of the thoracic spinal nerve. These official anatomical nomenclatures are obviously too long to use repeatedly, more so by including the medial or lateral branch descriptors.

Each of these terminal branches forms an acupoint, as shown in Figure 6.6. Because the pair of acupoints formed by a single posterior cutaneous can be regarded as a single point, it will be redundant to give each of them an anatomical name. They will be referred to as the posterior cutaneous point of a specific thoracic spinal nerve. In practice, they can be considered as a line of single points, as seen in the patient shown in Figure 6.7. Acupoints on this line will be referred to as the paravertebral points, which are very useful in acupuncture practice if there is a need to suppress hyperactivity of the sympathetic nervous system.

One paravertebral point requires additional attention. This is, the posterior cutaneous point of the sixth thoracic spinal nerve, as shown in Figure 6.6. Out of all paravertebral points, this one always becomes tender sooner than the rest. With respect to dermatomes, the visceral branch of the sixth thoracic spinal nerve is distributed to the gallbladder region. Tenderness in the posterior cutaneous point of this thoracic spinal nerve could reflect something wrong, an abnormality in the internal organ of the same dermatome. It is unknown why this particular acupoint should become tender earlier than other acupoints formed by other posterior cutaneous nerve branches.

**62** Acupuncture: An Anatomical Approach

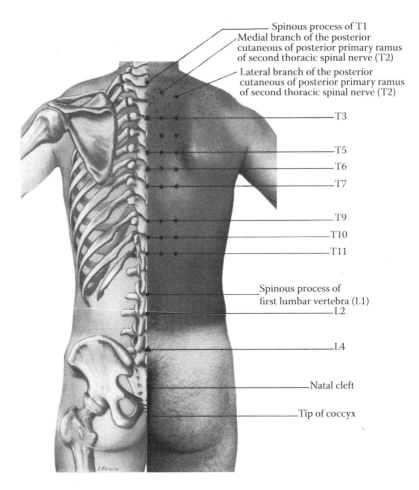

**FIGURE 6.6** Acupoints on the dorsal surface of the chest.

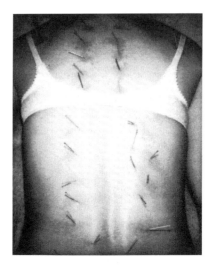

**FIGURE 6.7** A photograph of a female patient with a number of needles placed in the dorsal surface of the chest and in the lumbar region to activate the paravertebral acupoints. Atopic erythroid (reddish) reactions can be seen to be more obvious in the thoracic region than in the lumbar region, indicating a difference in the quantity of sympathetic nerves.

Acupoints in the Body Trunk

### 6.5.2 ACUPOINTS OF THE THORACIC SPINAL PROCESS

We have 12 thoracic vertebrae. Each vertebra has one spinal process pointing backward and downward. As can be seen in Figure 6.6, out of all the spinal processes, eight have an acupoint sitting on the tip of the process. These are the first, third, fifth, sixth, seventh, ninth, tenth, and eleventh. No acupoints are found on the spinal processes of the second, fourth, and eighth thoracic vertebrae. Acupoints in this group will be simply named as T1, T3, T5, T6, T7, T9, T10, or T11 spinal process point. This group of acupoints is very useful when we want to quantify pain in acupuncture. Pain quantification will be discussed in a later chapter. Here, it is appropriate to say that the T7 spinal process is a primary point, T5 a secondary, T3 a tertiary, whereas all others are nonspecific points.

## 6.6 ACUPOINTS ON THE LUMBAR AND SACRUM

All acupoints that we are going to cover for the lumbar and sacral regions can be found in Figure 6.8. From this figure, it is appropriate to group acupoints into four localities: the lumbar area, the tips of the spinal processes of the lumbar vertebrae, the sacral area, and along the iliac crest. The acupoints in each of these localities are described separately below.

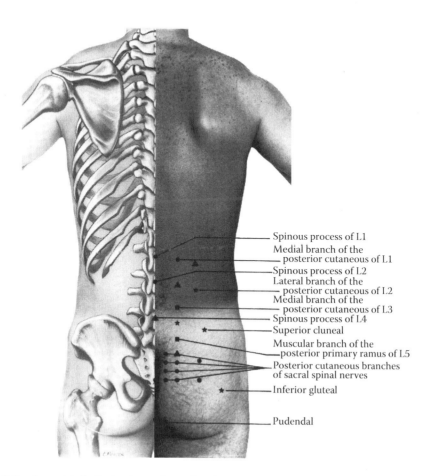

**FIGURE 6.8** Acupoints in the lumbar and sacral regions.

### 6.6.1 Posterior Cutaneous of the Lumbar Spinal Nerves

The distribution of the posterior cutaneous nerves in the back of the thorax is slightly different from that in the lumbar region. In the thoracic region, most nerve fibers in the lateral branch of the posterior cutaneous are distributed to the muscles. Only a few of them reach subcutaneously. Most nerve fibers in the medial branch of the posterior cutaneous manage to reach the skin to form acupoints. This is the reason that acupoints in the thoracic region are located closer to the midsagittal line than acupoints in the lumbar region. Both terminal branches of the five lumbar spinal nerves, the medial and lateral of the posterior cutaneous (Figure 6.9), reach to the skin. However, more fibers in the medial branches go to the muscles of the lower back, giving the lateral branches a more prominent role as the cutaneous nerves. That is why there are two acupoints for each posterior cutaneous branch in the lumbar region.

The easiest acupoint to detect is the posterior cutaneous of the second lumbar spinal nerve. The acupoint formed by the lateral branch of this cutaneous is located right at the lateral margin of the erector spinae muscle. The lateral margin of this muscle can be palpated in a person thin enough to lack fatty tissue in the superficial fascia. If a waistline is drawn across the narrowest point of the lumbar region, that point will be at the lateral border of the erector spinae where the lateral branch of the posterior cutaneous nerve penetrates the thoracolumbar fascia to form the acupoint. This will be the posterior cutaneous of L2. The posterior cutaneous of L1 is 1 inch above, and the posterior cutaneous of L3 is 1 inch below. A further inch below is the posterior cutaneous of L4. Acupoints for the posterior cutaneous L4 and L5 are also motor points. Branches from the posterior primary ramus of these two lumbar spinal nerves provide nerve fibers to the muscles in this area. Acupoints of the posterior cutaneous L2 and L4 are always detected as tender in people suffering from all kinds of lower back pain.

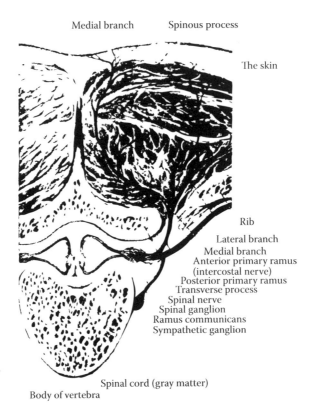

**FIGURE 6.9** A drawing of the back of the body trunk, showing the origin of the posterior primary ramus from a spinal nerve and two terminal branches of the posterior cutaneous nerves.

Acupoints in the Body Trunk

### 6.6.2 ON THE LUMBAR SPINOUS PROCESSES

Just as there are acupoints sitting on the tip of eight thoracic spinous processes, there are also acupoints located on the tip of three lumbar spinous processes, as shown in Figure 6.6. These spinous processes belong to the second, third, and fifth lumbar vertebrae. Very occasionally, an acupoint can also appear at the spinous process of the fourth lumbar vertebra. One or two of these acupoints on the spinous processes, particularly the third and fifth, will become tender in patients with chronic lower back pain.

### 6.6.3 POSTERIOR CUTANEOUS OF THE SACRAL SPINAL NERVES

Each of us has five pairs of sacral spinal nerves. Only four of them are shown to form acupoints on the sacral region from the posterior cutaneous nerve, as shown in Figure 6.8. One suspected reason is that the last or fifth sacral spinal nerve is too small to have substantial fibers going to the posterior primary ramus, and consequently, the posterior cutaneous becomes insignificant. How many acupoints there are in the sacrum does not really matter because acupuncturists have no chance to use them. In our more than 35 years of practice, not one patient was encountered with pain in the sacrum. Even pain in the tail bone seems to have no effect on the sacral region. The acupoints in the lumbar region described above and in the superior cluneal point, which will be discussed below, are different. They are important in acupuncture practices, specifically to manage lower back pain. Proper use of acupoints in the lumbar region will be the key to successfully taking care of lower back pain.

### 6.6.4 SUPERIOR CLUNEAL

This acupoint formed by the superior cluneal nerve is isolated from the rest of the acupoints in the lumber and sacral region because of its significance in the formation of acupoints. We have three cluneal nerves: the superior, middle, and inferior. Branches of the posterior cutaneous from the posterior primary rami of the first three lumbar spinal nerves form the superior cluneal nerve. This nerve pierces the thoracolumbar fascia at the lateral border of the erector spinae muscle, crosses the iliac crest a short distance in advance of the posterior superior spine of the ilium, and distributes to the skin of the gluteal region as far as the greater trochanter [5]. The middle cluneal nerve is formed by the posterior cutaneous of the upper three sacral spinal nerves. The inferior cluneal is the gluteal branch of the posterior femoral cutaneous nerve, which belongs to the lower limb. We will deal with acupoints in the lower limb next. In gross anatomy, practically no attention is paid to dissecting out these three cutaneous nerves. Very few medical graduates will even remember seeing them; much less know what and where the cluneal nerves are. There is no need to identify the middle and inferior cluneal nerves but it is very important to know the acupoints formed by the superior cluneal nerve. The superior cluneal point is the key to unlocking pain in the lower back. To locate this point (Figure 6.9), one need only palpate the margin of the iliac crest. The superior cluneal is at the highest point of the crest.

## 6.7 ACUPOINTS IN THE FRONT

### 6.7.1 ANTERIOR CUTANEOUS

Acupoints distributed in front of the thorax and abdomen are shown in Figure 6.3. There is only one acupoint for each dermatome, making a total of 12 points along a line approximately 20 mm lateral to the sternum in the thorax and lateral to the linea alba in the abdomen, where the branches of the anterior cutaneous nerves are located. Each anterior cutaneous nerve has two terminal branches, medial and lateral, which can be presented as one single acupoint. Acupoints formed by the anterior cutaneous are rarely used in acupuncture for the management of pain. One physiological function should be reiterated: the connection between the anterior cutaneous points externally and the visceral organs internally through splanchnic nerves. This connection can generate cutaneo-visceral reflexes [1–3].

Needle stimulation to the anterior cutaneous points has been reported to induce vascular dilation in the gastrointestinal tract. This cutaneo-visceral connection may also be the reason that acupuncture can occasionally treat irritable bowel syndrome effectively. Irritable bowel syndrome is defined as abdominal discomfort or pain associated with altered bowel habits for days over a period of months [6], with the absence of organic disease. Abdominal pain is the most common symptom and is often described as a cramping sensation. From our experience, by placing acupuncture needles in acupoints of the abdomen, cramping pain can be reduced or stopped for a period longer than months. Here, we choose three anterior cutaneous nerves as examples to demonstrate this relationship of interconnection between acupoints externally and visceral organs internally.

### 6.7.2 Xiphoid Point

The acupoint right under the xiphoid process indicates the location of the anterior cutaneous of the fifth thoracic spinal nerve. This acupoint is very easy to find and is noticeably tender in people who have a medical history of hiatal hernia. The hernia occurs at the esophageal–cardiac junction where the esophageal passage goes through the diaphragm. The splanchnic nerve to this part of the esophagus is the visceral branch of the ventral primary ramus of the fifth thoracic spinal nerve. The pain caused by the hernia is often expressed at the xiphoid point (Figure 6.3).

### 6.7.3 Angle of the Chest Cage Point

The costal cartilages of the sixth and seventh ribs join together, and then bend posteriorly and inferiorly. At the junction of this bending, known as the angle of the chest cage, is the location of the anterior cutaneous of the sixth thoracic spinal nerve. This angle is also easy to palpate because it is the lowest point of the ribs. This angle of the chest cage point (Figure 6.3) is the place where the anterior cutaneous of the sixth thoracic spinal nerve penetrates the deep thoracic fascia to become superficial. The visceral branch of this spinal nerve is distributed to the gallbladder area. Pain caused by stones in the gallbladder can manifest in the angle of the chest cage region.

### 6.7.4 Umbilical Point

The anterior cutaneous branches, which appear on either side of the umbilical, are from the tenth thoracic spinal nerve. We will name these points the umbilical (Figure 6.3). The visceral branch of this spinal nerve innervates the duodenal portions of the small intestine. Irritation in this part of the small intestine can result in pain around the umbilical area.

## 6.8 LATERAL SIDE OF THE CHEST CAGE

Acupoints on the lateral side of the chest cage occur because of the lateral cutaneous nerves in this region and are called lateral cutaneous points, with one exception—the intercostobrachial point. Thus, acupoints in the lateral side of the chest cage can be described under two headings.

### 6.8.1 Lateral Cutaneous

The distribution of the lateral cutaneous nerves has a similar pattern to that of the anterior cutaneous, as can be seen in Figure 6.2. Each of them is divided into terminal branches. In the case of the lateral cutaneous, the names of these two terminal branches are the anterior and posterior. Thus, we can expect to have two acupoints formed by each of the two branches. In actual cadaver dissections, the lateral cutaneous nerves are not as conspicuous and consistent as shown in Figure 6.2. Most of the time, they are rather difficult to see in a gross dissection. For this reason, acupoints on the lateral side of the chest cage do not appear as regularly as many other acupoints in other regions of

# Acupoints in the Body Trunk

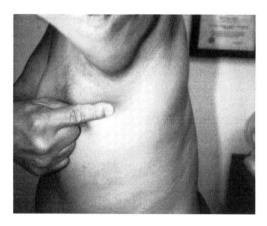

**FIGURE 6.10** The patient's finger indicates the intercostobrachial.

the body, and they are not used frequently in acupuncture. Out of all the possible acupoints that can appear along the distribution of the lateral cutaneous nerve, we describe one below.

### 6.8.2 INTERCOSTOBRACHIAL

This is the lateral cutaneous branch of the second thoracic spinal nerve. The branch penetrates the deep fascia at the second intercostal space. The patient complained of pain in the armpit. When asked where the pain was located, he pointed at the spot shown with his index finger (Figure 6.10).

In this book, we will describe pain as active, positive, or obvious if it is perceivable by the patients who complain of the sensation. There is another kind of pain, which we describe as passive, negative, or hidden. Most passive pain is found to be detectable in the acupoints. We will regard acupoints having tenderness as trigger points. Using this definition, a number of acupoints can sometimes appear in a rather limited area as shown in Figure 6.4, which is a photo taken from a patient suffering a herpesvirus infection in the axillary region. The number of passive acupoints or trigger points in this area can range as high as eight to 12.

## REFERENCES

1. Kuntz, A. and L.A. Haselwood. Circulatory reactions in the gastro-intestinal tract elicited by local cutaneous stimulation. *American Heart Journal* 20:743, 1940.
2. Kuntz, A. Anatomic and physiologic properties of cutaneo-visceral vasomotor reflex arches. *Journal of Neurophysiology* 8.421, 1945.
3. Lee, G.T.L. A study of electrical stimulation of acupuncture locus Tsusanli (St-36) on mesenteric circulation. *American Journal of Chinese Medicine* 2:53, 1974.
4. Dung, H.C. Acupuncture points of the typical spinal nerves. *American Journal of Chinese Medicine* 13:39, 1985.
5. Woodburne, R.T. *Essentials of Human Anatomy.* Oxford University Press, New York, 1965.
6. Wilkins, T. et al. Diagnosis and management of IBS in adults. *American Family Physician* 86:419, 2012.

# 7 Acupoints in the Lower Limb

## 7.1 REGIONAL ANATOMY

The lower limb is connected to the abdomen anteriorly by the inguinal ligament. Posteriorly, the gluteal region of the lower limb is demarcated from the lumbar region by the iliac crest. Below the inguinal ligament and gluteal fold, the lower limb can be divided into the thigh, knee, leg, ankle, and foot. A thigh has four compartments: anterior, lateral, posterior, and medial. The knee is a joint, the configuration of which is the patella anteriorly and the popliteal fossa posteriorly. The leg has three compartments: anterior, lateral, and posterior. The ankle joint has two bony prominences, the medial malleolus of the tibia and the lateral malleolus of the fibula. A foot has two surfaces, dorsal and plantar. In spite of so many regions, compartments, and surfaces, nerve supplies to the lower limb can be simplified into two plexuses, the lumbar and the sacral. Branches from the lumbar plexus innervate the inguinal region, the anterior and medial compartments of the thigh, the patella of the knee, and the skin that covers the medial surface of the leg. Branches from the sacral plexus take care of all other regions of the lower limb, including the gluteal, lateral and posterior compartments of the thigh, popliteal fossa, lateral and posterior compartments of the leg, and the entire foot. Thus, the quintessential point of this chapter is to become acquainted with the organization and distribution of the lumbar and sacral spinal nerve plexus. All acupoints that we need to know that appear in the lower limb are attributed to nerve branches of these two plexuses.

## 7.2 LUMBAR PLEXUS

The lumbar plexus is formed by the interconnection of branches of the ventral primary rami of the first four lumbar spinal nerves. Figure 7.1 is a schematic drawing of these interconnections. Six nerves are labeled with anatomical names. Out of these six, four are cutaneous branches. These are the iliohypogastric, ilioinguinal, genitofemoral, and lateral femoral cutaneous. The other two, the femoral and obturator, are muscular.

Each of the four cutaneous branches forms an acupoint in the inguinal region and proximal region of the anterior surface of the thigh, as shown in Figure 7.2. The femoral and obturator are muscular nerves that innervate quite a few muscles. Most of them are deep in the anterior and medial compartments of the thigh. Their motor points rarely appear superficially. Therefore, there are only a few acupoints discernible in the anterior and medial surfaces of the thigh, despite their relatively large skin area.

The femoral nerve descends to below the knee on the medial surface of the leg and becomes the saphenous, which is an important cutaneous nerve with respect to the formation of acupoints. More about the significance of acupoints formed by the saphenous nerve will be explained later in this chapter.

## 7.3 SACRAL PLEXUS

The sacral spinal nerve plexus is the interconnection of branches of the lumbosacral trunk and the ventral primary rami of the first three sacral spinal nerves. The lumbosacral trunk consists of a portion of the ventral primary of the fourth lumbar spinal nerve and the entire ventral primary ramus of the fifth lumbar spinal nerve. There are more than 20 different nerve branches coming

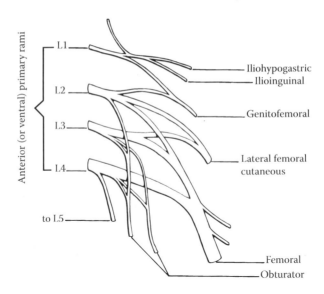

**FIGURE 7.1** A schematic drawing of the lumbar spinal nerve plexus.

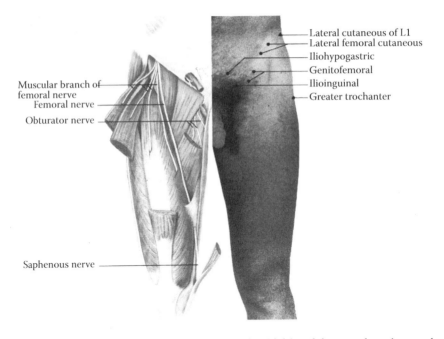

**FIGURE 7.2** Acupoints distributed around the inguinal region (right) and the nerve branches nearby (left).

either directly or indirectly from this plexus [1]. Not all of these nerve branches contribute to form acupoints. The branches that do play a role in forming acupoints are the inferior gluteal, pudendal, posterior femoral cutaneous, and the sciatic and its terminal branches. The division of the branches from the plexus can be seen in Figure 7.3.

As shown in the figure, the sciatic nerve is divided into two branches, the common peroneal and the tibial. The common peroneal then further subdivides into two terminal branches, the deep and superficial peroneals. The tibial nerve gives off a cutaneous branch, the sural nerve, in the posterior surface of the leg. After that division, the tibial turns medially to enter the plantar side of the foot

# Acupoints in the Lower Limb

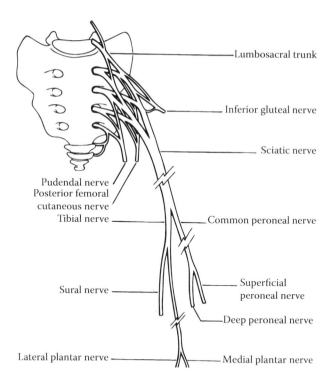

**FIGURE 7.3** A schematic drawing of the sacral plexus and terminal branches that contribute to the formation of acupoints in the lower limb.

and become the lateral and medial plantar nerves. Thus, it is clear that the sacral plexus supplies innervation to the gluteal region, the lateral and posterior compartments of the thigh, the popliteal fossa, the lateral and posterior compartments of the leg, and the entire foot.

## 7.4 ACUPOINTS OF THE LUMBAR PLEXUS

It is convenient to present the acupoints formed by nerve branches of the lumbar plexus as two groups, cutaneous and muscular. There are eight cutaneous and six muscular nerves identifiable. All acupoints formed by these 14 nerves are depicted in Figures 7.2, 7.4, and 7.5. These acupoints have been reported in a previous publication [2].

### 7.4.1 Cutaneous Branches

#### 7.4.1.1 Iliohypogastric

This is one of the three branches that divide from the ventral primary ramus of the first lumbar spinal nerve. As shown in Figure 7.1, the ventral primary ramus of each of the first four lumbar spinal nerves is divided into three branches. The upper branch of the first ventral ramus becomes the iliohypogastric nerve, the middle branch becomes the ilioinguinal, and the lower branch joins with the upper branch of the ventral ramus of the second lumbar nerve to become the genitofemoral nerve. These last two nerves will be described next.

The iliohypogastric nerve runs inside the posterior abdominal wall and penetrates the three abdominal muscles to reach the superficial fascia at the pelvic area at a site superior to the spermatic cord and lateral to the suspensory ligament of the penis in the male, and superior to the round ligament and lateral to the suspensory ligament of the clitoris in the female (Figure 7.2). An acupoint is

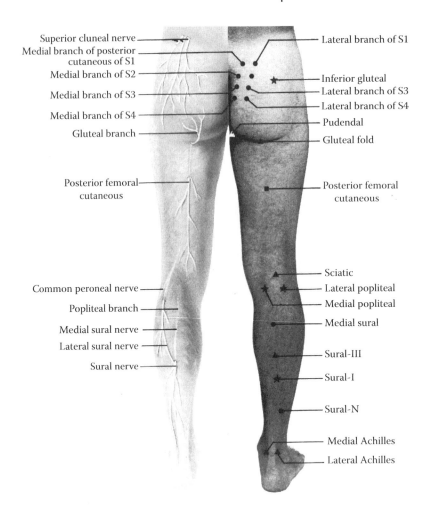

**FIGURE 7.4** Some cutaneous nerves of the lumbar plexus in the right lower limb and some acupoints formed by these nerves in the left.

formed at the spot where the nerve pierces the deep fascia of the abdomen or anterior layer of the rectus sheath. This iliohypogastric point is not often used, yet it has one useful aspect in judging whether pain has its origin from the first lumbar spinal nerve. Most often, pain originating from the lumbar region will begin at a herniated disc between the fourth and fifth lumbar vertebrae. The herniation has a tendency to expand and extend upward to the third, then the second, and then reach the first lumbar vertebra. By the time an intervertebrate disc is involved, the pain will already have been in the chronic stage for many years. Another useful indicator function for the iliohypogastric point is that it will become a trigger point with tender sensation in young female patients who have dysmenorrhea, or cramping pain during menstruation. Once menses stop, the trigger point disappears.

#### 7.4.1.2 Ilioinguinal

This is another branch that divided from the ventral primary ramus of the first lumbar spinal nerve. It initially runs parallel to the iliohypogastric. When it reaches the inguinal region, it passes through the inguinal canal and emerges through the superficial inguinal ring. Thus, the ilioinguinal point is located right at the opening of the superficial inguinal ring along the inguinal ligament immediately lateral to the tendon of the pectineal muscle at the superior border of the femoral triangle. Like the iliohypogastric, the ilioinguinal is not a frequently used point. Both of them are categorized as

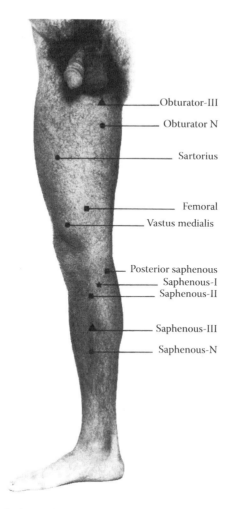

**FIGURE 7.5** A medial view of a lower limb, showing the locations of some acupoints.

tertiary points. Pain at the ilioinguinal point is very seldom described by patients younger than 45 years of age. When pain appears at this point, patients will not fail to tell their physicians precisely where the pain is located in the groin. Sometimes, the pain can be mistaken as originating from an inguinal hernia.

### 7.4.1.3 Genitofemoral

This nerve is formed by the lower branch of the ventral primary ramus of the first lumbar spinal nerve and the upper branch of the ventral primary ramus of the second lumbar spinal nerve, as can be seen in Figure 7.1. The nerve pierces the deep fascia immediately below the inguinal ligament and lateral to the superficial inguinal ring. The genitofemoral point is almost never used because practically no one receives acupuncture treatment due to pain in the testicles or labium major. The only possible cause for having pain in the scrotum is due to surgical removal of cancer in the testicles.

### 7.4.1.4 Cutaneous of Obturator

This is a variable offshoot of the anterior branch of the obturator nerve [3]. Its anterior branch is mainly muscular and articular nerves. Its cutaneous branch becomes superficial between the gracilis and adductor longus muscles in the location shown in Figure 7.4. This nerve varies in size. It is distributed, when present, to the skin of the distal one-third of the thigh on its medial side. The acupoint formed by this cutaneous branch of the obturator nerve is not important and is rarely used in practice.

### 7.4.1.5 Lateral Femoral Cutaneous

This nerve derives from the first three lumbar nerves, from which it courses across the anterior surface of the iliacus muscle where this forms a part of the wall of the false pelvis, and enters the thigh between the lateral border of the iliacus and the upper end of the inguinal ligament; thereafter, it pierces the fascia lata, commonly just below and medial to the anterior superior iliac spine. The larger part of the nerve runs downward on the lateral side of the anterior aspect of the thigh to supply skin here as far as the knee. A smaller posterior branch runs more laterally, supplying the skin below the greater trochanter but usually not reaching the knee [4].

First, we need to define the fascia lata. This is the deep fascia wrapping around the thigh superficial to the muscle mass. On the lateral side of the thigh, the fascia becomes thickened, and this thickening portion of the fascia lata is known as the iliotibial tract. The tract is an extension of the aponeurosis, which encloses the muscle of the tensor fasciae latae. The iliotibial tract runs downward on the lateral side of the thigh and blends into the ligaments and tendons on the lateral aspect of the knee joint. The iliotibial tract is a very important structure in acupuncture because many patients complain of pain right over and along the area covered by the tract. It is obvious that conventional medical wisdom has very little to offer for mending this condition of pain perceived under the iliotibial tract, clinically described as meralgia paraesthetica. The etiology of this disease is not clearly understood. Various things have been blamed for it, including being overweight, having a job as a waiter or waitress for too many years, etc. Anatomically, the nerve that is believed to be the culprit in producing meralgia is, in the descriptions of all experts, the lateral femoral cutaneous [5]. In a medical dictionary, meralgia paraesthetica is defined as "Bernhardt's disease; tingling, formication, itching, and other forms of paraesthetica on the outer side of the lower part of the thigh in the area of distribution of the external cutaneous branch of the femoral nerve. There may be pain, but the skin is usually hyperesthetic to the touch" [6]. In this context, "the external cutaneous branch of the femoral nerve" means the lateral femoral cutaneous. The lateral femoral cutaneous is not a branch of the femoral nerve. It is a blatant anatomical mistake.

Second, if meralgia paraesthetica is indeed neuralgic pain in the lateral femoral cutaneous nerve, then this nerve will be important in acupuncture. The problem with respect to pain in the lateral side of the thigh is that it does not come from the lateral femoral cutaneous, but from the sciatic nerve. After careful and thorough dissection of the iliotibial tract, we are able to trace cutaneous nerves that penetrate the tract to branches divided from the sciatic nerve. More will be said about cutaneous innervation to the lateral side of the thigh when we describe the acupoints formed by the sacral plexus next. The acupoints formed by the lateral femoral cutaneous nerve are not of much use to us.

Third, Bernhardt disease is a rather common occurrence among people seeking acupuncture treatments. Acupuncture seems to be very effective in reducing or even eradicating symptoms described in meralgia paraesthetica, particularly at the early stages of having the disease. In time, patients with Bernhardt disease will have difficulty sleeping on their sides because pressing the hip on the bed will cause pain to appear in the greater trochanter and wake up the sleepers. Also, pain caused by meralgia paraesthetica can be a precursor of eventual hip joint replacements for the patients encountered in our acupuncture clinic.

### 7.4.1.6 Anterior Femoral Cutaneous

This nerve has multiple branches that originate from the femoral nerve. As shown in Figure 7.4, there are three acupoints that appear in the distal region of the anterior surface of the thigh. They are formed by the anterior femoral cutaneous nerves. The places where these cutaneous nerves pierce the deep fascia vary from individual to individual. Acupoints of the anterior femoral cutaneous nerves are rarely found to become tender. For this reason, they are rarely needed in acupuncture.

## 7.4.1.7 Parapatellar

This refers to acupoints located in the area of the kneecap (Figure 7.4). Each knee has two acupoints in front of the joint. They appear like two eyes, right and left. We know that there are cutaneous nerves to the knee joints. They innervate structures like the lateral and medial meniscus. We suspect that the parapatellar points are formed by the cutaneous nerve branches from the femoral nerve to the knee joint. Parapatellar points are very useful for deciding whether pain in the knee can be effectively managed with acupuncture. Pain in the knee is very common because of osteoarthritis. More about parapatellar points will be presented when osteoarthritis comes up for discussion in later chapters.

## 7.4.1.8 Saphenous

This is the most important point in the entire lumbar plexus. The nerve that forms this acupoint is a cutaneous branch as well as the terminal branch of the femoral nerve. Arising from the femoral nerve in the femoral triangle, it enters the adductor, or Hunter's canal, where it crosses the femoral vessels anteriorly from their lateral to their medial side. It emerges medioinferiorly from underneath the sartorius muscle, becoming very superficial just immediately below the medial side of the knee under the medial condyle of the tibia. Immediately after penetrating the deep fascia under the medial condyle, the saphenous nerve divides into three branches: the anterior, middle, and posterior. The area covered by these three branches of the saphenous nerve is very important with respect to the formation of acupoints. Sometimes, more than four acupoints will appear in this area (Figures 7.4 and 7.5). Depending on how early these saphenous points appear, they can be categorized as primary, secondary, tertiary, or nonspecific acupoints. Tenderness in at least one saphenous point is almost universal for patients seen in our acupuncture clinic.

## 7.4.2 Muscular Branches

### 7.4.2.1 Obturator

This nerve leaves the pelvis via the obturator foramen to supply the skin and muscles in the medial compartment of the thigh. One acupoint formed by the cutaneous branch of the obturator nerve has been described previously. Two acupoints formed by the muscular branches of the same nerve are offered here (Figure 7.5). Obturator points are rarely used because pain in the medial compartment of the thigh is not common at all. Pain in the medial compartment can occur when one or more muscles become torn or otherwise injured in recreational sports such as speedboat racing or waterskiing. Accidents in these types of sports are known to happen because the thighs are pulled outward too fast and too hard, resulting in tearing or damage to the hamstring (the semimembranous and semitendinosus). In such cases, tender acupoints will appear in the muscular branches from the obturator nerve.

### 7.4.2.2 Rectus Femoris

This is one of the four heads belonging to the quadriceps femoris muscle. The entire thigh contains many muscles. They overlay one another, and most of them are buried deep inside the muscular compartments. Thus, their motor points don't have any strong possibility to serve as acupoints. Three of the four heads of the quadriceps—the rectus femoris, vastus lateralis, and vastus medialis—are the outermost layer of the muscles in the anterior compartment of the thigh. Their motor points are situated relatively superficially at the locations where the muscle mass (rectus femoris) is relatively thin, or right at the sites where the tendons of the vastus lateralis and vastus medialis spread out to continue as the patellar ligament to attach to the tibial tuberosity.

### 7.4.2.3 Vastus Lateralis

This point is illustrated in Figure 7.4. Locating it is relatively simple; it sits right on top of the lateral epicondyle of the femur. This point will become tender in people who have arthritis in the knee for a certain period. We suspect that the reason for vastus lateralis and medialis points becoming tender is a diminishing in the synergistic activities of muscular movement in the thigh. The extent of wear and tear in the quadriceps femoris muscle may increase under ordinary circumstances.

#### 7.4.2.4 Vastus Medialis

This point can be found in Figures 7.4 and 7.5. It is located right on the tip of the adductor tubercle of the medial epicondyle. As with the vastus lateralis point, the vastus medialis will become tender in people who suffer from knee pain. If both points demonstrate painful sensation, the arthritis in the knees is in an advanced stage and will be difficult to manage, even with the use of acupuncture. The sequence for these two points to turn passively painful is not predictable. Sometimes, the vastus lateralis point will become tender first, then the vastus medialis, and sometimes vice versa.

#### 7.4.2.5 Sartorius

The longest ribbonlike muscle in the body, the sartorius has a motor point that becomes an acupoint (as shown in Figure 7.5) because it is right under the skin in the medial compartment of the thigh. A slip of the aponeurosis of this muscle blends above with the capsule of the knee joint. Therefore, functional abnormalities in the knee can have a detrimental influence on the activity of the sartorius muscle, turning its motor point into an acupoint. Even so, this acupoint is very rarely called into use in acupuncture.

#### 7.4.2.6 Femoral

This enters the Hunter's canal (Figure 7.2) to become the saphenous nerve. At this location, it gives away branches to a number of muscles. None of them happen to cover the nerve, making directly pressing it possible when the acupoint formed by this nerve becomes tender. Young women experiencing menstrual cramping will notice that their femoral point can become sensitive during the arrival of menstruation.

### 7.5 ACUPOINTS OF THE SACRAL PLEXUS

Acupoints of the sacral plexus have been reported previously [7]. The distribution of acupoints formed by the nerve branches of the sacral plexus is more complicated to describe than that of branches formed by the lumbar plexus. Some of them are found in the posterior of the thigh and leg. Some are in the anterior and lateral, or located in the knee, popliteal fossa, and foot. For the sake of convenience, we will describe acupoints of the sacral plexus according to where they can be located. The localities are divided into the thigh, popliteal fossa, leg, and foot.

### 7.6 DISTRIBUTIONS TO THE THIGH

The acupoints in the thigh are found in the posterior and lateral compartments. There are two acupoints in the posterior compartment, and three in the lateral. One acupoint, the inferior gluteal, is placed in this group, simply because no other place is more appropriate for it.

#### 7.6.1 IN THE POSTERIOR COMPARTMENT

As can be seen in Figure 7.4, there are only two points shown in the posterior compartment of the thigh, the gluteal fold and posterior femoral cutaneous points. In fact, both of them are formed by the same nerve, the posterior femoral cutaneous. The third acupoint, the inferior gluteal, is not in the posterior compartment of the thigh, but in the gluteal region. We view the gluteal region as the upper extension of the thigh.

#### 7.6.1.1 Gluteal Fold Point

This is so named because it appears right in the middle of the gluteal fold. The cutaneous nerve that forms this acupoint is a branch of the posterior femoral cutaneous. The term "posterior femoral cutaneous" is actually something of a misnomer because it is a mixed nerve rather than purely cutaneous. The nerve receives posterior branches from the first and second sacral spinal nerves, and anterior branches from the second and third sacral spinal, as described by Woodburne [3]. The posterior femoral cutaneous thus includes both cutaneous and muscular branches.

Running parallel with the posterior femoral cutaneous is the pudendal nerve, which passes into the pudendal canal. This is a fascial canal formed by a split in the obturator internus fascia on the lateral wall of the ischiorectal fossa. The pudendal nerve has three branches: the inferior rectal, perineal, and dorsal nerve of the penis (or clitoris). At the location these three branches divide from the pudendal nerve is an acupoint, as indicated in Figure 7.4. This point can become very tender in patients who have a painful condition known as coccydenia. Otherwise, there is no chance to use this point in acupuncture treatments. The point is too close to the external genitalia, too sensitive an area to place needles. It is not necessary to describe this point separately as an entity of acupoints.

### 7.6.1.2 Posterior Femoral Cutaneous

The nerve keeps running distally along the midline of the thigh. At the center point of this midline between the gluteal fold and popliteal fossa, the nerve penetrates the deep fascia to go superficial. This is the location of the posterior femoral cutaneous point (Figure 7.4). Both the gluteal fold and the posterior femoral cutaneous points can become trigger points in people with a long history of chronic lower back pain. The opportunity to use them in treating pain is rather good.

### 7.6.1.3 Inferior Gluteal

This nerve is a muscular branch. It arises from the posterior branches of the anterior primary rami of the fifth lumbar and the first two sacral spinal nerves, then leaves the pelvis through the greater sciatic foramen below the piriformis and enters the gluteus maximus muscle. The motor point formed between the inferior gluteal nerve and the gluteus maximus muscle is the inferior gluteal point (Figure 7.4). There are many muscles in the gluteal region. Some of them are large, and some deep. None of them has a motor point that will turn into an acupoint, except the gluteus maximus. This muscle is the most superficially spread out in the gluteal region. This acupoint is the only point present in the entire region. The point is located right in the center of the gluteal region, where the nerve enters the muscle. The motor point of the gluteus maximus muscle has a rich vascular bed, covered by the inferior gluteal artery and vein. Pain in the inferior gluteal point can be very stubborn. Clinically, the pain is referred to as piriformis syndrome because it is believed that the inferior gluteal nerve is pinched by the piriformis muscle. Such an etiology of pain in the buttock is questionable for the very simple reason that the piriformis is a small muscle and sits deeply inside the gluteal. The inferior gluteal point is important because it will seem tender in anyone who has lower back pain.

### 7.6.2 IN THE LATERAL COMPARTMENT

Acupoints in the lateral compartment are important in acupuncture. Painful conditions such as Bernhardt disease are rather frequently encountered in the practice of acupuncture. Acupoints in the lateral compartment are necessary for treating pain in this area. Two controversies or dilemmas have come up for discussion: which nerve plays the necessary role to form acupoints in the lateral compartment of the thigh, and how many acupoints are there in the same anatomical localities? As explained briefly above, the cutaneous innervation to the lateral side of the thigh is said to be from the lateral femoral cutaneous nerve, according to conventional texts of gross anatomy. Our own research, through careful and thorough dissections of cadavers, proves otherwise. The cutaneous branches to the skin in the lateral compartment are derived from the sciatic nerve. Usually, there are four of them. These four cutaneous nerves penetrate the iliotibial tract to become superficial. We have no appropriate anatomical nomenclatures for these cutaneous nerves. The best choice is to name them as iliotibial points. Besides the iliotibial points, there are the greater trochanter and biceps femoris points to discuss.

### 7.6.2.1 Greater Trochanter Point

There can be just one or multiple greater trochanter points. Although there is no figure here to indicate where the greater trochanter point is located, it is (or they are) not difficult to find. The greater trochanter of the femur is a bony projection on both hips. As we sit down, this bony process is easy to palpate. If there is any acupoint appearing in this location, it will be easy detecting its presence. Anatomically, we don't know which nerve should be responsible for having acupoints over the trochanter. We do know that there is a large bursa, the largest in the body, covering the greater trochanter. We suspect that the bursa may play a role in causing pain over the trochanteric region.

### 7.6.2.2 Iliotibial Tract Point

There can be anywhere from one to four iliotibial tract points (Figure 7.6). Some people will have only one acupoint detectable in the lateral side of the thigh. This first appearance makes it the primary acupoint. This first point always appears in the center of the midlateral line. Some will have two, three, or four acupoints along the same line in the lateral compartment. The point that appears second is located approximately 2 in. superior to the first point. The third point is located 2 in. below the first. The fourth and last is 2 in. lower than the third point. As such, the iliotibial tract points shown in Figure 7.6 are designated as the primary, secondary, tertiary, and nonspecific.

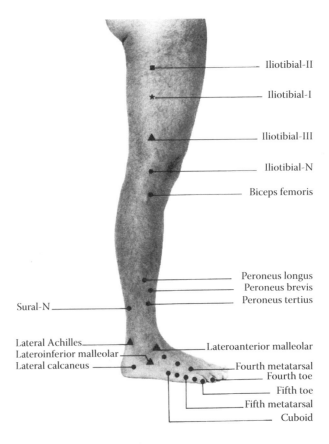

**FIGURE 7.6** Acupoints along the ilitibial tract, in the lateral compartment of the leg and the dorsal surface on the lateral side of the foot.

### 7.6.2.3 Biceps Femoris Point

This point is formed by two muscular branches to this muscle. One comes from the tibial nerve to the long head, and another from the common peroneal to the short head. The tendon of the biceps femoris muscle joins that of the quadriceps to become part of the fibular collateral ligament. This collateral ligament has the potential to be damaged, or even torn apart, because it is immediately beneath the skin. Tenderness in the biceps femoris point can be an indication of an injured fibular collateral ligament.

## 7.7 DISTRIBUTIONS IN THE POPLITEAL FOSSA

There are three acupoints that can appear in the popliteal fossa, as shown in Figure 7.4. These three points are the sciatic, lateral popliteal, and medial popliteal.

### 7.7.1 SCIATIC POINT

As the name indicates, this acupoint is formed at one locality along the course of the sciatic nerve. The sciatic is the biggest nerve trunk in the body. In most cadavers, the trunk is about the size of the little finger. In spite of it being the largest in diameter, no acupoint is attributed directly to this nerve because of its deep position. The sciatic nerve descends down in the posterior compartment of the thigh and divides into two terminal branches—the tibial and the common peroneal—toward the distal end, as indicated by the location of the sciatic point (Figure 7.4). Before becoming the tibial and common peroneal nerves, it gives away a few cutaneous branches, some of which have been described previously, including four branches along the iliotibial tract.

### 7.7.2 LATERAL POPLITEAL POINT

The popliteal fossa lies behind the knee and is covered by the popliteal fascia. The space is diamond-shaped. On each end of the diamond is a shallow pit forming a small concavity. Between the two concavities, as can be seen in Figure 7.4, is a slight elevated bulge in the middle of the fossa. Immediately inside the skin at the lateral pit runs the common peroneal nerve, which is the location of the lateral popliteal point (Figure 7.4). The lateral popliteal is a primary acupoint.

### 7.7.3 MEDIAL POPLITEAL POINT

Underneath the medial popliteal point (Figure 7.4) runs the tibial nerve. As the tibial nerve continues the course of the sciatic from the thigh, it travels through the fossa in a direction from latero-superiorly to medio-inferiorly. Both the common peroneal and tibial originate from the sciatic nerve, which plays an important role in the pain of sciatica. They also provide genicular branches to the knee joint, which is one of the main sources of pain in the body. Such anatomical and pathological facts make the lateral and medial popliteal points important. Almost every patient received in the clinic has tenderness in one of the two points. Such acupoints are used in every acupuncture session when the occasion permits.

## 7.8 ACUPOINTS ON THE POSTERIOR COMPARTMENT OF THE LEG AND ANKLE

Acupoints in the posterior compartment of the thigh are all related to the sural nerve. The sural nerve is constructed by joining the medial and lateral sural nerves. They are all cutaneous branches. No muscular branch forms an acupoint in the posterior compartment. The lateral sural is a branch of the common peroneal and is the smaller of the two nerves. The nerve does not participate in the formation of any acupoints. Thus, it will not be further described.

### 7.8.1 MEDIAL SURAL

The medial sural nerve arises from the tibial nerve in the popliteal fossa. It descends immediately under the deep fascia in the groove between two heads of the gastrocnemius muscle as far as the middle of the leg. Here, it pierces the deep fascia and is joined by the lateral sural from the common peroneal to become the sural nerve. This kind of arrangement is rather unusual. Most nerve branches become smaller in size as they are further divided when distributed more peripherally. The sural nerve is more distal to both the lateral and medial sural, and yet it becomes larger than both of the nerves that contribute to its formation. This may be the reason that the sural point serves as an important acupoint.

### 7.8.2 SURAL

The formation of the sural point (Figure 7.4) is explained in the previous subsection. There are three additional acupoints distributed along the medial sural nerve. We have no appropriate anatomical nomenclatures to name them, save for deriving names from the sural. Thus, these acupoints are named sural-III, sural-N, and medial sural, as indicated in Figure 7.4. The star in the figure indicates the primary or sural-I point, the triangle shows the tertiary or sural-III, and the black circles note the nonspecific or sural-N and medial sural points.

### 7.8.3 MEDIAL ACHILLES

The calcaneal tendon, commonly known as the Achilles tendon, is the thickest and strongest in the body. Two large muscles, the soleus and gastrocnemius, contribute to forming this tendon. It begins at about the middle of the leg. Narrowing below, it inserts into the middle part of the posterior surface of the calcaneus bone. A bursa lies deep to the tendon and separates it from the upper part of the posterior surface of the calcaneus. An injury to the muscles, to the tendon itself, or inflammation in the bursa can possibly cause the formation of tender points on each side of the Achilles tendon. Thus, there is a medial and a lateral Achilles point.

### 7.8.4 LATERAL ACHILLES

The lateral and medial Achilles points are very easy to check by rubbing the tendon between the thumb and the index finger. If there is tenderness on either side of the tendon, the indication is that either or both of them have become trigger points and are ready for acupuncture treatment. Immediately adjacent to the medial Achilles is the tibial nerve, which is along the plantar side of the foot. Immediately adjacent to the lateral Achilles is the sural nerve, which goes to the lateral side of the foot.

## 7.9 ACUPOINTS ON THE LATERAL COMPARTMENT OF THE LEG

Cutaneous innervation to the skin covering the lateral compartment of the leg belongs to dermatomes of the fifth lumbar and first sacral spinal nerves. Herniation of the intervertebral disc between the fifth lumbar and first sacral vertebrae has the potential to compress the dorsal root of the fifth lumbar spinal nerve. Such a condition, in an early stage of nerve root compression, can result in tingling and numbing sensations without much pain in the distal segment of the lateral compartment of the leg. This sensation indicates abnormal activities in the motor points formed by the muscular nerves. There are three muscles in the lateral compartment: the peroneus longus, peroneus brevis, and peroneus tertius.

### 7.9.1 PERONEUS LONGUS

This muscle is the most superficially located of the three. The common peroneal nerve passes through a gap between the attachments of the muscle to the head and the shaft of the fibula, winds around the neck of the fibula deep to the peroneus longus, and here divides into the deep peroneal and superficial peroneal nerves. There are usually branches to the peroneus longus from both the common peroneal and superficial peroneal nerves. Both of them contribute to form the peroneus longus point, as shown in Figure 7.6.

### 7.9.2 PERONEUS BREVIS

Deep to the peroneus longus is the peroneus brevis muscle. It is the shorter and smaller of the two. This muscle is innervated by a branch of the superficial peroneal nerve, which enters the posterior margin of the muscle where the peroneus brevis point is formed (Figure 7.6).

### 7.9.3 PERONEUS TERTIUS

This is a small muscle, a lateral slip of another extensor muscle. This larger muscle is the extensor digitorum longus, from which it is seldom completely separated. Two branches of the deep peroneal nerve innervate the extensor digitorum longus. One of the two branches sends a small nerve to form the peroneus tertius point, which is insignificant in acupuncture.

## 7.10 ACUPOINTS ON THE ANTERIOR COMPARTMENT OF THE LEG

Acupoints in the anterior compartment are formed by the common peroneal nerve (Figure 7.7). In the gluteal region, the common peroneal portion of the sciatic nerve is more superficially placed.

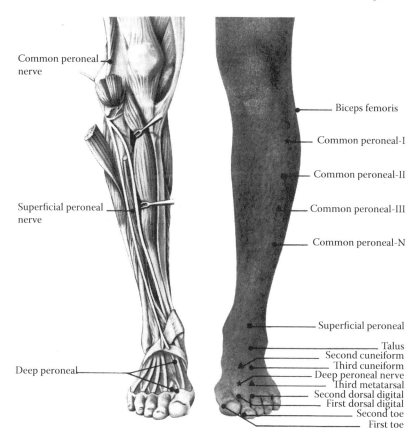

**FIGURE 7.7** Acupoints in the anterior compartment of the leg.

Thus, it is more easily injured by an instrument, such as a long hypodermic needle used for buttock injection. Such an incident occurred in a patient. A few days after the injection, she began to feel pain in the anterior compartment of one leg. The pain ran along the lateral border of the tibia where the common peroneal nerve is located, and reached the superficial and deep peroneal nerves to the dorsal surface of the first three medial toes. She felt no pain in her other leg.

The common peroneal nerve is separated from the tibial nerve at the superior angle of the popliteal fossa. It then follows the medial border of the biceps femoris muscle, the tendon of which forms the superolateral boundary of the fossa. The nerve leaves the fossa by passing superficially to the lateral head of the gastrocnemius muscle. It then passes over the back of the head of the fibula before winding around the lateral surface of the neck of the same bone, as shown in Figure 7.7. The nerve finally runs beneath the upper portion of the peroneus longus muscle to enter the anterior compartment of the leg. At the head of the fibula and posterolateral to its neck, the nerve can be palpated by rolling it against the bone. Here, the nerve lies very superficially, immediately under the skin, but there is no acupoint that can be attributed to the nerve at this location, possibly because the nerve lies deep inside the deep fascia without any dividing or accompanying major blood vessels. The common peroneal bifurcates into the superficial and deep peroneal nerves in the upper region of the anterior compartment. Anatomically, the common peroneal and the deep radial nerve in the forearm develop analogically. Both of them have four acupoints along their courses of distribution, as shown for the common peroneal nerve in Figure 7.7. The common peroneal-I is the primary point, the common peroneal-II is secondary, the common peroneal-III is tertiary, and the common peroneal-N is nonspecific.

## 7.11 ACUPOINTS ON THE FOOT

Three nerves situated in the leg—the common peroneal, sural, and tibial—and their branches provide the structural elements for having acupoints in the foot. The acupoints on the dorsal surface of the foot are formed by the superficial and deep peroneal nerves distributing to the medial four toes (Figure 7.7), and the sural nerve to the fifth toe (Figure 7.6). The acupoints on the plantar surface of the foot are formed by the terminal branches of the tibial nerve (Figure 7.8).

### 7.11.1 DORSAL SURFACE OF THE FOOT

Anatomically, the foot is a very complicated structure. Many bones, muscles, tendons, ligaments, and retinaculi make up a foot. Two bones are connected together by muscle tendons and ligaments to form a joint. All joints are innervated by nerves, and nerves have the potential to form acupoints. We will not be able to list all the potential acupoints in the foot because there are far too many to

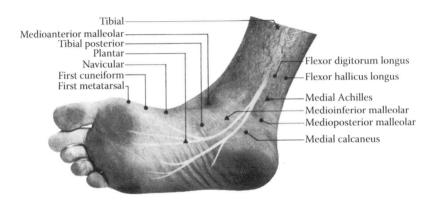

**FIGURE 7.8** Acupoints formed by the terminal branches of the tibial nerve on the plantar surface of the foot.

count. All we can do is select the most useful and important acupoints as examples to present to the readers. Ten acupoints are listed here to represent those located on the dorsal surface of the foot.

### 7.11.1.1 Superficial Peroneal

This becomes a cutaneous nerve after piercing the deep fascia immediately lateral to the tendon of the extensor digitorum longus in the anterior ankle to form the superficial peroneal acupoint (Figure 7.7). It is a secondary acupoint. The acupoint formed by the deep peroneal nerve is the primary point, meaning that the deep peroneal point becomes tender sooner than the superficial peroneal point.

### 7.11.1.2 Deep Peroneal

This nerve becomes cutaneous after running through the deep fascia at approximately 2 cm rostral to the web between the great and second toes. This is a very important acupoint, belonging to the group of the primary points. Smaller branches from the superficial and deep peroneal contribute nerves to form acupoints described subsequently.

### 7.11.1.3 Metatarsal

This describes five bones in the foot, which form joints with the toes. These joints are potential locations for having acupoints. The metatarsal point between the third and fourth toes is a good example. This point can become tender in people who have Morton neuroma. We have four metatarsal points in each foot.

### 7.11.1.4 Talus

The talus is one of the seven tarsal bones. It connects to the navicular and calcaneus. The junctions between these bones can become acupoints.

### 7.11.1.5 Cuneiforms

There are three cuneiforms. The same acupoint potential applies to their junctions with other tarsal bones adjacent to them.

### 7.11.1.6 Dorsal Digital

This refers to interphalangeal joints. The acupoints formed by these joints are useful when treating people who have the conditions known as hammer toe or bunions. Hammer toe is a deformity caused by permanent angular flexion, and a bunion is an inflammation that develops in the big toe.

### 7.11.1.7 Lateroinferior Malleolar

This is located below the lateral malleolus of the fibula, as its name indicates. There are a few ligaments in this area. Tearing or damage to one or more of these tendons is possible when the ankle is twisted due to overeversion or overinversion. The damage can lead to the appearance of acupoints in the lateroinferior malleolar point.

### 7.11.1.8 Lateroanterior Malleolar

The name is derived in the same fashion as that of the lateroinferior malleolar point. The appearance of either or both of these two points will depend on which ligaments are damaged. More ligaments injured with greater severity will have more acupoints appearing in the inferior region of the lateral malleolus.

### 7.11.1.9 Lateral Calcaneous

This is the point right on the lateral surface of the calcaneous bone, the largest and strongest of the foot. It is long, flattened from side to side, and bulbous posteriorly and inferiorly where it forms the heel. Acupoints can appear on each side of the flattened surface and the heel, particularly for people who suffer from chronic pain, such as diabetic peripheral neuropathy.

### 7.11.1.10 Cuboid

This tarsal bone is on the lateral side of the foot between the calcaneus (behind it) and the fifth metatarsal bones (in front). Its dorsal surface is rough and nonarticular, making it easy to palpate. Occasionally, an acupoint can be found in the dorsal surface of the cuboid. All of the last four acupoints mentioned previously located on the lateral side of the foot can exist because of the sural nerve.

## 7.11.2 PLANTAR SURFACE OF THE FOOT

All of the acupoints on the plantar surface of the foot are produced by the tibial nerve and its branches. The plantar surface can become very sensitive in some patients. Consequently, every point in the plantar will appear tender on proper pressing. Twelve acupoints are selected for demonstrative purposes.

### 7.11.2.1 Tibial Point

The tibial point is not located on the plantar surface, but toward the distal end of the medial side of the leg, as shown in Figure 7.8. This is one of the most important acupoints. It will be used every time the point is possible to reach. After branching from the sciatic nerve, the main trunk of the tibial nerve remains in the posterior compartment of the leg and gives off muscular and cutaneous branches. The cutaneous branches of the tibial contributing to the formation of acupoints are the sural and the plantar. The location of the sural nerve and the acupoints formed by it are shown in Figure 7.4. The tibial nerve comes close to the skin, approximately 7 to 8 cm above the medial malleolus. The skin surface over this area can become very sensitive in people with chronic pain. This is the location of the tibial point. At this point, the tibial nerve gives away branches to several structures, such as the deltoid ligament, before running into the plantar to become the medial and lateral plantar nerves.

### 7.11.2.2 Medioanterior Malleolar

This anterior acupoint is right under the medial malleolus. Under this bone projection, there are four ligaments that connect the tibia to the tarsal bones. The ligaments, from anterior to posterior, are the tibiotalar, tibionavicular, tibiocalcaneal, and posterior tibiotalar. They are collectively known as the deltoid ligament. If the tibiotalar ligament is injured, the medioanterior malleollar point will appear.

### 7.11.2.3 Medioinferior Malleolar

This point can appear immediately below the medial malleolus if the tibionavicular or tibiocalcaneal (or both) ligaments are damaged.

### 7.11.2.4 Medioposterior Malleolar

This point can be a short distance from the medial malleolus. If a ligament behind the ankle is torn, the medioposterior malleolar acupoint can appear there. All of the described acupoints in the ankle joint are more or less anatomical speculation. We don't really know for sure if these acupoints exist because of injury or damage to a particular ligament. Such injury or damage is not easy to verify in the first place.

### 7.11.2.5 Medial Calcaneous

This is analogous to the lateral calcaneous point on the lateral side of the calcaneous bone. These two points can become tender in patients with a history of chronic pain. Once the calcaneous points appear, the pain can become difficult, if not impossible, to manage. By then, amputation might be the best outcome for diabetic peripheral neuropathy in the foot.

### 7.11.2.6 Navicular Point

This acupoint can appear at the tuberosity of the navicular bone. The navicular, first cuneiform, and first metatarsal points are on the medial side of the foot. The nerves contributing to form these points are both from the tibial and peroneal on the dorsal side of the foot.

### 7.11.2.7 First Metatarsal Point

This point is on the head of the first metatarsal, and can become sensitive on feet that have been wearing shoes that are too tight. If the friction between the big toe and shoe is maintained long enough, the area can develop to become a bunion, as mentioned previously. Some bunions can be treated using acupuncture.

### 7.11.2.8 Flexor Digitorum Longus

Both this and the flexor hallucis longus point are examples showing that acupoints formed by motor points of the muscles in the leg and foot can appear when the conditions are appropriate. However, acupoints formed by such motor points are not commonly detected in the patients that we have encountered.

### 7.11.2.9 Plantar Point

This point appears right in the center of the plantar surface. Here, the tibial nerve splits into several branches, including the medial plantar and lateral plantar nerves. The plantar point will become tender in patients experiencing pain on the bottom of the foot. Clinically, the pain is diagnosed as tarsal tunnel syndrome, or calcaneus fasciatis.

### 7.11.2.10 Medial Plantar Point

This point is located under the head of the second metatarsal bone and is formed by the medial plantar nerve. Some patients with tarsal tunnel syndrome or calcaneus fasciatis can experience tenderness at this acupoint.

### 7.11.2.11 Lateral Plantar Point

This is located under the head of the fourth metatarsal bone. At this point, the medial plantar nerve divides into digital branches. Such divisions make the webs between the toes sensitive. The best and most obvious example of such sensitivity is between the third and fourth toes, where Morton neuroma can occur.

### 7.11.2.12 Calcaneus

This point is at the bottom of the calcaneus bone. Tenderness in the calcaneus point is typical for all patients who come in with a diagnosis of calcaneus fasciatis. It is not clear to us exactly which nerves contribute to the formation of this calcaneus point because under the calcaneus bone there is no conspicuous cutaneous branch identifiable as clearly coming from the tibial, peroneal, or sural nerve. However, the plantar has a relatively high sensory field. Its skin is rather difficult to penetrate because more severe pain can be felt by the patients when their plantar surface is punctured. We suspect this is the reason that there is only one acupoint described on the plantar surface of the foot in traditional books of acupuncture, because everyone hates to have needles piercing the bottom of the foot.

## REFERENCES

1. Warwich, R. and P.L. Williams. *Gray's Anatomy*. W.B. Saunders, Philadelphia, 1973.
2. Dung, H.C. Acupoints of the lumbar plexus. *The American Journal of Chinese Medicine* 13:133, 1985.
3. Woodburne, R.T. *Essentials of Human Anatomy*, 6th ed. Oxford University Press, New York, 1978.
4. Hollinshead, W.H. *Anatomy for Surgeons*, Vol. 3, *The Back and Limbs*. Harper and Rowe, New York, 1969.
5. Dyck, P.J. et al. *Peripheral Neuropathy*, vol. II, 2nd ed. W.B. Saunders, Philadelphia, 1984.
6. Asimov, I. et al. *Stedman's Medical Dictionary*, 21st ed. Williams and Wilkins, Baltimore, 1966.

# 8 Physiology in Acupuncture

Anatomy is the science of structures. The only facts of acupuncture are acupoints. We have explained and demonstrated the anatomical identity of each of the acupoints. There is no doubt that nerve fibers are anatomical bases for acupoints. Now that we know their anatomy, we will need to know their physiology. Physiology refers to the knowledge of the function of a living organism or its parts [1]. In case of acupuncture, the quintessential matters we shall discuss are how the nerves function and what kinds of activity they have in physiological terms. However, there is not much information available with respect to physiological research for acupuncture. The few reports found in the literature about the physiology of acupuncture are related to the electrical nature of acupoints. Thus, our attention will have to turn to the electrical phenomena of acupoints in the body.

## 8.1 ELECTRICAL PHENOMENA OF THE BODY

The human body is a good electrical conductor. Because of this electric nature, it is possible to measure electrical activities in certain organs in our body. Electrocardiograms, electroencephalograms, and electromyograms are just three good examples. Electrical activity in the acupoints is also measurable. The anatomical elements that have this electrical activity are the nerve fibers. Nerve fibers have a number of physiological characteristics that will be useful to briefly review here.

### 8.1.1 EXCITABILITY

Nerve tissue is an excitable structure. This excitability distinguishes life from death. Not everything in our body has the same degree of excitability. Hair and nails are less excitable than nerves. For that matter, the nerve is probably the most excitable structure in a living organism. Because of this excitability, nerves, as well as acupoints, are capable of producing action potential upon adequate stimulation.

### 8.1.2 POLARIZATION AND ACTION POTENTIAL

Nerve fibers are electrically conductive because they carry electrons. There are electrons lining inside every nerve fiber as negative ions. Outside the fiber are positively charged ions that represent chemical elements such as sodium. The arrangement of positive ions outside and negative ions inside the nerve fibers is known as polarization. Neural stimulation can come from heat, cold, touching, pressing, pinching, nipping, cutting, stabbing, etc. When a nerve fiber is stimulated, the positive ions will move inward and negative ions outward, resulting in depolarization. The switch of ions in depolarization creates an electric signal or impulse so that we feel a certain sensation. Once the sensation ceases or disappears, the negative and positive ions will move back to their original positions. This restoration of ion position is known as repolarization. Movement of the ions during the depolarization and repolarization is known as transport of ions. This sequence of the events—depolarization, transport of ions, and repolarization—constitutes an action potential. Action potential is a physiological activity by which the nerve fibers are capable of initiating and propagating sensory and motor messages or impulses. Action potential varies from nerve to nerve or from acupoint to acupoint. Higher action potential makes depolarization easier than does lower action potential. One anatomical characteristic that contributes to having higher or lower action potential is the difference in the size of the nerves. Larger A fibers will depolarize more quickly than will smaller C fibers. Nerves or acupoints that are easier to depolarize are described as having a lower threshold, and vice versa.

### 8.1.3 Threshold

To generate an action potential for a nerve or acupoint, the stimulation has to reach the threshold required. The threshold is the specific point in time when stimulation reaches sufficient intensity to put a nerve or acupoint to work or excite it. With respect to the threshold of pain, one practical example can be demonstrated by anyone. Use a thumb and index finger to squeeze gently and gradually any part of the flesh. Initially, no pain is perceived. As the force is gradually increased, the squeezing can turn into pain at a given time. At that time, the squeezing can be considered to have reached the point of threshold. Physiologically, the larger the nerve fibers are, the lower the threshold for an action potential will be. In contrast, the smaller the nerve fibers are, the higher the threshold will be.

High and low thresholds are important concepts in this book. It should be understood that the threshold can change under different physiological and pathological conditions. Some acupoints will have a low threshold to become painful, whereas other acupoints will have high pain threshold under the same physiological conditions.

### 8.1.4 Conductivity

Once a nerve is stimulated and becomes excited to begin an action potential, this potential will spread along the same nerve fiber, following the mechanism of the depolarization by transporting negative ions out of and positive ions into the fiber. This mechanism to propagate depolarization is described as the conductivity of nerve fibers. Conductivity enables nerve impulses or messages to be transmitted from one area of the body to another. The speed of nerve impulse conduction is different from fiber to fiber. Larger A fibers will have higher speed of conductivity than smaller C fibers. This difference in conductivity has significance in the physiological function of acupoints. Briefly stated, all acupoints are formed by nerve fibers of different sizes. When an acupoint is stimulated, larger nerve fibers in the acupoint will be fired sooner to become depolarized and produce action potential than will smaller fibers. After the impulse is conducted by the larger fibers into the spinal cord, the gate in the spinal cord will be closed to prevent the impulse transmitted by the smaller fibers from entering. This is the well-known gate control theory proposed by Melzack and Wall [2]. This gate control mechanism explains why acupuncture is able to reduce or stop the pain, but not sensations such as numbness. Numb sensations are conducted by large A fibers, whereas pain is conducted by small C fibers.

### 8.1.5 Fatigue

If a nerve is repeatedly stimulated, eventually it will not be able to respond to that repeated stimulation. This is another physiological phenomenon of the nerve fibers known as fatigue. Fatigue can also occur at acupoints. Thus, it is not desirable to stimulate the same acupoints too frequently within a short interval. It is not uncommon to see press needles placed in the ears of patients for months.

## 8.2 ELECTRICAL ACTIVITY IN ACUPOINTS

Measuring electrical activity in the nerves is a well-established medical practice. Patients who suffer from carpal tunnel syndrome are known to have abnormal electrical activity in the median nerve. This fact indicates that electrical activity of the nerves can be quantified. Scientific reports to measure electrical activity in acupoints have been found in the literature. Here, we will cite three articles as examples to show electrical activity in acupoints. These three articles were all published in the *American Journal of Chinese Medicine*, which is a nonpeer review periodical.

The first article was authored by Drs. Brown, Ulett, and Stern [3], and is entitled "Acupuncture Loci: Techniques for Location." The original purpose of the research was not to prove any electrical activity at the loci of acupoints. Rather, they used skin potential recording techniques to identify the accurate locations of acupoints. Their findings can be summarized into two sentences: First, electrical conductivity at an acupoint is higher than that of the skin surface away from an acupoint. Second, electrical resistance at the same acupoint is lower than that of nonacupoints. Differences also existed between the different known acupoints they tested and measured. In other words, electrical conductivity and resistance are not uniform throughout our skin surface. This observation suggests that electrical activity such as conductivity and resistance can be quantified to be different at different acupoints by using an appropriate recording technique. This quantifiable difference is an indication that not all acupoints are equal or function the same physiologically. Physiological functional differences must be related to anatomical discrepancies, such as the size of nerve bundles or trunks, whether they are cutaneous or muscular branches, and how deep their locations are. Thus, it should be apparent that acupoints that are formed by a larger nerve branch located superficially will have more electrical activity for recording. Our conclusion is that because of the variability in anatomical structures, some acupoints will have lower thresholds for undergoing depolarization in generating action potential than others.

The second article was reported by Kano and his coworkers [4]. Their study involved using "an electrical probe for the localization of superficial sensory nerves." No acupoints are mentioned in the entire article. Nevertheless, what is described in the study could be properly applied in interpreting the electrical phenomena of acupoints. What they intended was a continuous effort to produce a local anesthesia in the arm, solely by the application of electrical currents. The article says, "best results are produced when the currents are applied over the points where the superficial sensory nerves enter the underlying fascia in the skin." Their superficial sensory nerves are the cutaneous nerves described in this book. The words "enter the underlying fascia" obviously are intended to mean that the cutaneous nerves penetrate the deep fascia. It is clear that the points on which Kano et al. used the electrical probe to stimulate the nerves are the acupoints formed by the cutaneous nerve branches going through the deep fascia. The points they used possess certain anatomical features described previously to contribute to the formation of acupoints. Their study also showed that electrical stimulation to acupoints is quantifiable.

The third article was reported by Lee [5]. The acupoint that Lee used in his report is known in traditional acupuncture as *Tsusanli*. The same point is described in Chapter 7 of this book as the common peroneal. It is located on the lateral side of the leg below the lateral condyle of the tibia. Lee observed that electrical stimulation at this acupoint produced a significant change in the blood flow of mesenteric arteries. A remarkable vasodilation in the arterioles was seen in the mesentery. This observation demonstrates a relationship of somato-visceral reflex. There are other reports [6–14] available for more studies of electrical phenomena observed in acupoints. That acupoints have electrical properties reveals to us that they are physiologically dynamic in nature.

## 8.3 DYNAMIC NATURE OF ACUPOINTS

Physiologically, acupoints have dynamic functions. The dynamic nature of acupoints is supported by the fact that they appear and disappear at whim. One dependable and reliable way to demonstrate if they appear is to check for the existence of certain sensitivity at a point. This sensitivity is universally present as aching or tenderness. The appearance and disappearance of acupoints will depend on the physical and physiological conditions of each individual. People who suffer from any kind of injury, whether occurring internally, such as infections, or sustained externally, such as severe flesh damage, will have acupoints appear in time as a result. Generally speaking, when acupoints seem to have tenderness, the individuals with the acupoints will not perceive that tenderness. The uncomfortable sensations of aching, tenderness, or pain can only be felt upon adequate stimulation, such as fingertip pressing. We will consider pain of this nature as passive. Passive pain has to be induced or provoked by external stimulation to be perceived. It is like a pain hidden in the body. Normal individuals can have it, but will not know that their acupoints have this hidden pain unless they know where acupoints are located.

Acupoints with tenderness were observed by Sola et al. [15] in 1955. Dr. Sola was the chief of Physical Medicine Service at Lackland Air Force Base, San Antonio, Texas in the 1950s. As a military physician, he most likely encountered freshly recruited young airmen coming to his clinic complaining of aches and pains in different parts of the body after a few weeks of intensive, strenuous basic training. Those aches and pains appeared over certain muscles in which a number of tender points were detectable. He used the term "trigger points" to describe these tender points. His opinion was that "trigger points can be most easily accounted for on the basis of mechanical stress" [15]. No doubt that mechanical stress is one of the important factors that contribute to the occurrence of aches and pains in the muscles that are overused. The question is why so many recruits went through the same mechanical stress, yet only some of them suffered from aches and pains in the muscles. Here lies another aspect of the quantitative variations of acupoints. Clearly, it is possible to quantify who does and who does not have tender or trigger points after an equal quantity of stressful exertion on the same muscles. The number of tender or trigger points is likely quantifiable. The locations of tender or trigger points turn out to be identical to those of acupoints. We begin to realize that all acupoints have different physiological functional phases.

The most revealing word used in Sola's report is "latent." He said, "these observations led to the question of the possible existence of the latent trigger points in asymptomatic individuals, where upon being subjected to the physiological insult of strain, chronic fatigue, chilling, or other irritating stimuli, they might serve as the source of clinical symptoms" [15]. The word latent adequately connotes the concept of the dynamism of acupoints. The implication is that, physiologically speaking, acupoints can exist in our body under different functional states or phases. Taking this thought into acupuncture practice, patients coming with pain symptoms were tested to determine if their acupoints had tenderness. The conclusion from the tests is unequivocal that all acupoints must have at least three different functional phases. By adapting Sola's opinion, the three functional phases of acupoints can be described as latent, passive, and active.

## 8.4 THREE PHASES OF ACUPOINTS

### 8.4.1 Latent Phase

Anatomically speaking, each person is born with acupoints in the latent phase. Individuals at an optimal state of health should have most or all acupoints in the latent phase. The word latent is intended to describe a state of dormancy. Acupoints in the latent phase are structural entities that lurk undetectably within the body. People with all acupoints in the latent phase are least likely to experience pain, particularly chronic pain. Acupoints in the latent phase seem to have a relatively high threshold because they seem to have less of a tendency to be depolarized in generating action potential. Acupoints in young and healthy people without much illness or physical injury tend to be latent. The concealment of the latent points will diminish or disappear when physical and physiological conditions ripen, as suggested by Sola et al. [15]. As acupoints change their functional phase in lowering the threshold to become more easily depolarized, their latent status will turn to the next phase, which is passive.

### 8.4.2 Passive Phase

Passive in this context means submissive. Passive also implies existence without explicit awareness. The objective existence of passive acupoints can only be discovered by ones who have sufficient knowledge of the location of acupoints. One has to know the right anatomic locations of acupoints to be able to detect them in the passive phase. Any acupoint in the passive phase must have an unfailing quality, which is the sensation of aching, pain, or other forms of possible discomfort. This quality can be elicited upon adequate stimulation.

It is still beyond our knowledge why and how the acupoints can be turned from latent to passive. Physiologically, it is obvious that an acupoint in the latent phase has a higher threshold and is harder to be depolarized under the same mechanical stimulation than the same acupoint in the passive phase. There is no scientific evidence to explain how acupoints are able to change from latent to passive phase. Speculations based on medical knowledge available will be offered at the appropriate times later in this book. For the time being, we just accept that acupoints exist.

Having acupoints in passive phase is a fact for practically all people who have experienced pain in the body for a certain time. How long this period should be is difficult to say. You don't have to be a trained physician to discover passive acupoints in your own body. All you need is to know where acupoints are located, which can be learned easily within this book. Acupoints may not be familiar to everyone. Trigger points certainly are known widely among nonmedical professionals. It will be definitely appropriate and accurate to say that acupoints in the passive phase are all trigger points. From now on, when trigger points are mentioned, we mean acupoints in the passive phase.

Two important aspects relating to the dynamic nature of acupoints and their changes in functional status deserve attention. The first aspect is the transition from latent to passive in a rather orderly sequence. One undeniable phenomenon is that certain acupoints invariably become passive more easily and sooner than others. The reasons for the sequential order can be attributed to the anatomic features described in Chapter 1. The second aspect is that acupoints turning from latent to passive phase can be statistically quantified. The quantity of passive or trigger points is in direct proportion to the chronicity of the pain. A person with a longer period of enduring pain symptoms will have more trigger points than another with a shorter period of pain suffering or none at all. That is to say, the number of trigger points is a reliable indicator for judging the duration of the pain present in the body. This observation provides a useful guideline for quantifying pain in a relatively objective manner. More will be said concerning pain quantification and its implications in pain management later in the book. Using trigger points to quantify pain gives a unique and unprecedented way to diagnose and predict a dependable outcome in the clinical practice of acupuncture.

### 8.4.3 ACTIVE PHASE

As the duration of pain increases, a few passive acupoints can develop into the active phase. Patients with acupoints in the passive phase may have pain in a particular region of the body for a considerable time, and acupoints in that region can become active. Individuals with active acupoints will know where the points are because pain in the active acupoints is subjectively perceivable. Indeed, an active acupoint can be defined as a trigger point that can be readily identified by the person who has it. Only a small percentage of patients will show acupoints in the active phase.

The locations of active acupoints vary from time to time and from individual to individual. However, only a limited number of areas will have active points. These are the areas where the passive points are more likely to appear sooner, following the conditions of the anatomic features that contribute to the formation of acupoints. These anatomic features include the size of nerve branches, where they are situated, and whether they are muscular or cutaneous nerves. Acupoints formed by the spinal accessory, superior cluneal, and posterior primary ramus of the second lumbar spinal nerve are a few good examples. The appearances of active acupoints don't follow any sequential order. We cannot predict when or where they will be in whoever has them. Some active points can appear near the sites of disease or injury. In acute and traumatic injuries involving extensive tissue damage or bone fractures, active points can appear randomly, without discernible order. In most patients who are found to have active points, the number is just a few, one or two. Only very occasionally, the number of active points presented can be more than three or four. Clinically known examples are tennis elbow, or lateral epicondylitis, and calcaneous fasciatis. To treat pain with active acupoints, the needles have to be placed in such a way that the patients will subjectively feel the sensation produced at the sites where the needles are inserted.

## 8.5 PHYSICAL PROPERTIES OF ACUPOINTS

Thus far, what has been said about anatomic structures and the physiologic functions of acupoints have all been learned from observing patients who have come to the clinic. Data collected from clinical observations could be subjective. To be accepted as bona fide scientific fact, control studies are required. However, we have no way to conduct such clinical investigations (if anyone is able to reproduce the results offered in this book, then that will support our claims). Any phenomenon that is possible to reproduce may be trusted as having scientific viability.

An undeniable circumstance in acupuncture is that every person attends because of pain, mostly chronic pain. Each of them is carefully examined and tested on a number of selected acupoints. Over a period of approximately 6 months, 250 patients were examined. For comparison, 16 individuals were recruited as control subjects. They were either dental or medical students. One hundred and ten acupoints were chosen, 20 from each of five regions in the body. These five regions are the head, neck, upper limb, thorax and abdomen, and lower limb. For each selected acupoint, we recorded its sensitivity, the sequence in which it became passive, and the specificity in the area where the acupoint became a trigger point. The sensitivity, sequence, and specificity are the "three S's." We view these three S's as the physical properties of acupoints. Each of them is further defined and explained below.

### 8.5.1 Sensitivity

The word "sensitivity" in this context indicates the amount of pain, aching, tenderness, or other uncomfortable feeling produced when finger pressure is applied. The existence of sensitivity is determined by observing the patients' responses, both verbal and otherwise (wincing, grimacing, etc.). It should be remembered that the locations of acupoints are clearly known to examiners, but the tested individuals didn't have the slightest idea why a particular area chosen was or wasn't an acupoint.

It could be said that the examination is a simple blind test. Nonacupoints are used to make sure that no false response will be given by the tested individuals. The belief is that no person will be able to intentionally mislead the examiners because the examined people don't know how to. This assumes that all people who are tested are honest in responding to the question of whether or not they feel sensitive at the points tested.

The testing resulted in the following summarized observations:

1. All patients complaining of pain were found to have a number of acupoints with sensitivity. In other words, everyone tested had passive acupoints or trigger points. The numbers varied from a few, four or five, to more than a hundred.
2. Most control individuals had no detectable trigger points. In other words, their acupoints were in the latent phase. In those few with some sensitivity, the number of trigger points was very small, one or two at the most. The sensitivity at the passive acupoints was often described as minimal.
3. The degrees of sensitivity varied in different acupoints, and reactions from individuals who received the tests were not uniform. Certain passive acupoints were so sensitive that the persons tested winced or grimaced. Sometimes, the body parts involved, such as the arm, forearm, or hand, were withdrawn because of pain caused by the tests. Very often, patients could distinguish a passive acupoint that was more or less sensitive than the next acupoint or another acupoint tested.

4. The passive acupoints with more intense sensitivities were the ones that became trigger points more often and sooner. The number of acupoints turning from latent to passive could increase as the duration of pain was extended. Patients suffering from pain in multiple locations of the body had more passive acupoints or trigger points.

In summary, sensitivity in the acupoints indicates that they are functionally in the passive phase, and that they are categorized as trigger points.

### 8.5.2 Sequence

The word "sequence" refers to the order by which acupoints become passive. The sequence has both qualitative and quantitative connotations. An acupoint that becomes sensitive sooner is considered to be at a higher order in sequence, and vice versa. The sequential order of acupoints becoming passive is clearly determined by the anatomic features they have. An acupoint formed by a larger nerve branch will have a higher order than one formed by a smaller nerve, even if they are located at the same depth under the skin. The infraorbital point is at a higher order than the supraorbital point. Both acupoints are formed by the cutaneous nerves in the face, and the depth of both cutaneous nerves under the skin is the same. Because the infraorbital nerve is bigger than the supraorbital, the infraorbital point becomes passive sooner than the supraorbital point. The same situation applies to the lateral antebrachial cutaneous point and the medial antebrachial cutaneous point. The lateral antebrachial point is formed by a larger cutaneous nerve branch than that of the medial antebrachial, and turns to become passive sooner than the medial antebrachial point. Similar examples can be found for many other acupoints.

Because acupoints turn from the latent to passive phase in a predictable order, it is possible to physically count how many trigger points any person may have. The number of trigger points provides a reliable way to objectively measure how much pain we may have at the time of examination. The quantity of pain measured in this way seems to have very little fluctuation over a reasonable period, if no therapeutic intervention is provided to manage the pain. Much more will be discussed with respect to pain quantification in Chapter 12. Essentially, what we have found is that having more trigger points will indicate having more objective pain in a person. Once it is possible to quantify pain by the physical calculation of existing trigger points, the manageability of pain will become predictable.

### 8.5.3 Specificity

The word "specificity" refers to the precise location and the size of the trigger points. The size of the sensitive area for a trigger point is very small, not much wider than a fingertip (estimated as 0.5 cm in diameter) in the beginning when acupoints turn passive. The area of the sensitivity will enlarge, and can reach 3 to 4 cm in diameter in some patients with chronic pain. The higher the specificity, the harder it is to locate the trigger points. As the specificity diminishes, the trigger points will become easier to detect: In short, sensitivity and specificity seem to be inversely related. As the sensitivity of passive acupoints increases, the specificity decreases. One good example is the saphenous point right below the medial condyle in the knee. The specificity of this acupoint can become so low that the whole area may turn passive in some patients, particularly if they happen to be female with gynecological problems.

In conclusion, we will summarize our findings in relation to acupoints. Physiologically, all acupoints have three functional phases: the latent, the passive, and the active. Conversion of acupoints from latent to passive is demonstrated by three physical properties of acupoints, described as the "three S's" (sensitivity, sequence, and specificity). Having sensitivity indicates that acupoints have turned from the latent to passive phase. They convert from the latent to passive phase in a predictable sequence, which enables counting how many acupoints are in a passive phase for each individual who is in pain or not. The quantitative evaluation of how many passive acupoints a patient has provides a useful criterion for making a reliable prognosis in pain management. Predictions in pain management will be thoroughly explained in a later portion of the book.

## REFERENCES

1. Bell, G.H. et al. *Textbook of Physiology.* Churchill Livingstone, New York, 1980.
2. Melzack, R. and P.D. Wall. Pain mechanism: A new theory. *Science* 150:971, 1965.
3. Brown, M.L. et al. Acupuncture loci: Techniques for location. *American Journal of Chinese Medicine* 2:67, 1974.
4. Kano, T. et al. An electrical probe for the localization of superficial sensory nerves. *American Journal of Chinese Medicine* 2:75, 1974.
5. Lee, G.T. A study of electrical stimulation of acupuncture locus *Tsusanli* (St-36) on mesenteric microcirculation. *American Journal of Chinese Medicine* 2:53, 1974.
6. Frost, E. and W.R. Orkin. Localization of acupuncture loci. *Proceedings of the NIH Research Conference.* DHEW Publication No. 74:165, 1973.
7. Matsumoto, T. and M.F. Hayes. Acupuncture, electric phenomenon of the skin and postvagotomy gastrointestinal atony. *American Journal of Surgery* 125:176, 1973.
8. Bergsmann, O. and A. Wooley-Hart. Differences in electrical skin conductivity between acupuncture points and adjacent areas. *American Journal of Acupuncture* 125:176, 1973.
9. Flech, H. and S. Spring. Acupuncture points: Study of events. *New York State Journal of Medicine* 6:1060, 1974.
10. Becker, R.O. et al. Electrophysiological correlates of acupuncture points and meridians. *Psychoenergetic System* 1:105, 1976.
11. Reichmanis, M. et al. D.C. skin conductance variation at acupuncture loci. *American Journal of Chinese Medicine* 4:169, 1976.
12. Farden, J. Active acupuncture point impedance and potential measurements. *American Journal of Acupuncture* 2:137, 1979.
13. Zhu, Z.X. Research advances in the electrical specificity of meridians and acupuncture points. *American Journal of Acupuncture* 9:203, 1981.
14. Rosenblatt, S.L. The electrodermal characteristics of acupuncture points. *American Journal of Acupuncture* 10:131, 1982.
15. Sola, A.E. et al. Incidence of hypersensitive areas in posterior shoulder muscles. *American Journal of Physical Medicine* 34:585, 1955.

# 9 Biochemistry in Acupuncture

## 9.1 BIOCHEMISTRY IN RELATION TO ACUPUNCTURE

Biochemistry is possibly the most important key to opening the secrets of acupuncture. Essentially, acupuncture is a useful tool to manage pain. How the pain is produced in the body, how the pain is transmitted from location to location, and how pain can be reduced or stopped will eventually have to be based on how much understanding there is with respect to the chemical substances that mediate the activities of pain. To keep acupoints in function, it is obvious that some biochemical media are required. These biochemical media are known as neurotransmitters. A great deal is known about neurotransmitters. However, their relationship to acupuncture is not totally clear. We know that if an acupoint is stimulated and the nerve that forms that acupoint is depolarized to generate an action potential, the depolarization is propagated and transmitted from nerve to nerve by certain neurotransmitters. The contents of this chapter are about the neurotransmitters that have a functional relationship to acupuncture.

## 9.2 TERMINOLOGIES IN NEUROTRANSMITTERS

There are a few terms that we need to describe neurotransmitters. For review purposes, they are briefly defined and explained below.

### 9.2.1 Neuroreceptor

The concept of a receptor in biochemistry was introduced at the beginning of the twentieth century [1]. There are receptors for drugs, hormones, and neurotransmitters. Our concern is mainly for the receptors of the neurotransmitters. They will be referred to as neuroreceptors [2], or simply receptors for our purposes. We don't know how many receptors there are. All that can be said is that each neurotransmitter discussed in this chapter has its own receptor. All receptors are located on the surface of the neurons. How important the receptors are in acupuncture is not well known. The search and research for various kinds of receptors is one of the most intensively investigated areas for the nervous system. It will remain so in the foreseeable future, and more receptors will be discovered in future studies of the nerves. There is no doubt that receptors must play some role to lead to a better future understanding of how acupuncture works.

### 9.2.2 Agonist and Antagonist

The agonists and antagonists are two enemies because they work against each other in a chemical sense. If an agonist works for one neurotransmitter, an antagonist will work against the same transmitter. Receptors are said to be a major factor in determining whether something will be an agonist or antagonist. An agonist can enhance a particular neurotransmitter and an antagonist will suppress or prevent such a potential. The terms agonist and antagonist are often used in a pharmacological sense or in the study of drug action. However, they also appear rather frequently in acupuncture literature. In acupuncture, "agonist" implies something that can increase needle effectiveness, whereas "antagonist" is something that can minimize or block such effectiveness.

### 9.2.3 SYNAPSES

A specialized site of contact between neurons is defined as a synapse. There are numerous types of synapses, which are described in textbooks of histology as axoaxonic, axodendritic, axosomatic, chemical, and electrical synapses. Chemical and electrical signals pass from neuron to neuron through the synapses. Neurotransmitters are synthesized in one nerve cell, the presynaptic neuron. The neurotransmitters are then released into the microspace of the synapse and received by the receptors in the postsynaptic neuron. Thus, there are presynaptic and postsynaptic neurons. The relationship between synapses and acupuncture is entirely unknown. No report has been found in the literature to explain what role the synapses play in making acupuncture work or not work.

### 9.2.4 GRANULES

One reason to mention synapses is the presence of granules. Many neurotransmitters appear like granules when prepared and observed under an electron microscope. In presynaptic neurons, many granules containing neurotransmitters can be seen. These granules are described as synaptic vesicles. There are different forms of granules and vesicles. These differences in form are believed to represent different transmitters. There is no information to offer with respect to the form and shape of any neurotransmitter implicated in acupuncture mechanisms. Information such as what granule will be released when acupuncture is applied, and in which synapse, is all unknown.

### 9.2.5 NEUROMUSCULAR JUNCTION

Anatomically and physiologically, "neuromuscular junction" is a well-known term. We know how a neuromuscular junction looks microscopically, what it does physiologically, which transmitters its synaptic vesicles contain, and which diseases associated with pathological changes can occur at the junction. There is no direct relationship between neuromuscular junctions and acupuncture. However, one indirect relationship can occasionally be observed. When a needle is inserted into an acupoint that contains a muscular nerve to the motor point, and the motor point is formed by a large number of neuromuscular junctions, immediate twitching in the muscles can be easily seen. This immediate twitching muscle reaction is due to a simple nerve reflex. The neurotransmitter participating in this nerve reflex is acetylcholine, which is irrelevant in the actions of acupuncture.

## 9.3 RELEVANCE OF NEUROTRANSMITTERS

For all of the neurotransmitters we have learned, we come to conclude that some of them, such as endorphins, have significant physiological relevance to acupuncture. Others, such as acetylcholine, have little or no relevance to acupuncture. We will first take the example of acetylcholine to interpret the relevance of neurotransmitters in relation to acupuncture.

Acetylcholine has been known as a neurotransmitter for more than 100 years [3]. This chemical was the first neurotransmitter experimentally identified in the central nervous system. A great deal of information and knowledge has been accumulated about the chemical nature, physiological functions in the nervous system, and diseases associated with acetylcholine because of the enormous quantities of scientific research on this substance. There could be as many as a million scientific publications carrying the word "acetylcholine" reported by countless numbers of investigators.

The first person to point out that acetylcholine might be a chemical cellular mediator for modulating certain physiological function was Dr. Hunt [3]. In 1914, Dr. Dale provided clear evidence to show that acetylcholine was released in nerve stimulation. By 1984, this neurotransmitter had been purified chemically by a number of investigators [4,5]. Thus, the chemical structure of acetylcholine was firmly established.

# Biochemistry in Acupuncture

Acetylcholine is found in many locations in the body. It has broad functional effects in a number of tissues and organs. Acetylcholine is known to be able to dilate blood vessels in the skin and viscera so that blood flow will increase in that area. It can cause contraction of the eye's iris and play a role in the accommodation of our vision. Acetylcholine is a possible promotor of the secretion of the salivary and sweat glands. Release of acetylcholine from presynaptic neurons has been shown to slow down heartbeat, lower blood pressure, and speed up peristalsis of the alimentary canal. It can relax the urinary bladder and the erect penis. These are just a few examples to show what acetylcholine can do for and in the physiological system. By unraveling how acetylcholine is synthesized, stored, released, and metabolized, scientists have attained a fairly good idea of how acetylcholine causes all these functional changes in the system.

We go to such a great extent to speak of acetylcholine for one purpose: to show how much the scientific communities know about this neurotransmitter. Acetylcholine has many physiological activities and functions. Surprisingly, no evidence is available to indicate whether acupuncture is involved in the activity of this neurotransmitter. Nothing is known of whether acetylcholine plays any role in how acupuncture works. We do know that in the peripheral nerves, acetylcholine is very active in the skeletal neuromuscular junctions. This neurotransmitter is released at the end of the efferent nerve fibers that innervate the skeletal muscles. Acetylcholine is also found to be released from the preganglionic and postganglionic cells of the parasympathetic nerves. They are all in the group of efferent nerves (see Chapter 2). No acetylcholine has ever been found to be present in the afferent nerves. The efferent nerves play no beneficial role in the usefulness of acupuncture. Therefore, diseases such as myasthenia gravis, which is caused by a deficiency of acetylcholine in the neuromuscular junctions, will be impossible to improve much by acupuncture.

Parasympathetic nerves contain acetylcholine. One drawback is that these nerves are not readily available over the skin of the body. No definite evidence shows that acupuncture directly induces the secretion of acetylcholine. However, there are some indications that acupuncture changes certain functional activities in some visceral organs. These physiological changes are related to the activities of acetylcholine. Here are a few examples: acupuncture can momentarily reduce blood pressure. Certain incontinences can be improved by acupuncture. Patients have claimed that they can control the bladder better with decreased frequency of urination after acupuncture. Conditions of constipation seem to improve with acupuncture treatments. All these effects are manifestations of cholinergic nerve reaction with an increase in acetylcholine activities. All these effects are indirect actions of acupuncture. The results are often short-lasting and difficult to sustain for a long period of relief or improvement. There are many questions that need to be answered with respect to what effect acupuncture can have over the activities of the neurotransmitter acetylcholine.

## 9.4 IMPORTANCE OF ENDORPHIN

We all know that endorphin is an endogenous morphine. There are approximately half a dozen peptides that deserve to be named endorphin. The name refers to a number of neuropeptides, all of which are considered neurotransmitters. Two of them are most often mentioned when topics of pain and acupuncture come up for discussion. They are metenkephalin and leuenkephalin. Other neuropeptides have rather complicated and difficult-to-comprehend nomenclatures, such as proopimelanochortin and prodynorphin. To simplify matters, neuropeptides that constitute this family of endorphins will be referred to as opioid peptides. The term obviously derives from the fact that morphine is a powerful ingredient in opium. So the connection between opium, morphine, opioid peptides, and endorphin should be clear. Opium and morphine are very effective substances for pain management. It stands to reason that because endorphin or opioid peptides are endogenous morphines, they ought to have the property of relieving pain. In fact, there is evidence to suggest that endorphin is 100 to 200 times more potent in relieving the same pain than exogenous morphine. This fact makes endorphin the most important, popular, and relevant neurotransmitter in acupuncture research.

Endorphin is found in many areas of the central nervous system. Major organs believed to synthesize endorphin include the pituitary gland, dorsal root ganglia, and intestine. In animals, endorphin receptors are said to be found in the vas deferens, heart, and other locations. The data available seems to indicate that not all opioid peptides have the same analgesic potency. One peptide can be more potent than another at different locations and at different times. Different neurons with distinct morphological features may contain different peptides. The biochemical physiological complexities are unquestionably overwhelming.

We are incapable of repeating everything reported for endorphin. Only a few items in the relation between endorphin and acupuncture deserve our attention and are mentioned here.

One of the best known antagonists for endorphin is naloxone. In acupuncture research, naloxone is used to determine if a given phenomenon or manifestation is an endorphin-related reaction. Thus, naloxone is used to block the effects of acupuncture. To prove if a physiological activity, such as facilitating mitosis of lymphocytes, is a result of acupuncture, administer naloxone before acupuncture stimulation, and the division of lymphocytes will be seen to decrease. This observation leads us to believe that acupuncture can enhance the activity of the immune system. This suggests why acupuncture is useful in improving some conditions, such as nasal congestion due to allergies.

There are many articles available for us to read that report the results of studies in acupuncture. One of the most important findings is that acupuncture induces the production of endorphin, which is the reason that pain can be reduced or even stopped. This finding is useful to help us understand why acupuncture works. Nevertheless, it will not help anyone to become a better acupuncturist. The status of acupuncture stays the same. Some pain will be manageable by using acupuncture, other pain will remain impossible for acupuncture to do anything. Theories based on endorphin have been proposed to explain how acupuncture works. None of them either enhances or reduces the effectiveness of acupuncture.

## 9.5 OTHER NEUROTRANSMITTERS

There are several other neurotransmitters. They can be categorized into six groups: catecholamines, serotonin, histamine, neuroactive peptides, amino acids, and adenosine. What role these neurotransmitters play in acupuncture is not entirely clear. We will try our best to speculate whether acupuncture applications will involve the activities of any of these chemicals.

### 9.5.1 Catecholamines

The term "catecholamines" refers generically to all organic compounds that contain a catechol nucleus, which is a benzene ring with adjacent hydroxyl substituents [6] and an amine group. The compound from which the other catecholamines described here are derived is known chemically as dihydroxyphenylamine or dopamine. Dopamine can be converted into norepinephrine, and norepinephrine can be transformed into epinephrine or adrenaline. Adrenaline is produced in the adrenal gland. It is common knowledge that adrenaline is pumped out very quickly from the adrenal gland when we undergo stress. Therefore, it is easy to understand the relationship between the adrenal gland and pain. Pain in patients with a deficiency in the adrenal gland is harder to manage with acupuncture than in those with normal adrenal function. For example, acupuncture will not be of much use in handling reflex sympathetic dystrophy.

Norepinephrine is another catecholamine. This neurotransmitter is released at the nerve terminals of postganglionic sympathetic fibers. The postganglionic sympathetic nerves are widely involved in acupuncture treatments. A release of norepinephrine is expected each time acupuncture is performed. The relationship between norepinephrine and acupuncture is a temporal event. Immediately after needling, acupuncture seems to serve as an agonist for norepinephrine. In time, acupuncture becomes an antagonist to suppress the sympathetic nerve's activities. The suppression of sympathetic activity can be used to explain why acupuncture is able to reduce or minimize menstrual cramping. One hormone that has something to do with cramping is prostaglandin, which is a potent antagonist of norepinephrine. Acupuncture increases norepinephrine release, which in turn reduces the production of prostaglandin.

In the course of acupuncture treatments, a number of reactions to needling occur rather frequently. These needle reactions are clearly related to a surge in the activity of the autonomic nerves due to an increase in the secretion of catecholamine neurotransmitters. These reactions will be further mentioned in the last part of this chapter, after we finish our discussion on neurotransmitters.

The third neurotransmitter in the catecholamine group is dopamine. In the central nervous system, dopamine is found in the red nucleus of the medulla oblongata. In the peripheral nerves, it is known to be present in the carotid body and the superior cervical ganglia. A deficiency in dopamine can result in Parkinson disease. Acupuncture is not of much use for improving the symptoms of the disease, possibly because it is an abnormality in the function of efferent or motor nerves, in which acupuncture does not provide much effect.

### 9.5.2 Serotonin

This neurotransmitter can inhibit neural firing. Nerves become harder to depolarize. Yet, serotonin has the potential to increase dopamine and norepinephrine release, which means that it can act like an agonist for dopamine and norepinephrine, and an antagonist for acetylcholine. The reason serotonin is an antagonist to acetylcholine is because sensitivity to acetylcholine at postsynaptic nicotine receptors is depressed or suppressed. That being true, serotonin must be an antagonist for acupuncture.

Serotonin has been found in many areas of the brain and the spinal cord. Neurons containing serotonin are known as serotonergic nerve cells. Nerve terminals of serotonergic neurons are known as serotonergic fibers or pathways. Some serotonergic neurons and pathways contain not only serotonin but also other groups of neurotransmitters, namely, substance P and enkephalin. Substance P, enkephalin, and serotonin have all been implicated in the transmission or modulation of pain impulses in the central nervous system [7]. Substance P is thought to be an excitatory neurotransmitter for neurons in the dorsal horn of the spinal cord to transmit pain signals, whereas enkephalin and serotonin seem to suppress pain transmission in various parts of the spinal cord and brain. Thus, substance P is an agonist for pain, and enkephalin and serotonin are antagonists as far as the central nervous system is concerned in the perception of pain. Just why substance P and enkephalin should be present in serotonergic neurons and possibly be released with serotonin remains a mystery. Can the relationship between serotonin and acupuncture not be the same?

Serotonin is found in two more central nervous system locations: preganglionic sympathetic neurons in the lateral intermediate cell column and motor neurons in the ventral horn of the spinal cord. Axons of motor neurons form efferent fibers to skeletal muscles, and as noted previously, acupuncture is not very useful for problems in efferent fibers. Whether serotonin in preganglionic sympathetic neurons has anything to do with acupuncture is not known. From our clinical observations, we conclude that serotonin plays no significant role in the practice of acupuncture.

### 9.5.3 Histamine

Histamine is found in mast cells, which are ubiquitous in connective tissue. Connective tissue is right underneath the skin. When the skin is irritated, either by a simple act of finger scratching or acupuncture stimulation, a histamine reaction can be seen. Histamine plays an obvious and important role in acupuncture. It is arguable whether histamine is a real neurotransmitter. First, mast cells are not neurons. Second, no mast cell is found in the central nervous system. Third, very few nerve cells can be identified as histaminergic. Yet, no one argues that histamine is not a neurotransmitter. Histamine is found in the brain. Antihistamines, which are histamine antagonists, are commonly consumed drugs. Consumers know very well how they feel after taking antihistamines. It is well known that antihistamines can induce drowsiness. There are occasions in which acupuncture can produce similar results. Thus, it is reasonable to think that acupuncture is an agonist of antihistamines. This assumption explains why acupuncture is useful for relieving allergic symptoms due to excessive histamine activity.

The histamine released by the mast cells in connective tissue has certain biochemical and physiological differences from histamine in the nervous system. Histamine in the mast cells is high in quantity and slow in turnover. It can be depleted by antihistamine drugs. In the nervous tissue, histamine acts in a different manner. We don't know if such a functional difference plays any role in the applications of acupuncture. If histamine serves any purpose in the utility of acupuncture, this usefulness can be only in the peripheral nerves and not in the central nervous system. In the smooth muscles, two types of histamine receptors have been identified. Smooth muscle is an essential structural element for many organs, including the blood vessels, sweat glands, sebaceous glands, and the arrector pili attached to hair follicles. They all contain smooth muscles, and they all are found under the skin. Smooth muscles in these structures have histamine receptors. Acupuncture stimulation activates mast cells to release histamine, which is accepted by its receptors. After receiving histamine, the smooth muscles undergo certain functional changes. These changes are frequently seen in patients receiving acupuncture treatments. Examples of the changes are presented in the last section of this chapter.

### 9.5.4 Neuroactive Peptides

Neuroactive peptides are produced by the neurons. Their activities are in the specific target nerve cells, which are neuronal, glial, smooth muscular, glandular, or vascular in nature. Not much is known for us to report on what functions neuroactive peptides serve as neurotransmitters in the use of acupuncture; except for endorphin and substance P. Endorphin has been presented. Here, substance P deserves some mention.

Substance P is frequently described as playing a role in relation to the neuronal functions of pain. The relation of substance P to acupuncture is unknown. We do know that substance P is a very potent neurotransmitter that depolarizes afferent fibers in the spinal cord. Morphine can serve as an antagonist to substance P, whereas naloxone is its agonist. Substance P causes pain; it is released from the cut ends of sensory neurons. Substance P is thought to be responsible for neurogenic pain and inflammation. It is an agent that can bring vasodilation in time after injury as well as release histamine from mast cells. It is not synthesized at either the efferent or afferent terminal ends of the peripheral nerves. Therefore, substance P cannot have a direct influence on acupuncture stimulation.

### 9.5.5 Amino Acids as Neurotransmitters

After afferent fibers in the peripheral nerves are activated, as in acupuncture, the depolarization becomes a signal to excite secondary neurons in the substantia gelatinosa in the dorsal horn of the spinal cord. The same signal can also inhibit the secondary neurons from becoming excited. This is the basis for the formulation of the gate control theory. The inhibition of secondary neuronal firing is designated as presynaptic inhibition. Presynaptic inhibition is an imperfectly understood event [8]. We know it takes place in the presynaptic terminals of afferent fibers. We select one amino acid, γ-aminobutyric acid (GABA), to illustrate what relationship presynaptic inhibition can have with acupuncture.

Explaining presynaptic inhibition is not easy. The hypothesis was initiated by Eccles in the 1960s. The neurotransmitter assumed to play the role of inhibitor was believed to be released from so-called axoaxonic synapses located on, or close to, the synaptic terminals of afferent fibers. Eccles and his coworkers postulated that GABA was the amino acid acting as the responsible neurotransmitter. After extensive testing over 30 years, some provisions of the hypothesis have been fully accepted, but certainly not all of them. There are still some disputes among the experts in this field of research.

Biochemists and pharmacologists distinguish afferent fibers as the primary and secondary sensory nerves. Neurons for the primary afferent fibers are in the dorsal root ganglion. Neurons for the secondary afferent fibers are in the substantia gelatinosa. No such distinction is known in anatomy. A great deal of research for GABA has been done in the dorsal root ganglia, sympathetic chain, and collateral ganglia near the intestine. Reports of the studies seem to indicate that GABA as a neurotransmitter might act by inhibiting pain signals from entering the central nervous system. This presynaptic inhibition could help acupuncture to reduce or stop pain, because acupuncture might enhance GABA production in the terminals of the primary and secondary afferent fibers.

### 9.5.6 Adenosine

The last neurotransmitter introduced is adenosine. The adenosine receptor, which mediates the local antinociceptive effects of acupuncture, was reported in 2010 [9]. It was then used in a study for pain control [10]. A group of investigators found that "adenosine was released during acupuncture in mice and that its antinociceptive actions required adenosine A1 receptor expression. Direct injection of an adenosine A1 receptor agonist replicated the analgesic effect of acupuncture. Inhibition of enzymes involved in adenosine degradation potentiated the acupuncture-elicited increase in adenosine, as well as its antinociceptive effect. Their observations indicate that adenosine mediates the effects of acupuncture and that interfering with adenosine metabolism may prolong the clinical benefit of acupuncture." In the study of pain control, "the endogenous adenosine has various modulatory effects in the peripheral and central nervous system, mediated through specific cell surface-associated receptors." The view is that "adenosine receptors of the A1-subtype are associated with a modulatory effect on pain transmission at the spinal cord level. Animal studies have repeatedly demonstrated adenosine- and adenosine analog-mediated inhibitory influences on presumed nociceptive reflex responses. These examinations in rodents have tested acute pain models involving tactile, pressure, and heat stimulations. More recently, animal lesion models, presumably reflecting chronic pain, have shown that adenosine analogs can suppress nociceptive behavior through both systemic and intrathecal administration. Consequently, there is substantial evidence that adenosine can modulate nociceptive input. Further, it has been proposed that endogenous adenosine formation is involved in opioid antinociception."

Two important questions arise from this information: Will adenosine replace acupuncture? And will adenosine become the next panacea to manage pain? We are not familiar with pharmaceutical markets. It is not known if adenosine has been manufactured as a pain control medication available in drug stores. Adenosine may be able to suppress nociceptive behavior, but it is doubtful that it will totally replace acupuncture. We expect that acupuncture will be kept in use for managing pain regardless of what happens with adenosine. We remember well that when endorphin was first found to be a powerful analgesic, it was thought that acupuncture would just disappear. Instead, the use of endorphin as a pain control agent disappeared. We have one expectation for adenosine: We wish that further research will determine whether adenosine turns out to be the common denominator acting as the antagonist of subjective and objective pain detectable in the body.

## 9.6 IMMEDIATE ACUPUNCTURE REACTIONS

It is a fact that interactions and interrelations between acupuncture and neurotransmitters occur. Inserting needles into the body will induce certain changes in the activity of neurotransmitters. However, what changes occur, such as which transmitters increase and which decrease, is not precisely known. Many of these changes are observable by the practitioners and comprehensible by the patients in the course of acupuncture treatments. Observable changes can occur while needles are still *in situ*. Such changes are considered to be immediate acupuncture reactions. Some changes were noticed by patients days after the acupuncture was carried out. These were described as latent acupuncture reactions. Three examples of immediate reactions are offered here.

### 9.6.1 ATOPIC ERYTHROID SKIN CHANGE

Figure 9.1 is intended to show this atopic erythroid skin change. The photo was taken roughly 5 min after the needles were inserted into the skin. By then, the skin reaction was complete. There was a clearly visible pink halo surrounding each needle. The pinkish hue was caused by the dilatation of capillary beds under the skin. One neurotransmitter that might be acting on the postganglionic sympathetic nerves would be histamine. Histamine release by acupuncture varies from individual to individual. Even in the same person, the quantity of histamine resulting from one acupuncture stimulation is not equal every time. Atopic erythroid skin reaction can be more intense in one area, such as the upper region of the back, than another, such as the lower lumbar area, as seen in the figure. This difference may indicate differentiated innervation of postganglionic sympathetic nerves, denser in the upper back and less so in the lower back. To exhaust histamine release, as in the case of improving allergic conditions, it will be more effective to place needles in the upper back than in other locations.

### 9.6.2 SWEATING

Physiologically, there are two kinds of sweating, hot and cold. Hot sweat is produced by either physical or environmental increase in temperature. Cold sweat is a consequence of mental stress. Some sweat glands, such as the apocrine in the armpits, are said not to participate in thermoregulatory sweating, but are thought to secrete in response to mental stress. Sweating is controlled by the sympathetic nerves. Parasympathetic nerves don't directly participate in regulating the activity of the sweat glands. No parasympathetic nerves reach peripherally to the glands. The sympathetic supply to sweat glands is cholinergic. Epinephrine exerts a major influence on cold sweat. During acupuncture, sweating in patients is not uncommon. The sweating produced during acupuncture has to be of the cold type, because there is no objective thermal change, either physically or environmentally. Needle insertions in the course of acupuncture can undeniably cause a small degree of mental stress. Nevertheless, mental stress cannot be the sole physical cause of

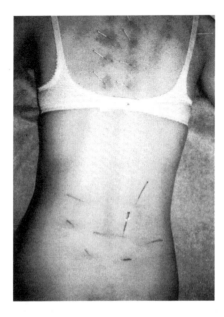

**FIGURE 9.1** A photograph of a patient showing immediate atopic erythroid reaction induced by a number of acupuncture needles.

sweating in acupuncture. Such sweating seems to only occur in certain patients, and it may not occur every time that needles are inserted in the same individual. The quantity of sweat produced is different from one person to the next. The amount of sweat can be so little as to be practically invisible on the paper placed on top of the clinic table, or so profuse that the entire sheet of paper becomes soaking wet. The degree of hyperhidrosis most likely depends on how much of the relevant neurotransmitters are involved. We do not know what kinds of neurotransmitters are involved in having sweating reactions. Patients who have hyperhidrosis during acupuncture are most often young, between the ages of 25 and 45 years old. More males than females are found to have a sweating reaction during acupuncture. Having this reaction often indicates that acupuncture is going to be useful. Thus, neurotransmitters that promote sweating must be agonists for acupuncture treatments.

### 9.6.3 Syncope

Syncope is a fancy physiological term that means fainting. In a small pamphlet by R.T. Ross [11], only 3% of the adult population is reported to have the potential to develop syncope. Fainting is not a harbinger of brain or heart disease. Why only a small percentage of the general population will develop syncope is still a wonder to us. The physiological mechanism for syncope is well-defined and understood medically. It is a reversible, temporary loss of consciousness due to a qualitative and quantitative disturbance of the cerebral blood flow.

In most instances, syncope induced by acupuncture needles is a mere nuisance; it is inconvenient and embarrassing for acupuncture practitioners. Yet, it can be dangerous if the patients having syncope are not properly dealt with and cared for. The dangers can range from broken bones to premonitions of death. In fact, patients dying from incidences of syncope while in the hands of acupuncturists is nothing new. Coughing, sneezing, micturition, vomiting, defecation, and profuse sweating have been encountered in patients during the course of acupuncture treatments that cause syncope to happen. On very rare occasions, if needles are not removed quickly enough, the body could become rigid and stiff as in death. The appearance of patients in a state of syncope can be frightening. Fortunately, it is rather easy to wake up patients with a very simple technique, by inserting a needle into a fingertip or immediately under the nasal septum. Which neurotransmitter is involved in creating syncope is not clear. Patients who have syncope reactions are believed to have poor homeostasis. Their physiological systems are less stable. Female patients are more likely to have syncope than males. The ages during which syncope occurs are 30 to 50 years old. They often have a medical history of low blood pressure with symptoms of dysmenorrhea, such as painful menstruation, irregular periods, and long menstrual bleeding. For male patients, syncope most often occurs for those between 20 and 40 years of age. They appear to be physically strong. Their pain is in the acute stage. Patients having syncope during acupuncture always respond well to needle treatments.

## 9.7 REACTIONS AFTER ACUPUNCTURE

A few reactions can occur after acupuncture. The duration of their occurrence range from hours to days. In some incidences, this period can be as long as a week. These are considered to be latent reactions. Three examples are described here as typical of latent reactions. These have to be more than mere neural phenomena. Nerve reactions are always rapid in manner, like electrical activity. When a switch is turned on, the light appears in an instant. Upon stimulation, a nerve becomes depolarized right away, and the impulse will be transmitted very quickly along the nerve fibers, as in the propagation of the electricity. Thus, the idea of neural phenomena is incapable of explaining the occurrence of latent reactions, which takes hours or days after needling to realize. The factors to produce latent reactions have to be humoral in blood circulation, such as the neurotransmitters.

### 9.7.1 FLARE-UP OF PAIN

Flare-up means to burst into sudden intensity, like an abrupt flame. With respect to pain, a flare-up brings heightened perception of discomfort. The pain is exacerbated. Ironically, the flare-up of pain doesn't have to be the same as the original pain being suffered. It can be discomfort outside the pain perceived before receiving acupuncture treatments.

Flare-up of pain is rather common among patients undergoing acupuncture. In truth, flare-ups can be produced artificially. Two main factors determine if the flare-up will occur: the number of needles inserted and the intensity of needle stimulation. The number of needles is quantitative, and the intensity of stimulation is qualitative. Thus, the flare-up has quantitative and qualitative aspects in acupuncture therapy. The quantitative aspect can be easily shown by giving needles to the patients at sites exceeding the number of primary acupoints at the initial session of acupuncture treatments, or at the first session after an interval of sufficient time, such as four or more months since the last needling session. The quantitative aspect of the flare-up is rarely observed if the needles are placed in only one small skin area, or after a patient is repeatedly given a number of acupuncture treatments in a limited time interval. The qualitative aspect of the flare-up can be purposefully demonstrated by continuously manipulating a few needles for a minute or less, once every 2 to 3 min during the entire therapy session, with the needles turned being those at the location where pain was actively and subjectively perceived by the patients. It should be accurate to say that a latent reaction with a flare-up of pain must be related to the freshness of the nervous system in the persons involved.

The sensation of worsened pain is often described by patients as occurring suddenly 8 to 12 h after the initial session of acupuncture treatments. This flare-up can last from a few hours to a day. Some patients will become anxious. They might call to report what is happening. Most of them experience a kind of relief within 48 h, which is the time interval between two acupuncture sessions. By the time they come for the second treatment, the flare-up will have subsided, with the pain perceived originally before receiving acupuncture being reduced or disappearing.

There are speculations on how acupuncture might evoke flare-ups. One of these is related to the sensory homunculus shown in Figure 9.2. According to the sensory homunculus, every part of the skin surface is represented in the postcentral gyrus of the cerebral cortex. The representative area can be relatively small or large, depending on the density of sensory receptors or sensory field, in the skin. The palms of the hands and plantar surfaces of the feet have a relatively larger area represented in the postcentral gyrus, because the skin in them has a denser sensory field with more receptors. This is the reason that inserting needles in the palm or plantar surface is almost always more painful than doing the same to other skin surfaces. There are more representations in the sensory cortex for the palm and plantar than other peripheral regions of the body [12]. All nerve impulses from peripheral locations have to reach centrally for the cerebral cortex to process to give away proper reactions. The response from the cerebral cortex will be lesser if only a few skin sites are stimulated with acupuncture needles, and the response can be expected to be greater when we use acupuncture to stimulate many different locations in the skin. Activation of the postcentral gyrus in the cerebral cortex is neural. Responses from the cortex to provoke flare-ups have to be hormonal through certain neurotransmitters.

### 9.7.2 DROWSINESS AND SLEEPLESSNESS

The second example of latent reaction in acupuncture is drowsiness. Such feelings can occur within 30 min after acupuncture, or as long as 3 to 4 h afterward. Most patients come for treatments in the late afternoon or early evening. Whether the time of day has anything to do with drowsiness is difficult to say. The fact is that patients will claim that they were tired and sleepy after the initial visit. The sleepiness can be so bad that they have a tough time driving home after their treatment. On the other hand, we have patients who swear that they had the best night's sleep in a long while

# Biochemistry in Acupuncture

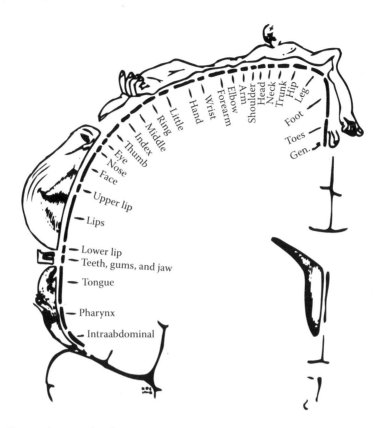

**FIGURE 9.2** Sensory homunculus drawn overlaying a coronal section through the postcentral gyrus.

after their first acupuncture treatment. The sleep can be so profound (the words "slept like a log" are often used) that the patients didn't wake up to go to the toilet for urination throughout night, which is unusual for them.

It is also not uncommon to hear the comments by patients who complain of an increase in irritability and sleeplessness after acupuncture. Such an opposite reaction often comes from patients who experience a flare-up in pain after needle stimulation. Both reactions, sleepiness or sleeplessness, take time to develop. Again, having this kind of latent reaction indicates that acupuncture doesn't affect the nervous system alone. It has to involve factors such as hormones or neurotransmitters. Which neurotransmitter is the most likely candidate for producing drowsiness or sleeplessness from acupuncture? The answer clearly is endorphin. Endorphin behaves like morphine, which can seduce or excite our physiological functions. Seduction leads to drowsiness and sleepiness. Excitation causes agitation, arousal, and awakening. From a pharmacological point of view, seduction and excitation have to be dose-dependent. Adequate amounts of morphine may be beneficial in inducing sleep. Excessive quantities can overstimulate the nerves, resulting in difficulty in sleeping. Inciting sleepiness or sleeplessness also depends on the number of needles given. If more needles than needed are used, sleeplessness can occur. But it is impossible to induce sleepiness if not enough needles are used. Similar to flare-ups, drowsiness and sleeplessness also have quantitative and qualitative aspects of acupuncture.

Because of the potential for needles to induce sleepiness temporarily, acupuncture has been widely claimed to be able to cure insomnia. Such a claim lacks scientific support. Insomnia is clinically a chronic problem with rather complicated psychological and physiological backgrounds as underlying causes. Just because acupuncture occasionally makes patients become sleepy for a few nights, it doesn't qualify as a panacea to solve the problem of insomnia.

### 9.7.3 Parasympathetic Enhancement

Anatomically, acupuncture is unlikely to have direct action on the parasympathetic nerves. However, there are indications that indirect actions do occur. These indirect actions have to be mediated through neurotransmitters. Some patients report improvements in their incontinence or impotence after acupuncture. The same applies to irregular bowel movements or constipation. Among the elderly, particularly in female patients over 70 years of age, incontinence can be a problem. To claim that acupuncture can cure diseases of such nature is unjustifiable. However, in the course of acupuncture treatments with the primary purpose of managing pain, occasionally there are patients who insist that their bladder control improved. Such improvement is possible not through direct nerve stimulation but by indirect action of certain neurotransmitters. Which neurotransmitters these can be is not known. We do know that the autonomic nervous system must be involved. Hypersympathetic activity is more prevalent in the autonomic nervous system. When sympathetic nerves become hyperactive, parasympathetic nerves will be suppressed and hypoactive, resulting in indigestion, poor bowel movements, constipation, or weak bladder control (or all of the above). Acupuncture has a tendency to reduce tension from the sympathetic nerves. Consequently, the activity of the parasympathetic nerves will be enhanced.

## REFERENCES

1. Ariens, E.J. and A.J. Beld. The receptors concept in evolution. *Biochemical Pharmacology* 26:913, 1977.
2. Kuriyama, K. *Neurotransmitters and Neuroreceptors.* International Congress Series 785, Excerpta Medica, Tokyo, Japan, 1987.
3. Siegel, G.J. et al. *Basic Neurochemistry: Molecular, Cellular and Medical Aspects.* Raven Press, New York, 1989.
4. Dale, H.H. The action of certain esters and ethers of choline and their relation to muscarine. *Journal of Pharmacology* 6:147, 1914.
5. Changeux, J.P. et al. Acetylcholine receptor: An allosteric protein. *Science* 25:1335, 1984.
6. Cooper, J.R. et al. *The Biochemical Basis of Neuropharmacology,* 5th ed. Oxford University Press, New York, 1986.
7. Basbaum, A.I. Descending control of pain transmission: Possible serotonergic enkephalinergic interactions. In *Serotonin Current Aspects of Neurochemistry,* edited by B. Haber, et al. Plenum Press, New York, 1981.
8. Rogawski, M.A. and J.L. Barker. *Neurotransmitters in the Vertebrate Nervous System.* Plenum Press, New York, 1985.
9. Goldman, N. et al. Adenosine A1 receptors mediate local anti-nociceptive effects of acupuncture. *Nature Neuroscience* 13:883, 2010.
10. Sollevi, A. Adenosine for pain control. *Acta Anaesthesiologica Scandinavica Supplementum* 110:135, 1997.
11. Ross, R.T. *Syncope.* W.B. Saunders Company, Philadelphia, 1988.
12. Kruk, Z.L. and C.J. Pycock. *Neurotransmitters and Drugs,* 3rd ed. Chapman & Hall, New York, 1991.

# 10 Pathology in Acupuncture

## 10.1 CONVENTIONAL WISDOM IN PATHOLOGY

Pathology can be defined simply as any abnormality that occurs in the body. The abnormalities can be in anatomical structures, in physiological functions, or in biochemical substances. They can be due to changes in molecules, cells, tissues, organs, or systems. One common indication of pathology is pain, which is the primary concern in acupuncture. It would be accurate to state that the overwhelming majority of people seeking acupuncture, if not all, suffer from some kind of pain. Their pain, in our opinion, is subjective, obvious, and perceivable. They know where the pain is located. However, in acupuncture, there is another form of pain. For this book, this pain will be described as objective, hidden, or unperceived pain. Much more about subjective and objective pain will be presented in Chapter 12. The main purpose of this chapter is to explain how objective pain appears in acupoints. Objective pain is always discernible in passive acupoints, which are also known as the trigger points. Pathology in acupuncture will mean what diseases, damage, or injuries in the body are capable of converting acupoints from the latent phase to the passive phase, as known and observed in the patients received in our own acupuncture clinic.

## 10.2 PATHOLOGICAL ORIGINS

In Chapter 8, we stated that each acupoint has three functional phases, which are described as latent, passive, and active. Acupoints in the latent phase can become passive, and then go from passive to active. In the latent phase, acupoints have no discernible sensitivity, such as aching, pain, or tenderness. Once they are converted into the passive phase, discernible sensitivity will be present, but not subjectively perceivable. This unperceived pain is what we described as objective pain. Objective pain will help us determine whether pain can be managed with the use of acupuncture, and how to use acupuncture therapeutically. Thus, it is vital that we know what causes acupoints in the latent phase to be converted into the passive phase and become trigger points. The mechanism for this conversion is unknown. No reports are available because no one ever makes any effort to study the phenomenon. What we have is all derived from empirical observations in clinical experiences. Clinically, it is clear that pathological changes are behind the reason for acupoints to convert from the latent to passive phase.

To date, we have received a total of more than 24,000 patients in our clinic. The data and studies presented here come from this number. Demographically, there are more females (57.3%) than males (42.7%). All these patients had a number of passive acupoints or trigger points detected in their bodies. A small group of these patients also had a few acupoints in the active phase. We decided to theorize that passive acupoints or trigger points are an expression of somatic pain, which we describe as subjective pain. In the process of taking medical histories, or asking for medical diagnoses given by their respective physicians, we have discovered the pathological causes of the patients having objective pain in passive acupoints. The pathologies can be categorized into two origins, which will be simply described as endogenous and exogenous.

## 10.3 ENDOGENOUS ORIGINS

"Endogenous origins" mean that the pathology starts from the internal milieu of our physical environment. How many endogenously originated pathologies are there that are capable of transforming acupoints from latent to passive? We do not know the answer to this question. We do know that a large number of patients can suffer from the same kind of pain with similar pathological causes. Here, it is only possible to give a few examples as an illustration.

### 10.3.1 HORMONAL IMBALANCES

Among female patients, one of the most commonly noticed pathologies in relation to having trigger points is hormonal imbalances. The suspected cause is derived from the menstrual cycles that females have in their life. To maintain normal menstrual function, a delicate balance of hormone production and consumption is required. Many times, this delicate balance can be disturbed. Disorders that result from such disturbances include dysmenorrhea, diabetes, and abnormal thyroid activity. Here, we will first focus on dysmenorrhea.

Dysmenorrhea can be caused by a variety of diseases, including endometriosis, pelvic inflammatory illness, uterine leiomyomas, or adenomyosis [1]. To us, dysmenorrhea is defined as having one or any combination of the following three conditions. The first condition is menstrual cramping, or pain in the pelvic region during the monthly periods. The second is irregular periods. Normal periods occur once every 29 or 30 days. If the periods are less than 27 days or longer than 32 days apart, or variable out of this time interval, they will be considered as a symptom of dysmenorrhea. The third condition is menstrual bleeding of less than 2 days or longer than 5 days. It is not unusual for menstruation to last more than 7 days among the patients seen in the clinic.

We divided all the female patients into three age groups: premenopause, which includes from age at menarche to the time of menopause (generally before 40 years of age), menopause (41–60 years of age), and postmenopause (61 years or older). The respective percentages are 25.5%, 40.3%, and 34.2%. Most patients were in the menopause age group, followed by the postmenopause and premenopause age groups. Of the premenopausal women, 98.9% said they had experienced some degree of dysmenorrhea, and 66.9% had had their uterus removed surgically. Among the patients in the menopause group, 95.2% reported that they had suffered from dysmenorrhea at some time during their reproductive lives, and 88.6% had already had a hysterectomy. Among the postmenopausal patients, menstrual cramping was their common experience (88.2%) when they were young, and 90.1% of them had had a hysterectomy. The most commonly cited reason for having a hysterectomy was fibroid tumors (67%), followed by endometriosis or prolonged bleeding (21%), prolapsed uterus (8%), and other diseases (4%). From these statistics, we concluded that the subjective pain perceived by all the female patients may have certain causes originating in hormonal imbalances. One fact holds true for all of them: they all had acupoints in the passive phase, or trigger points, present. Their subjective pain varied widely, ranging from headaches, neck pain, or trapezius muscle spasms in the shoulder to lower back pain, arthritic knee, restless leg, or tarsal tunnel syndrome. You name a subjective pain, and some of them were found to have it. Almost none of them suspected a connection between their subjective pain and the dysmenorrhea they had experienced.

There are clear relationships between age groups and the number of trigger points detectable. Premenopausal females between 15 and 25 years of age usually are found to have few acupoints in passive phase throughout the entire body, generally eight to 24 in number. Dysmenorrhea in this young age group can be very effectively treated using acupuncture [2,3]. However, there were very few young patients with dysmenorrhea who sought acupuncture treatments to stop their menstrual cramping. Most patients didn't even bother to mention that they had dysmenorrhea. To them, menstrual cramping was part of being feminine, and nothing to be concerned about. They certainly didn't realize that their subjective pain originated from the dysmenorrhea they'd had years ago.

As patients grow older, their number of trigger points tends to increase. Patients between 25 and 45 years old with a history of dysmenorrhea would have 24 to 50 trigger points on one half of their body. By the time they reached 65 years or older, the number could increase to more than 100. Many of them suffered from lower back pain, osteoid or degenerative arthritic knees, headache, neck and shoulder pain, carpal tunnel syndrome, spastic colon, hiatal hernia, leg cramping, diverticulitis, fibromyalgia or myofascial pain syndrome, or indigestion with excess stomach acid. One wonders whether there is any connection between these seemingly disparate problems and dysmenorrhea or diagnoses ending in hysterectomy.

There are other diseases involving some sort of hormonal imbalances that result in acupoints becoming passive. Diabetes and abnormal thyroid functions are two examples. Among our patients, only 3.2% can be considered as having these types of hormonal imbalances. People with diabetes can have the potential to develop pain in the extremities—the hands and fingers, feet, and toes. The pain is diagnosed as a peripheral neuropathy. Patients with abnormal thyroid function had either undergone a thyroidectomy or were taking synthetic thyroid hormones. One reason for them to seek acupuncture treatments was pain in different locations of the body. They might also have hypoglycemia. Their hope for acupuncture was that it could "energize" them, as they felt a constant tiredness and lack of energy required to perform their daily routines. These patients were all found to have passive acupoints, even when no subjective pain was perceived at the time of their visits to the clinic. Thus, we speculate that hormones may play some role in converting acupoints from the latent phase to the passive phase.

### 10.3.2 Poor Blood Circulation

For one reason or another, blood supply to certain regions of the body can become insufficient for maintaining normal metabolic activities. The regions we know of that are susceptible to poor blood circulation include the palmar side of the hands, the calf of the leg, and the trapezius muscle in the shoulder bridges. Pain in the trapezius muscle is used here as an example.

Approximately 15% of our patients complained specifically of having pain in the trapezius and the suboccipital triangle regions. The trapezius region medially includes the base of the neck and laterally extends to the acromion. The suboccipital triangle region is just behind the occipital bone. Subjective pain perceived in these regions was believed to be due to poor blood circulation because these patients invariably had low blood pressure. Generally, their systolic pressure was 110 mm Hg and their diastolic pressure was 70 mm Hg. The lowest diastolic pressure on record was 59 mm Hg, and the lowest systolic pressure was 94 mm Hg. Most patients with this kind of low blood pressure were female. Their medical records reflected a history of dysmenorrhea, most prominently prolonged days of menstrual bleeding, as long as 7 to 8 days for each monthly cycle. It is obvious that the hemopoietic capacity of the patients was not sufficient to replenish the blood needed for normal circulation. For reasons unknown to us, poor blood circulation seems to convert acupoints from the latent to the passive phase. The specific affected region would display a higher than normal proportion of passive acupoints in that specific region. This phenomenon is described as regional appearance, which will be discussed next in this chapter. Poor circulation in the hands can turn them cold, with passive acupoints detectable in the palm. Poor circulation in the calf can create restless legs, which have many passive acupoints along the sural nerves. Of course, all these patients had trigger points in other parts of their bodies as well.

### 10.3.3 Degeneration

Aging is followed by degeneration. There are many abnormalities known as degenerative diseases. Nephropathy, asthma, emphysema, and arthritis are just a few examples. Some degeneration is not visible because it happens inside the body, whereas some can be seen physically. When kidney function is weakened, patients often are found to have edema in the lower limbs, particularly around the ankles. Swollen ankles inferior to the medial and lateral malleolus will have obvious trigger points. Another sign of degeneration is easy to notice in patients who have a history of respiratory diseases, such as asthma and emphysema: they will frequently run out of breath. Trigger points are always detectable in the anterior, lateral, and posterior thoracic wall along the distributions of the cutaneous nerves in the body trunk.

The most prevalent example of degenerative disease in relation to the production of trigger points would have to be degenerative arthritis in the knees. There are all too many knees with degenerative arthritis, most obviously among females older than 60 years. We are convinced that degeneration and the appearance of trigger points must be related. What we don't know is which comes first, degeneration or trigger points? Every knee with a medical diagnosis of degenerative arthritis invariably had a number of passive acupoints or trigger points. These points would appear in a predictable sequential order. The more trigger points an arthritic knee had, the harder it would be to manage the pain in that knee. We have observed that when the trigger points exceeded a certain number, even after the knee was replaced, the pain would not disappear. The same principle can be applied to other points with degenerative arthritis, such as the shoulder, hip, and lower back, even after surgery.

### 10.3.4 Infections

We have no idea how many infectious diseases there are in this world. With regard to infections as the pathology of endogenous origin for producing trigger points, we do know that some infectious diseases are mundane and insignificant, whereas others are vicious and toxic. One speculation we have about these two extremes is that if the infection is mild, the conversion of acupoints from latent to passive will be slow in speed and number. However, if the infection is strong, passive acupoints will quickly become numerous in the body. The common cold and influenza are forms of infection. How potent these infections are in converting latent acupoints to passive is not known because we have not had the chance to systemically study people with colds or influenza. We have had sufficient opportunities to examine and test patients with rheumatoid arthritis. Patients with rheumatoid arthritis always came with a clear and firm diagnosis from their physicians. Among infectious diseases, rheumatoid arthritis (or Still's disease in young individuals) is probably the most invasive and vicious with respect to generating passive acupoints. Patients with rheumatoid arthritis almost always were found to have a high number of trigger points in a relatively short period after they began to notice pain in various joints. There are other kinds of infectious diseases, such as postherpetic neuralgia, trigeminal neuralgia, and other forms of neuropathies, which are also found to have a massive number of trigger points. How quickly patients with these diseases acquired a high number of passive acupoints is not known because an insufficient number of patients are available for reliable studies.

## 10.4 EXOGENOUS ORIGINS

Pathology originating from outside the body is defined as exogenous. Therefore, all external injuries inflicted on our body can be said to have exogenous origins. They can be sports injuries, automobile accident injuries, gunshot wounds, job-related diseases, other ailments caused by stress, and more. In general, pathologies of endogenous origin contribute to abnormal functions in physiological systems. Pathologies of exogenous origins always begin as localized problems, occurring in a limited region of the body. Such pathologies are not as potent as those of endogenous origin. It takes a longer period for a pathology of exogenous origin to convert the same number of acupoints from the latent phase to the passive phase.

There are several ways to categorize injuries of exogenous origins. We all know that injuries can occur during a sports competition, while on the job, in the battlefield during a war, or just by sheer accident without any justifiable reason. What is important in acupuncture is the intensity and extensiveness of the injuries. Some injuries are only minor scratches or skin lacerations. Some involve torn tendons and muscles. Some result in bone fractures. Some involve severe damage to visceral organs. For the convenience of our presentation, we will simply divide exogenous injuries into three categories: minor, moderate, and monstrous.

Minor injuries involve only soft tissues. The pain resulting from these injuries is short-lasting. The wounds will heal on their own within weeks without medical intervention. However, if the injury is substantial enough, the pain can linger for a relatively long period. Examples include tennis elbow, carpal tunnel syndrome due to long hours of typing at work, or neck stiffness after excessive viewing of computer screens. Pain of this nature can be taken care of effectively because most patients with such injuries have a low number of passive acupoints.

Moderate injuries include cuts deep into the muscle mass and hard tissue damage, such as bone fractures, joint dislocations, and concussions to the head. Pain produced by moderate injuries is commonly seen in the clinic. Examples include baseball players with wrist pain, football players with lower back injury, and basketball players with ruptured cruciate ligaments or menisci in the knees. Many of these injuries can cause pain lasting for months.

Shelby is a good example of such an injury. Here is the history provided by her mother. "In the summer of 2001, my daughter was a healthy 9-year-old girl who suffered a concussion in a sports injury. No physical damage, not even a skin laceration, was found. After the accident, she experienced dizziness, nausea, vomiting, blurred vision, and severe headaches. We took her to the emergency room, where she had a CAT scan. She was released that day and given instructions to restrict her activities for a few weeks. The following spring, she started to experience severe headaches. They would start in the front, just above the eyebrows, and move to the back either in a halo effect or all over the head. After several episodes, I took her to our family doctor, who prescribed adult-strength Aleve. The medicine seemed to help, and she had headaches roughly every 2 to 3 weeks until the early fall, when the headaches appeared to stop on their own. However, a few months passed until the next spring, and the same headaches began to attack her again. On Mother's Day, 2003, Shelby had a classic migraine for the first time. She had vomiting, dizziness, and blurred vision. I called the doctor, who prescribed Zomig. It took several hours for the medicine to take effect. Two days later, she had another migraine. Since that time, she has averaged a headache approximately once a week. Often, the medicine the doctor prescribes does not work. The doctor has told me he has no idea why she has the headaches or what causes them and why the medicine prescribed wouldn't help stop the headache…" To the patient's doctor, there is nothing medically wrong with her. For us, the only pathology definable in Shelby was a high number of passive acupoints present in her entire body. Our firm opinion is that there is a cause-and-effect relationship between a high number of passive acupoints and migraine headaches.

Monstrous injuries include limbs being blown apart, extensive lacerations into the body, and puncturing of internal organs. Healing these wounds will require multiple surgical repairs. Clinical cases that have had monstrous injuries include patients suffering from phantom limbs, reflex sympathetic dystrophy, and causalgia. Their pain is not easy to manage even with acupuncture, simply because patients with this type of pain always have the highest number of passive acupoints that could possibly exist. One consoling fact in the practice of acupuncture is that patients experiencing pain because of monstrous injuries are rarely clinically encountered.

One conclusion from dealing with pain, with respect to its exogenous origins, is that there is a clear relationship between the kind of injuries sustained and the potential for the passive acupoints to grow physically. Minor injuries that don't provide latent acupoints the time and opportunity to reach the passive phase will not be harmful to people. When injuries are severe, involving intensive and extensive damage, they require a longer time to heal, providing latent acupoints the chance to be converted into the passive phase. We don't know what physiological functions and biochemical substances are involved in turning latent acupoints to the passive phase. We do know that injuries of exogenous origin will eventually make acupoints sensitive, with aching and pain detectable in the bodies of victims.

## 10.5 MODES FOR TRIGGER POINTS TO APPEAR

We have offered endogenous and exogenous reasons as pathological factors for acupoints to be converted from the latent to the passive phase. We have observed two methods for such a conversion. In other words, when trigger points begin to appear, they can do so in a systemic manner or in a limited region. What is systemic or regional can be best understood by using cases of patients seen in the clinic as examples for explanation.

### 10.5.1 Systemic

Because acupoints turn from latent to passive in an orderly sequence, it is logical to view such a phenomenon as being of a systemic nature. "Systemic" is also used to mean the entire body. Passive acupoints appear systemically in different loci of the body with an orderly and predictable sequence. This sequential appearance in a systemic manner occurs in patients whose pathology is endogenous in origin, such as hormonal imbalances, infectious diseases, or degeneration in physiological systems.

Acupoints can turn from latent to passive beginning at a young age. Nine-year-old Shelby is an example. Young patients often begin to have a small number of passive acupoints in comparison with adult patients examined and tested for their passive acupoints, although this is not always the case. Passive acupoints in some young patients can also be high. Here are six examples:

*Case 1*: Greta was a 14-year-old junior high student. She was brought to the clinic by her mother, essentially as the last available choice for her severe attacks of migraine headache. Greta began suffering from migraines when she was just over 10 years old, at the time she started her menarche. The headaches gradually worsened in the following 4 years. To overcome her problem, every conceivable drug believed to be effective for stopping headaches had been prescribed and taken. The attacks had recently become so severe that she had been hospitalized three times in 1 month, and even in the hospital, the headaches could only be stopped by doses of synthetic narcotics. The frequent usage of narcotics began to worry her parents and attending physician. Her father was a professor and chairman in the dental school department where the author worked, and her mother had been a good friend of the author's wife. Greta was a good example for showing the systemic appearance of passive acupoints in the initial stage. For approximately 120 acupoints tested, only 20 could be definitely identified as being in the passive phase. These 20 passive acupoints or trigger points were distributed systemically throughout the entire body (see Chapter 12 for the distribution of the primary acupoints). The trigger points in her face were more sensitive than those in other loci. The distribution of passive acupoints similar to Greta's were found among female patients who were younger than 20 years, and who had symptoms of dysmenorrhea.

*Case 2*: Theresa was a 23-year-old housewife. She came to the clinic because she wanted to see if auriculopuncture would be able to help her reduce her weight by about 10 pounds. She looked a little chubby, but certainly not obese. She claimed that she had always been very healthy. However, upon careful checking, approximately 12 acupoints seemed to be sensitive and exhibited tenderness. They certainly qualified to be considered in the passive phase. During the interview, Theresa revealed that she had irregular menstrual periods and suffered from menstrual cramping almost every month. She said that cramping could be so bothersome that she had to take medicine to ease her pain. Her cramping lasted for only 1 day, usually the day before or the first day of each period. She thought that it was normal to have some cramping, that it was a part of being feminine. Repeated menstrual cramping month after month might serve as the pathology of endogenous origins in turning latent acupoints passive. A great number of patients in the menopausal and postmenopausal age groups were found to have menstrual cramping as a symptom of dysmenorrhea. These older female patients always have a higher number of passive acupoints detectable, indicating that passive acupoints will grow in number as symptoms become prolonged in age.

*Case 3*: Randall was the youngest patient we had. He was only 7 years old. His mother wanted him to try acupuncture to see if it was possible to control his asthmatic attacks, which he had suffered from frequently since infancy. Not too long before his visit, he had almost drowned in a river not far from his family ranch. It was in midsummer, but despite the warm climate, the water in the river was cold. It was so cold that when Randall jumped in, he was unable to breathe because, as he described it, his chest became so tight that he was immediately choked up and almost suffocated right on the spot. He looked weak and seemed underweight for his age. We were surprised to find that this boy had so many trigger points throughout the body at such a young age, particularly in the neck and thoracic regions. These trigger points represent the anterior, lateral, and posterior cutaneous branches of the upper fourth thoracic spinal nerves. Acupoints formed by the same cutaneous branches of other spinal nerves didn't transform to become trigger points.

*Case 4*: Beverly was 24 years old. She had been diagnosed as having rheumatoid arthritis about a year earlier. The pain in her wrists and interphalangeal joints was so bad that she could barely perform her routine secretarial duties, such as typing, although her arthritis was said to be in a stable state under prescribed antiinflammatory drugs and analgesics. The medications taken were not of much help to easing her pain in the wrists and fingers when she attempted to work. Among pathologies of endogenous origins, rheumatoid arthritis can be considered as one of the most vicious diseases, turning acupoints from the latent to passive phase rather quickly in a relatively short time. When we tested her acupoints, our estimate was that more than 85% of them were already in the passive phase.

*Case 5*: Debbie was a 19-year-old senior high student. We had known each other for more than 4 years, since her family immigrated to the United States. Because of the language barrier, her family sought our assistance for various reasons. From the time we became acquainted, she appeared to be a healthy young girl, without any indication that one day she would become ill from systemic lupus erythematosus at such a young age. For a month, it seemed to her parents that she was unwarrantably gaining too much weight, because her face suddenly appeared puffy. In fact, her mother cautioned her to watch her diet. Then one day, she became sick with fever and felt weak. They thought that the symptoms were nothing but a common cold and assumed she would be all right in no time. However, her condition worsened, and she was unable to go to school because of her weakness and fatigue. Her parents turned to us for help because of our medical knowledge. Looking at this young girl closely, it was not hard to conclude that she needed to see a physician. After a preliminary examination and hematological tests, her physician suggested that Debbie be put in a hospital for a more thorough evaluation because of conspicuous abnormalities in her bone marrow. Three days later, she was positively diagnosed as having systemic lupus. Before she went to the hospital, we checked her acupoints. She said that she experienced no pain except occasional backaches if she was in bed for a long period. Yet, it turned out that Debbie had many passive acupoints in her body. All of the 24 primary points and most of the secondary points were tender upon testing. Even a few tertiary points were also passive, although no nonspecific acupoints were found to be in the passive phase. It was clear that lupus was capable of systemically turning acupoints from latent to passive in a rather short time. We cannot tell if the appearance of trigger points took place before the existence of lupus, or after the patient became sick with the disease. If the passive acupoints began to appear only after the onset of the disease, then systemic lupus erythematosus is indeed a very powerful endogenous factor for turning acupoints from latent to passive. The idea for using the word "systemic" in this book, in fact, was derived from the name of this disease. Not too long after the diagnosis, Debbie was sent back to Taiwan, and died there 6 months later.

*Case 6*: Lu Ann was a 17-year-old high school student. She had had rheumatic fever when she was 7 years old. Thereafter, she had suffered low-grade temperature elevation, increased sedimentation rate, and painful joints. According to her medical evaluation, the infection had not caused damage to her heart. Nevertheless, she suffered from occasional pain in the knees and hands. The intermittent pain got worse one winter after a strenuous cheerleading practice at school. She took aspirin to "kill" the pain in the knees; relief occurred approximately 30 min after taking the medicine. She took 4 gr. (or eight tablets) of aspirin a day for almost 2 weeks. By then, she had developed a ringing in the ears. When she stopped taking aspirin, her knee pain recurred in a short time. Her father brought her to the clinic to see if her knee pain and tinnitus could be managed with acupuncture. She looked pale, indicating the possibility of anemia. She complained of feeling weak and getting tired easily. It was approximately 10 years between the time of her rheumatic fever infection and her visit to the clinic. Upon examination, she was found to have all the primary and some of the secondary acupoints in the passive phase. Thus, it is clear that rheumatic fever is another powerful endogenous factor that can turn acupoints from latent to passive, although its potency for converting acupoints to trigger points may be not as effective as that of lupus.

### 10.5.2 REGIONAL

Regional is just the opposite of systemic. Instead of following the sequential order described in Chapter 8, acupoints in the latent phase will become passive in the locality where the pathology of exogenous origin occurs. The initial appearance of trigger points is always limited to the vicinity of the injury. The regional appearance of passive acupoints has no sequential order. They will appear randomly around the region of the injury. Tender sensitivity can be detected in the acupoints described in the book or at loci not traditionally recognized as acupoints. So-called nonacupoints can become tender or passive regionally. Most passive acupoints appearing regionally were observed in injured young patients with pain that could be viewed as acute in nature. Here are three examples.

*Case 1*: Carl was a 17-year-old high school student. He was a very enthusiastic soccer player and practiced the game almost weekly. During a game, he was kicked very hard in his left abdomen by another player. Carl claimed that the kick was so hard that he collapsed abruptly to the ground with a severe, sharp pain. Fortunately, the pain subsided after time, and he was able to continue in the game until the end. Not too long after the incident, he began to experience pain in his left lower abdomen either during or after each game or practice. The pain began to extend to the left hip region. It bothered him so often and so much that finally medical consultation was sought to determine if there was any serious injury that was causing the pain repeatedly. Three different specialists were visited: a gastroenterologist, a neurologist, and an anesthesiologist. Their final conclusion was that Carl was a perfectly healthy young man without any detectable pathologic changes that could be the source of his pain. The treatments offered included prescriptive analgesics to be taken for the pain, and advice to discontinue playing soccer for a time. Carl claimed that soccer was half of his life and he would not give it up. Unfortunately, the pain kept recurring, and the medications were not very helpful for his problem. His mother thought that acupuncture might be useful as an alternative. Upon careful and thorough examination, no trigger points were detected, except in the region where he was kicked in the abdomen. The region where tenderness appeared was approximately 1.5 in. (40 mm) in diameter on the skin under which the iliohypogastric nerve pierces the deep membranous layer of Scarpa's fascia to emerge subcutaneously. The tender region was approximately 3 in. (78 mm) superior to the inguinal ligament and 4 in. (102 mm) medial to the left anterior superior iliac spine. The whole area was tender upon palpation. The accidental kick was coincidentally right at a strategic locus of anatomy and acupuncture, where the iliohypogastric nerve is located. This is a typical case in which passive acupoints appear regionally.

*Case 2*: Ben was a 21-year-old college student. He had been healthy thus far except for being slightly overweight, and he'd decided to reduce his weight by jogging. One day, he stepped into a hole covered by grass in the sidewalk and sprained his right ankle. He thought it was nothing more than an innocent mishap and that nothing could be seriously wrong. By the following morning, however, his right ankle was swollen and so painful that he could hardly stand on his right foot. There was ecchymosis visible on the lateral surface of the foot, indicating tissue damage and internal bleeding around the ankle. He was taken to an orthopedic clinic, where a surgeon examined the injured foot. It was decided that there was no bone fracture but that he had torn one of the talofibular ligaments. A foot casting was made and a prescription was given for reducing his pain. I had the opportunity to closely follow this case because Ben is my son, and we lived in the same house at the time. The morning after the accident happened, I made a complete testing of all acupoints I could think of. The only passive acupoints detected were all around the injured ankle, particularly inferior to the lateral and medial malleoli. Some of the tenderness was at the known acupoints, but some were not. In other words, nonacupoints in the area of the injury seemed to become passive or trigger points. Ben's injured ankle is a typical case, demonstrating that passive acupoints can appear regionally after a specific injury in a limited locality. He had no other acupoints that could be found to be in the passive phase.

*Case 3*: Matthew was 25 years old and a freshman medical student in the Health Science Center. One day, during the laboratory in Gross Anatomy for which I was on the teaching staff, he asked if acupuncture would be able to help eradicate the pain in his right elbow. The pain had just started to bother him recently, and no formal medical consultation had been sought thus far. It was suspected to be a case of tennis elbow because the pain was located right on the lateral epicondyle. Excessive use of the muscles can produce the condition of tennis elbow, and Matthew played tennis very vigorously. His right elbow had never given him any problem before. The pain had occurred only about a couple of weeks earlier. He stated that he had had an automobile accident approximately 2 months before the pain started to appear in his elbow. As a consequence of the accident, he was diagnosed as having whiplash because of his neck pain and stiffness. Although a few nonprescriptive analgesics were able to take care of the neck pain and stiffness, it was difficult to determine if the whiplash and tennis elbow were related in this case. Upon testing, no acupoints were found to be in the passive phase except three tender points distributed over the lateral epicondyle, where the long extensor muscles of the forearm have their origins. In addition, acupoints of the deep radial and lateral antebrachial cutaneous were also tender. This appearance of tender points on the epicondyle and the two passive acupoints in Matthew is another example of the regional phenomenon.

Patients who have pain due to regional injury with passive acupoints found in a limited locality are not commonly seen in the clinic. However, there are a sufficient number of them to convince us that the pain mentioned above must be what we consider as acute. Most acute pain can subside on its own in time after the wound is healed. The question for which we would like to find an answer is— can acupuncture shorten the duration of acute pain? In the meantime, acupoints in the passive phase associated with the injury will disappear and return to the latent phase. If the exogenous injury is monstrous in degree and extensive, acupoints could linger in the passive phase for a long time, and the pain will have the potential to become chronic. As the pain develops to the chronic stage, the number of passive acupoints will grow throughout the body in time. This is our distinction between acute and chronic pain. More about acute and chronic pain will be expanded on in Chapter 12.

## 10.6 COMBINATION OF SYSTEMIC AND REGIONAL APPEARANCES

Demographically, typical examples of systemic or regional appearances of passive acupoints alone are relatively few in comparison with the total number of patients received. Most patient cases can be described as results of the convergence or combination of systemic and regional manifestations.

In the beginning, acupoints turn from the latent to passive phase systemically or regionally alone. If they keep in the passive phase long enough, other pathologies of either endogenous or exogenous origins have the opportunity to set in, and two modes of passive acupoints will appear. Thereafter, more passive acupoints will appear in the body. Inevitably, this will create a physical and physiological environment for the pain to become chronic and hard to manage. Four examples are provided for illustration (Figures 10.1–10.4). They are all from patients received in the clinic. Because we have the photos to prove their existence, their names have been withheld.

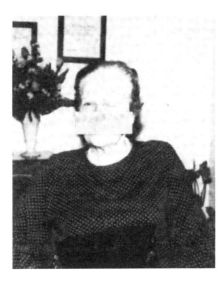

**FIGURE 10.1** This patient had postherpetic neuralgia affecting the ophthalmic division of the left trigeminal nerve. The pain in the left side of her face had been hurting for 18 years. We found that more than 85% of all her acupoints were in the passive phase. Furthermore, the entire left frontal forehead extending superiorly from the left eyebrow to the coronal suture line was tender practically everywhere it was touched. Systemically, all primary through tertiary acupoints in her body were passive. Regionally, even all nonspecific acupoints in the area where the herpes infection had occurred were passive. All patients afflicted with postherpetic neuralgia have been found to have a high number of passive acupoints, whether the infection occurred only a month previous or 18 years ago. This observation led us to conclude that the neuralgia developed from herpes in patients with sufficient numbers of preexisting trigger points in their bodies.

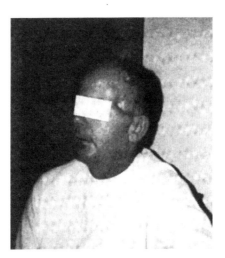

**FIGURE 10.2** This image shows a middle-aged man who had intracranial surgery to remove a meningioma from the left side of his brain. A surgical scar is clearly seen on the left parietotemporal region of his scalp. The area was soft because part of the cranium had been surgically removed, and it was also very tender in the whole region when adequate pressure was applied. His reason for coming to the clinic was to stop his headaches, which had been hurting him even before his surgery many months prior. Acupuncture was not much help for this patient and others like him because they had too many acupoints in the passive phase. Again, having so many passive acupoints is only possible with sufficient time permitted; passive acupoints need time to generate and increase in number.

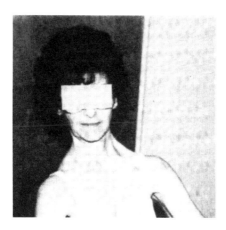

FIGURE 10.3  This middle-aged woman had a condition diagnosed as torticollis. She had had the condition for so long that she didn't remember how many years she had been suffering. Nor could she recall its cause. The result was visible; hypertrophy could be seen to have developed in the trapezius and sternocleidomastoid muscles. The patient had a lot of cervical stiffness and neck pain. Our guess was that the patient must have had some kind of injury to the neck that was exogenous in origin. The injury might not have been monstrous, but was substantial enough to involve some kind of abnormality in the cervical vertebrae. Damage to the vertebrae often takes a long time to heal, giving injury a chance to make pain chronic. Initially, only acupoints in the neck become passive. As time progresses, acupoints outside the neck will begin to turn from latent to passive. When she came for acupuncture, her systemically passive acupoints were only limited to the primary and secondary categories. In addition, tertiary and nonspecific acupoints in the neck region were in the passive phase, which was certainly understandable. Acupuncture was able to reduce her neck pain, but only for a short period. In a couple of weeks, the same pain would relapse, which was expected when the injury had resulted in an organic anatomical change, such as muscular hypertrophy.

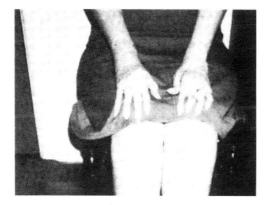

FIGURE 10.4  This shows the two lower limbs of a 73-year-old patient who had been suffering from rheumatoid arthritis for 25 years. This is an autoimmune disease that produces antibodies that invade one's own joints. The most vulnerable structures for the antibodies to attack include the finger joints, which can be deformed and become crooked. The disease can also affect kidney function. The kidneys of this elder patient were in poor condition, as indicated by the edema in her ankles, which appear swollen. Her ankles were shown to have many tender points surrounding the medial and lateral malleoli, as can be seen in the photo with needles inserted in them. The tender points appearing in the ankles, as seen in this patient, are nonspecific. They are there because the localities have endogenously originating pathological changes. Acupoints in patients affected by rheumatoid arthritis will turn from latent to passive rather quickly, most of them making the shift within 1 year's time. This is the reason that pain in patients afflicted by the disease is generally not easy to manage. The patient in the photo was no exception. Pain from rheumatoid arthritis is still possible to control within a year from the time the disease is first detected and diagnosed. It will be hopeless once the deformity is set in the fingers, wrists, toes, or ankles.

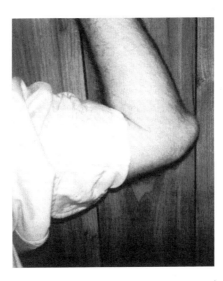

**FIGURE 10.5** The patient developed a hemangioma on his left elbow, projecting outward from the olecranon.

## 10.7 A SPECIAL CASE

The four individuals shown above were all senior patients. Here is one young person who may serve as an example to show that the convergence and combination of systemic and regional appearances of passive acupoints can also occur at a younger age. The name of this young individual is Fred. Fred is not a patient, he is a friend. We have known him from the time he was a child because he is the son of one of our graduate school professors. We estimate he was about 30 years old at the time of examination. As shown in Figure 10.5, Fred developed a hemangioma on his left elbow, projecting outward from the olecranon. He had noticed that something was growing in his elbow from the time he was in medical school. After graduation, he joined the military to become a naval surgeon. He had ended up at the Okinawa military base by the time we met again. We met because he came to Wilford Hall AFB Hospital for the operation to remove the tumor in his left elbow. Because he was an old friend, we were very happy to have the opportunity to entertain him and his wife. We became aware of this medical condition after lengthy conversations with him. Because he is a medical doctor, it was only natural for us to explain some aspects of acupuncture, and we showed him where he would have tender spots in his body. We expected, because of his young age, that he would not have a high number of passive acupoints systemically, but would have more passive acupoints regionally around his left elbow, and up and down his left upper limb. Our expectations turned out to be accurate in this case.

## 10.8 A FEW CONCLUSIONS

First, the appearances of passive acupoints are so common as to be universal, and yet very little—almost nothing, we could say—is known about how this can happen. This will remain unknown for some time to come because no one is doing anything to answer this perplexing question.

Second, acupuncture definitely is a very useful and effective tool for managing pain. Some pain is very easy to manage and eradicate. Some is impossible to reduce for even just a short time. Pain of an acute nature will subside and disappear on its own in time when and after the damage caused by pathology of endogenous or exogenous origins heal. If the injuries are severe enough and the damages are substantial, making healing and repair difficult or impossible, pain will become chronic. The physical and temporal extent of chronic pain is clearly related to the quantity of passive acupoints the patients have.

Third, as passive acupoints increase in number, the chances for pain to become chronic will be enhanced. Such occurrences provide a possibility for us to define what acute pain is and what chronic pain is. It will be a new way to differentiate the two types. More about defining acute and chronic pain is presented in Chapter 12.

Fourth, as far as we are aware, there is no objective way to measure or quantify pain. All we can attempt to do is to estimate how much subjective pain an individual has. Subjective pain changes from time to time, making measurement meaningless. There is another mode of pain that we describe as objective pain, which is stable and will stay the same in the body for a reasonable time. The pain reflects the quantity of passive acupoints one has. These are quantifiable.

Fifth, how much pain one has can be measured by quantifying how many passive acupoints one has. The objective pain measured is useful and reliable for predicting the outcome of managing the subjective pain. A pain with fewer passive acupoints is invariably easier to eliminate than similar pain with more passive acupoints.

Sixth, none of the statements given above require a double-blind control study to prove. Their results all can be repeated in any patient available in an acupuncture clinic. It is our hope that more physicians who are caring for patients suffering from pain will be willing to try the treatment methods offered in this book and to report their observations.

## REFERENCES

1. Lackritz, R.M. and P.C. Weinberg. Dysmenorrhea, premenstrual syndrome and dyspareunia. In *Gynecologic Disorders,* edited by C.P. Paurstein, Grune & Stratton, New York, 1982.
2. Walker, J.B. and R.L. Katz. Peripheral nerve stimulation in the management of dysmenorrhea. *Pain* 11:355, 1981.
3. Steinberger, A. The treatment of dysmenorrhea by acupuncture. *American Journal of Chinese Medicine* 9:57, 1982.

# 11 Psychology in Acupuncture

Does psychology play any role in acupuncture? There is no ambivalence in the answer to this question. It is an unequivocal "no." We know whether acupuncture is useful to manage pain, how much that pain can be managed, and even how long the relief can last if such pain has a probability to relapse. With this ability, there is no need to have psychology play a role in the practice of acupuncture. Our prognoses in predicting the outcome of pain management are not 100% accurate. Nothing in medicine works 100% of the time. However, we have the confidence to claim that our prognoses are 92% dependable and reliable. As such, there is no sense in making false claims. If acupuncture does not work, then it will not be of any help no matter how hard the patient believes that the pain will be eradicated. If acupuncture does work, the results of improvement will be difficult to deny, regardless of the patient's positive or negative psychology.

If psychology plays no part in acupuncture, why then do we spend time to discuss the subject? The answer is simple: Acupuncture is used primarily to deal with pain, and there is a great deal of psychology in pain. When medical professionals raise the issues of pain, psychological elements or factors are nearly always involved. Therefore, when we talk of using acupuncture to manage pain, certain psychological aspects need to be addressed. This chapter on psychology in acupuncture is included for this purpose.

## 11.1 PSYCHOLOGY OF PAIN

One reason that psychology is important in pain is because whenever someone writes about pain, psychological factors will be mentioned. There are far too many books available with some pain-related content for use in citation. The quotations provided here are randomly selected from among several such books that we have on hand in our bookshelves.

First, according to Walter B. Cannon [1]: "Closely related to fear is pain. Indeed, fear has been defined as the premonition of pain. As a rule, pain is associated with the action of injurious agents, a fact well illustrated in cuts, burns, and bruises. There are, to be sure, instances of very serious damage being done to the body—for example, in tuberculosis of the lung—without any pain whatsoever; and there are instances, also, of severe pain as in neuralgia, without corresponding danger to the integrity of the organism. These are exceptions, however, and the rule holds that pain is a sign of harm and injury. By experience, agents which injure and destroy, and which produce pain, become associated, so that our relations to them are conditioned by their effects. Thus, pain saves us from repeating acts which, in the end, might make and an end to life itself."

The word "psychology" is not used in this writing, but there is no doubt that in Dr. Cannon's opinion, psychology plays a part in pain because of our fear of this uncomfortable feeling.

In a book by Janet G. Travell and David G. Simons [2], we have the following: "A number of psychological factors can contribute to perpetuation of myofascial TPs (trigger points). Most important, the physician must be careful *not to assume* that psychological factors are primary. It is all too easy for the physician to blame the patient's psyche for the inability of physician to recognize all of the medical and neurophysiological factors that are contributing to the patient's myofascial pain. This wrong assumption can be—and often is—frightfully devastating to the patient. We have so much to learn about pain, especially referred pain. Patients who misunderstand the nature of their condition may be depressed, may exhibit anxiety tension, or may be victims of the 'good sport' syndrome; some may be exhibiting secondary gain and/or sick behavior; a few will evidence conversion hysteria. Each must be diagnosed on its own merits."

Our comments on those specific psychological factors to generate pain will be made later in this chapter.

Next, we hear from Robert P. Sheon et al. [3]: "Pain may cause temporary changes in personality. Psychologic evaluation of persons who suffer from chronic pain reveals several common deviations, including neuroticism and depression. These personality patterns do not, however, relate to future disability or disease outcome. In fact, these deviations tend to normalize following relief of the pain. Anxiety, hostility, denial, fear, guilt, hysteria, and depression are associated with changes in pain perception. In one study, six different personality patterns were defined, yet none of these related to chronicity or to illness behavior patterns. In another study, examining patients who were undergoing surgery for treatment of painful disorders, affirmative answers to two questions were useful as predictors of a poor outcome: (1) 'Has your appetite decreased recently?' and (2) 'Has your sexual interest lessened?' In other reports of patients treated nonsurgically, certain other characteristic features were also found that were predictive of an unsuccessful outcome. These included guilt, particularly if related to a supernatural reason given for the illness; projection of guilt onto others, particularly the therapist and pretreatment medication dependency; accident proneness; and expressed dissatisfaction with previous therapy. During care in a comprehensive pain center, these patients opposed psychologic approaches, used circumscribed delusions, and resisted many attempts at treatments. The pain center utilized formal and informal psychologic approaches in an effort to alleviate a 'negative–resigned' attitude in such patients."

This excerpt drags pain into a very complicated psychologic sphere.

The fourth quotation is made by Roy J. Mathew [4]. In the treatment of migraine headaches, Mathew describes in his book that there are "many emotional factors in the migraine patients' personality." They are found "to suffer from being anxious, (to be) striving, perfectionistic, order-loving, rigid. They become progressively more tense during periods of threat or conflict and show mismanagement and suppression of anger." Mathew also reports that "migraine sufferers tend to be tense and overconscientious. Their personality is described as sensitive, worrisome, perfectionist, chronically tense, apprehensive, and preoccupied by achievement and success. The migraine personality was also characterized by superficial interpersonal relationships, sexual maladjustment, and obsessive preoccupation with moral and ethical issues and was more neurotic than that of nonmigraine patients." One trouble with this quotation is that we don't believe any of these descriptions given to patients with migraine headache. We have met quite a few migraine patients, and none of them were known to have the personality described above. It is questionable whether the migraine personality is real. If it is, we certainly know nothing about such a personality.

Next, we excerpt from an article in *Time* magazine by Claudia Wallis [5]. In the article, chronic pain is said to come with anxiety, depression, and hopelessness. Throughout this short report, the terms "psychotherapy," "psychologist," and "psychological perspective" were repeated six times. One specific example was mentioned: a patient "for 2 years had been battling searing pain in his shoulder blade and armpit from shingles. Tried a variety of drugs, but they brought only temporary relief. Finally, he was referred to pain psychologists to learn techniques that would help him control his pain. The techniques include teaching patients relaxation exercises, breathing skills, guided imagery (focusing on pleasant mental images), and distraction techniques." According to Wallis, "pain psychologists play a vital role at most pain management centers, though patients are often reluctant to consult them. Patients hate to hear you offer them mind therapy, because they feel what you're doing is telling them they have a mental illness and you don't really believe they have a physical problem." She quoted an anesthesiologist, an internist, and a psychiatrist who is chief of pain medicine at a medical center, saying that "the mind is always actively involved in pain, especially in chronic cases. When we image the brain, the areas that light up when you experience pain include parts of the brain involved in emotions. That is why learning to relieve fear, anxiety, and depression related to pain actually helps bring relief, probably by activating the body's own pain-killing chemicals." Toward the end of her article, Wallis quoted the opinion of the then-incoming president of the American Academy of Pain Management on the question of why psychological therapy is less frequently used to manage pain compared with prescribing drugs. The answer was that "insurance companies prefer quick pharmaceutical fixes over the kinds of physical and psychological therapies that chronic-pain patients need. The bias toward drug treatment is not only bad medicine but is also expensive." The question here is what constitutes psychological therapy for pain management. In our view, what the psychological therapists use for the patients mentioned in this report is more neuromodulation than the dialectic oral consultation conducted in psychological therapy. Briefly, neuromodulation is defined as stimulation of the nervous system by whatever means to affect its function. As so defined, acupuncture is a mode of neuromodulation; and so are relaxation exercises, breathing skills, or biofeedback.

Finally, we hear from a book by Alice Park [6]. The author began by stating, "Pain is the human bodyguard, the cop on the beat racing to the scene, sirens wailing, shutting down traffic" and discussed "finding new ways to treat pain." The new ways include training the brain to ignore pain, using magnetic waves to reset neural circuits involved in pain, and using talking to cure pain, which is described as the talking cure. The talking cure is based on the fact that a "low-tech piece of the pain puzzle involves the psychological, social, and behavioral factors at play. Whether or not postsurgical pain becomes chronic certainly has a lot to do with a person's genetic sensitivity to activating pain pathways, but it may also depend in part on temperament and mental state. Because the brain chemicals that regulate mood and emotion, such as serotonin and norepinephrine, are closely linked to those that govern crisis response—including pain—it makes intuitive sense that their functions would be intertwined, and doctors see evidence of that all the time. Chronic pain really is a disease of the central nervous system. As such, it is a disease that affects the sensory, emotional, motivational, cognitive, and modulatory pathways. And the more we understand, in particular, the emotional pathways, the more we begin to understand that the traditional way we approach patients in pain may need to be revised. Patients with depression or anxiety, for example, often report a higher incidence of chronic pain, and their discomfort rises as their depression worsens. In addition, the opioid-based response to pain loops in the same reward and motivational systems that reinforce behaviors like addiction. Treat the depression and you may break the entire pathological cycle. New research into mental illness, genetic and molecular biology is giving researchers and patients new hope that pain may not have to remain so intractable and untreatable. And rethinking chronic pain as a disease, as a normally adaptive process gone awry instead of as a symptom, may be the key to finding safer and more effective ways of interrupting the hurt." To us, Alice Park's writing sounds more like fantasy than true scientific reality. Nothing she says about pain has any scientific proof to date, as far as we are aware.

## 11.2  TRUE OR FALSE

So much has been said about the psychology of pain. There may be questions on whether what has been said is true or false. However, we need not attempt to answer this question, because most, if not all, of what is said about the psychology of pain is inapplicable to the practice of acupuncture. The purpose of having acupuncture is to manage pain. If acupuncture is useful, pain will be manageable, and vice versa. Whether psychology is involved makes no difference to the outcome of acupuncture treatments.

However, a few issues related to psychology in acupuncture deserve our comments. One is the reality of psychological factors. What are these factors? Do these factors exist before or after the pain occurs? Does acupuncture treat the pain to make these factors disappear, or are these factors eliminated before pain is made to subside?

We begin by asking how many psychological factors we have. From what we have learned, medically mentioned terminology includes depression, anxiety, stress, tension, fear, hypochondriasis, worrisome, apprehension, and more. Conventional wisdom often is ambiguous in whether the factors or the pain comes first. We need to point out categorically that in the overwhelming majority of patients we have met, pain always precedes the factors. The patients have pain years before they begin to have depression and other psychological difficulties. We don't know if their psychological problems disappeared after acupuncture helped to eliminate their pain because none of our patients return to provide the opportunity for the follow-up studies once their pain is gone.

We cannot deny that once pain, particularly when it becomes chronic in nature, is set in the body, psychological factors of anxiety, stress, and tension will aggravate its intensity. We have never had patients come in purely for the treatment of stress and tension. Psychological derangement is very rare among our clientele. Out of more than 24,000 patients, we have encountered only a couple of cases of schizophrenia. There are more patients suffering for many years from chronic pain coming to complain of depression and anxiety. There is no question for us that after years of suffering pain, depression, as a consequence, is only to be expected.

## 11.3 HISTORICAL PROSPECT OF PAIN PERCEPTION

It is undeniable that psychology plays an important role in the perception of pain, as supported by the following example: A 46-year-old woman came to the clinic and declared that she suffered from fibromyalgia, because, for the last 4 days, she had had pain under the right armpit over the area covered by the latissimus dorsi muscle. Fibromyalgia is an illegitimate child in medicine. Even today, many doctors still don't recognize fibromyalgia as a genuine disease entity. There are doctors who think that the pain caused by fibromyalgia is all in the imagination of the sufferers. Most patients who suffer from fibromyalgia are female, and there are some six million of them. Six million is a substantial number, and to say that they are all "just crazy" or have something wrong in their heads would not merely be impolite, but insulting. The dismissive attitude stems from the fact that no pathology can be cited as the cause for having pain in fibromyalgia. Most patients with fibromyalgia have no obvious source of pain resulting from an injury of endogenous or exogenous origins. The symptoms they claim to have include chronic fatigue, insomnia, and depression without a substantive manifestation of psychological disorders. The psychological burden for the patients is aggravated when the pain they suffer is difficult to dispel. Therefore, it was imperative that we would be able to determine whether the woman really had the disease described as fibromyalgia. Otherwise, she would be regarded merely as having a psychopathic belief that she was suffering. Whether fibromyalgia is just a psychopathic symptom or a real pain symptom is beside the point of our discussion for the time being. The point here is that this is a useful case to help us look into why the mind is important in perceiving pain. We first have to look at it from a historical perspective.

Primitive people believed that the pain they sustained was inflicted by foreign objects. These foreign objects could be anything intruding into the body. To stop pain, besides extracting the intruding object, efforts also had to be made to ward off, appease, or frighten away any ill-intentioned spirits or demons with rings, talismans, amulets, tiger claws, or similar charms worn in the ears or nose. Figure 11.1 is one such example that is still in practice today. Even if the individual shown in the figure did not have his nose pierced for the sake of repelling pain, we do know that, in modern times, tattooing one's skin with exorcism symbols and wearing copper bracelets are accepted as ways to keep evil spirits and pain out of the body. Scientifically, practices of this nature are viewed as nothing but psychological make-believe.

It was an ancient belief in countries such as Egypt, India, and China that painful afflictions without injuries or wounds were caused by gods or evil spirits. Evil spirits usually arrived in darkness and could enter the body through the nostrils or the ears. Thus, pain clearly could carry religious overtones in different cultures. These overtones are another role that psychology plays in the perception of pain.

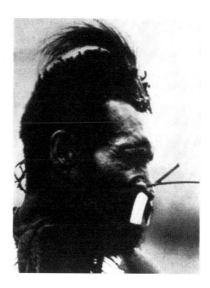

**FIGURE 11.1** Piercing the nose with certain objects is still a known practice among primitive tribes in our modern world. This picture is valid proof for such a custom, although there is no proof whether the ornament in the nose of this individual was for vanity or for repelling any evil which might bring pain through the nasal orifice.

## 11.4 MENTAL ATTITUDE TOWARD PAIN

By the Middle Ages, during the Renaissance, medical professionals began to think that pain was more than a psychological phenomenon and described 15 different types of pain due to different kinds of humoral presences. To relieve these different types of pain, they suggested exercise, heat, and massage. They also used natural compounds such as opium to control the pain. European cultures began to dominate the world, and scientific thinking was emerging among European medical schools. The center of sensory perception shifted from the heart to the brain. The Renaissance fostered great scientific advances in anatomy, physiology, and chemistry. The anatomy of the nervous system became the focal point for the understanding of pain. However, the scientific study of the sensation in general and pain in particular didn't take root in physiological experiences until the nineteenth century. It is accurate and fair to say that we now know much more about the anatomical, physiological, and biochemical aspects of pain. Nevertheless, it is also true and fair to say that old beliefs die hard; spiritual elements, including the mind and thought, still play a significant role in the perception of pain. Isn't it true that people suffering from chronic pain may wonder why they have to be punished with such terrible agony? Pain is still thought by some people to be supernatural, beyond secular control.

Besides the differences in cultural background and religious belief (Figure 11.2), there are other factors that are known to influence our psychology toward pain. The most commonly cited factors include financial gain, social pressure, judicial litigation, personality conflict, etc. We wonder whether religious devotees performing self-flagellation may understate the pain that they have inflicted on themselves. On the other hand, it is also a known fact that victims who stand to have financial gain can and will overstate pain suffering. Complaining of pain is also known as a tactic to attract attention and sympathy. More examples are available to show the interplay between our mind and pain. Further arguments over which mental attitude toward pain is beneficial for its relief or exacerbates suffering will serve no useful purpose. There are, and always will be, disagreements among medical experts in the study and care of pain in relation to psychology. Their disagreements indicate the uncertainty in our understanding of how psychology plays a role in the perception of pain.

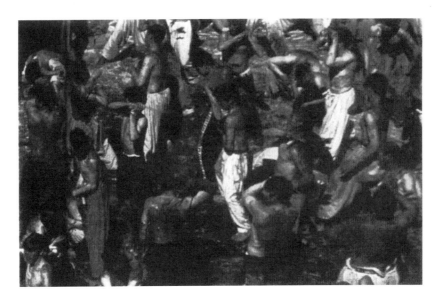

**FIGURE 11.2** Self-flagellation is a common religious practice. Do these faithful have a different psychology toward pain than ordinary individuals? (From *National Geographic*, November 2003, page 33, photographed by Steve McCurry.)

The biggest disagreement among the experts and pundits is that they don't have a uniform view of how much of a role psychology plays in pain. Is it 99% or only 1%, or somewhere in between? If so, just where in between does it fall? How important the mind is over pain depends very much on which school of thought we are willing to accept. There are many schools which have proposed different theories to explain pain. These include the specificity theory, the intensive theory, the pattern theories, the central summation theories, the fourth theory, the sensory interaction theory, the gate control theory, the psychological theory, and the behavioral theories.

A student of psychological and behavioral theories naturally will be more inclined to think that the mind is more important. Otherwise, how logical is it to explain that pain can occur in the absence of tissue damage or other organic pathology, as in case of fibromyalgia? Such pain is believed to be of a psychogenic nature. Psychogenic pain is said to occur in patients with a neurosis or psychosis. No demonstrable pathology can be found in these patients. The highest incidence of psychogenic pain is said to be found in patients with neurotic disorders, especially hysteria, and less frequently with reactive depression and other psychotic disorders. This view seems to imply that crazy people will suffer more pain, and the crazier they are, the more pain they will have. This theory has one inherent pitfall: How can we trust what crazy people tell us? They are known not to be trustworthy. Furthermore, if psychogenic pain is indeed less frequent in patients with depression than in hysteric patients, how can the difference in frequency be tangibly measured?

To avoid possible conflicts between the different theories promulgated by different schools and to cover any possible domain of psychological pain, when any questionnaires are designed to measure pain, they almost always turn out to require a thorough and total comprehension beyond that of ordinary intelligence. Like theories, there are many questionnaires used in clinical practices to estimate how much pain the patients might be suffering. Realistically, most of them cannot be considered as helpful for medical professionals to reliably understand the quantity of pain the patients might have. This is only to be expected if the patients themselves have no clear idea of their own pain.

## 11.5 THE VICIOUS CYCLE OF PAIN

Psychology is an undisputed factor in the perception of pain. However, we have to be aware of other factors that can also play a more substantial role than the mind. Medically speaking, each of these factors can be as complicated and intriguing as psychology. Discussing them all would be excessive for this book, which is intended to be brief and concise. One way to simplify their interactions and interrelationships is to use a conceptual diagram, such as in Figure 11.3, for an easy visualization. What is shown in the figure is not entirely our own imagination. The same vision has been proposed by many other well-known people in the study of pain. Here is a mere adaption of their ideas to put into use for our readers.

Understanding what role psychology alone plays in pain (and how) is mind-boggling enough. To tangle with all the factors listed in the figure of the cycle will certainly make it more difficult to better understand pain. However, from the diagram, we can imagine that pain operates like a wheel turning in a cycle. The axle of the wheel is the sensory nervous system. When the system is stable, as described in an optimal homeostatic state, the wheel remains sedate, without much need to move and become active. The wheel can and will turn on its own when the various factors included are stimulated. When the wheel of pain begins to turn, it will turn in two dimensions, larger in size and faster in speed. These two dynamic phenomena explain why pain grows in intensity and severity if permitted to perpetuate for too long. The size and speed dimensions of the wheels' turning will be determined by elements including hormones, nutrition, blood flow, infections, etc. All these factors can be fed into the cycle of pain, and it is this vicious cycle that is capable of exacerbating our pain.

The information provided above is intended to illustrate two simple and obvious facts. First, no one knows how to measure or quantify pain in a realistic and reliable way so that we are able to understand how much pain people are suffering. Clearly, we need to find such a way to quantify pain realistically and reliably. This is precisely what this book is intended to offer. The claim is not preposterous; we expect our readers to come to the conclusion that the promise offered is genuine.

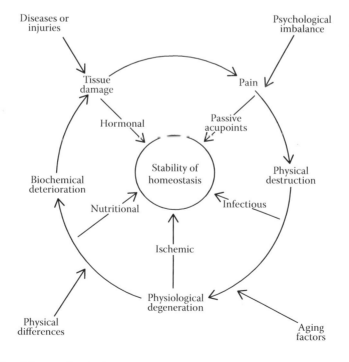

**FIGURE 11.3** The vicious cycle of pain.

By reading this book, one may discover that pain is culturally, politically, ethnically, economically, educationally, religiously, and socially neutral. How much pain each of us has is measurable and quantifiable. One can be atheistic or fanatic, and the pain measured will be the same. The results of the measurement turn out to be independent of our mood. Quantifiable pain is relatively constant whether we are happy or sad, depressed or exhilarated, angry or cheerful, provoked or pacified, rich or poor, during daytime or at night. A person will be shown to have the same degree of pain regardless of whoever conducts the testing as long as the identical procedures described are followed. There is definitely no psychology involved in our understanding of pain.

## 11.6 REBUTTING ACUPUNCTURE AS PLACEBO

To conclude the discussion of psychology in pain, one last item of controversy we face in acupuncture is whether the efficacy produced by needle insertion is real or just imaginary. Critics of acupuncture insist that the results from needle therapy are nothing but placebo. Acupuncture has been viewed as a product of placebo because the results of several clinical investigations have shown that the positive results of acupuncture were no greater than those of control or nonacupuncture groups. In other words, the difference between experimental acupuncture groups and control nonacupuncture groups is not statistically significant. There is no need to dispute whether the results produced by acupuncture are wholly or partly placebo. Even if the results are placebo, acupuncture is still undeniably useful in managing pain in some patients. The merit of having the potential to reduce or stop pain in one or more patients justifies keeping acupuncture in practice for the time being. Most clinical studies in acupuncture have not had much scientific meaning in determining whether the pain suffered indeed was reduced because we do not have a reliable method to measure how much there is to begin with. Thus, whether or not acupuncture is placebo does not mean much to us. If there is no way to reliably measure the pain in the beginning, how can we say for sure that the pain had been reduced at the end of the therapy? One of the missions set for this book is to show our readers how pain can be measured reliably.

## REFERENCES

1. Cannon, W.B. *The Wisdom of the Body.* W.W. Norton & Company, Inc. New York, 1963.
2. Travell, J.G. and D.G. Simons. *Myofascial Pain and Dysfunction: The Trigger Point Manual.* Williams & Wilkins, Baltimore, 1983.
3. Sheon, R.P. et al. *Soft Tissue Rheumatic Pain: Recognition, Management, Prevention.* Lea & Febiger, Philadelphia, 1982.
4. Mathew, R.J. *Treatment of Migraine: Pharmacological and Biofeedback Considerations.* SP Medical & Scientific Books, New York, 1979.
5. Wallis, C. The Right (and Wrong) Way to Treat Pain. *Time,* February 28, 2005.
6. Park, A. Healing the Hurt: Finding New Ways to Treat Pain. *Time*, March 7, 2011.

# 12 Pain and Measurement

## 12.1 A CHALLENGE AND A PUZZLE

In the study of pain, two renowned scientists, Melzack and Wall, wrote a book entitled *The Challenge of Pain* [1], which was published in 1982. In the book, the authors view pain as a puzzle. The reason that pain is challenging can be best described by Bonica [2]. He said that today, as then, proper management of pain remains one of the most important and most pressing issues of society in general, and of the scientific community and the health professions in particular. Demographically, one-third of all Americans have chronic discomfort due to pain. Medically, pain is the number one reason people seek medical care. Financially, medical care for pain is estimated to cost $100 billion a year in treatments, lost wages, and other expenses. Drugs used to treat pain are one of the leading causes of liver failure. Painkillers send more than half a million to the emergency room annually, and about 200 die from taking them each year.

Pain is a puzzle. No mentally sane individual wants to have pain, even though we all need it, because pain is protective. The sensation we seek most to avoid is, in fact, one of the most essential ones for our survival. We think that we know a great deal about pain, yet we still don't know what pain really is. We don't know when pain could go rogue. Pain can help us get well and stay safe. Yet, it can become an illness in itself, resulting in persistent torment. Pain can act like a thief. It breaks into your body and robs you blind. With lightning fingers, it can take away your livelihood, your marriage, your friends, your sanity, your joy, your happiness, your favorite pastimes, and big chunks of your personality. Left unapprehended, it will steal your days and nights until the world has collapsed into a cramped cell of suffering.

Pain is said to be gaining new respect at all levels of health care. It is even making its way onto the national political agenda. The U.S. Congress has declared that this is the decade of pain control and research. Pain is an important medical, political, and social issue. Yet, we still have a lot of unknown factors when facing pain: We don't know the exact cause of generalized pain disorders. We have no dependable method to measure pain. We don't have any agreeable, reasonable way to define acute and chronic pain. Can a pain grow? Does pain have memory? And these are only a few examples of questions we still have regarding pain. Our available space and time are far too limited to investigate even the small selection given above, much less all of them. Our intention in this book is to select three of the questions most urgently in need of answers. Can pain be objectively measured? Is it possible to differentiate acute pain from chronic pain? What is the relationship between acute and chronic pain? Finding reasonable answers for these three questions will be helpful in understanding how and why acupuncture is useful.

## 12.2 MEASUREMENTS OF PAIN

There are four commonly used procedures to measure pain in patients: psychophysical, rating scale, magnitude estimation, and measurement of performance behavior on laboratory tasks. A good example of the psychophysical method is the McGill Pain Questionnaire. There are many rating scale methods available for both clinical research and daily routine practice. The magnitude estimation method uses direct judgments of stimulus intensity or quality made by number assignment or cross-modality matching techniques such as hand grip force. The fourth method obtains indices of discrimination ability or detection. These four methods are not inclusive; there are other methods described in the literature.

It will not serve much purpose to evaluate the different methods used conventionally in pain measurement. However, to be informative, we will just point out one disadvantage for each of these methods. For example, the McGill Pain Questionnaires are very tedious and lengthy. Answering all the questions alone takes hours, not to mention how long it requires to evaluate all the answers provided. Results obtained from rating scale methods can vary from time to time, reading eight out of a possible 10 in one hour, and then dropping down to two the next hour. The third and fourth methods involve elaborate procedures that require too much time, manpower, and expensive facilities to perform. They are not suitable for routine use in ordinary clinical setups.

Any method for measuring pain must have several feasible aspects to be clinically useful. It should be applicable to every patient coming to the clinic. Its procedures should be usable anytime by people trained in acupuncture as promulgated in this book. For experienced acupuncturists, pain in a patient should be measurable in less than 5 min. Measured pain should be recordable with integers to designate its degree of intensity. The measurement must be reproducible for any patient with any possible painful condition. Most importantly, the data on the degree of pain collected must be applicable for prognostic purposes in determining whether the pain in that particular patient can be managed. If the pain can be managed, how many acupuncture sessions are required to achieve a substantial relief? And, indeed, once the pain has subsided, what is the possibility for it to relapse? To medical professionals who provide care in pain management, the claims offered here could sound outlandish. I recommend they try out my methods for themselves before drawing a final conclusion.

Pain has to be quantifiable. As the prelude to his book [3], Dr. Bond quoted Lord Kelvin: "…when you can measure what you are speaking about, and express it in number, you know something about it, but when you cannot measure it, when you cannot express it in numbers, your knowledge is of a meager and unsatisfactory kind; it may be the beginning of knowledge, but you have scarcely in your thoughts, advanced to the stage of science whatever the matter may be." This quotation is quite applicable to the scientific status of pain. When we speak of pain, there is not much science involved because we don't have a reliable way to numerically express pain measured in the bodies of patients. Until it is possible to measure what degree of pain there is in every patient, pain research will remain meaningless to all of us.

## 12.3 SUBJECTIVE PAIN VERSUS OBJECTIVE PAIN

Why is pain impossible to measure? The reason is very simple. We have two kinds of pain: subjective and objective. To this day, when we want to measure pain medically, we invariably will target subjective pain. Why do we always focus on subjective pain? Because subjective pain is perceivable; it is the unpleasant sensation produced after injuries of either endogenous or exogenous origins. We know where subjective pain is located. This kind of pain is mutable; it changes frequently from time to time. This mutability makes the assessment of subjective pain difficult, if not impossible. Subjective pain is capricious in nature. It hurts now, but a few hours later, the hurting will disappear on its own. If we use a scale rating of one to 10 to measure how much pain a patient has, and the answer is eight right at this moment, it could change to one a few hours later. Subjective pain can appear randomly in any part of the body. Where there is an injury, the injured location will have subjective pain. Subjective pain provides no clue for us to determine if the pain is acute or chronic in nature.

In contrast, there is objective pain. Objective pain is measurable. It is our main focus of pain measurement. Objective pain is not perceivable. People who have objective pain will not know they have it. The pain is relatively stable, meaning without noticeable variation in the intensity of hurting sensation over a rather long period of time, such as months. Objective pain serves as a useful indicator to differentiate chronic from acute pain. All objective pain is found to occur in acupoints in the passive phase, or trigger points. In other words, trigger points are acupoints where objective pain is stored. How many trigger points one has will indicate the quantity of objective pain one carries. The method for counting trigger points will be explained subsequently. All we want our readers to know right now is that the manageability of a subject's pain depends on how much the objective pain the subject has.

## 12.4 RANKING THE TRIGGER POINTS

Almost all of our patients have been found to have trigger points. The trigger points appear in an orderly sequence, as described in an earlier chapter of the book. The sequence appears to be predictable, as shown from our study. Over an approximately 4-month period, 221 patients were studied. The sex and age distribution of these patients is summarized in Table 12.1. Of the patients studied, 130 (58.8%) were female, and 91 (41.2%) male. There were fewer young patients than older ones. Only two were younger than 19 years of age. One of the two was 12 years old and came not because of pain, but because of asthma. Patients between 40 and 69 years of age made up 63.8% of the total.

The pains these patients complained of suffering varied widely. They included lower back pain, arthritis of different types, headaches, and pain at various joints. Most of the patients (95%) had received conventional medical treatment without substantial benefit in terms of pain relief. They often confessed that acupuncture was their final recourse.

A total of 110 acupoints were selected for study. That number is approximately a third of the total number of acupoints described in this book. The acupoints selected for the study were chosen to represent the head, neck, upper limb, body trunk, and lower limb proportionally. The time required to test all 110 acupoints in each patient was less than an hour, giving the opportunity to schedule two patients per hour. Generally, three to four patients were available for the study per night.

A checklist with all 110 acupoints was prepared. After testing if tender sensation was present, a functional phase of latent, passive, or active was recorded for each acupoint. All the tests were conducted by the author. Acupoints on the anterior side of the body were tested first, followed by those on the posterior surface. After completing the study, we determined how many patients had a given number of passive phase acupoints. As can be seen in Table 12.2, out of a total of 221 patients, 220

### TABLE 12.1
### Sex and Age Distributions of Patients Examined for Passive Acupuncture Points

| Age in Years | Female Patients | | Male Patients | | Total Patients | |
|---|---|---|---|---|---|---|
| | No. | (%) | No. | (%) | No. | (%) |
| 10–19 | 0 | 0 | 2 | 2.2 | 2 | 0.9 |
| 20–29 | 8 | 6.2 | 7 | 7.7 | 15 | 6.8 |
| 30–39 | 17 | 13.1 | 14 | 15.4 | 31 | 14.0 |
| 40–49 | 25 | 19.2 | 11 | 12.1 | 36 | 16.3 |
| 50–59 | 32 | 24.6 | 18 | 19.8 | 50 | 22.6 |
| 60–69 | 31 | 23.9 | 24 | 26.3 | 55 | 24.9 |
| 70–79 | 15 | 11.5 | 14 | 15.4 | 29 | 13.1 |
| 80–89 | 2 | 1.5 | 1 | 1.1 | 3 | 1.4 |
| | 130 | 100.0 | 91 | 100.0 | 221 | 100.0 |

**TABLE 12.2**
**Names of the Primary Trigger Points in Sequence of Appearance**

| Sequence | Acupuncture Points (Anatomical Nomenclature) | Passive Phase Frequency | (%) |
|---|---|---|---|
| 1 | Deep radial-I | 220 | 99.5 |
| 2 | Great auricular | 219 | 99.1 |
| 3 | Spinal accessory-I | 217 | 98.2 |
| 4 | Saphenous-I | 216 | 97.7 |
| 5 | Deep peroneal | 215 | 97.3 |
| 6 | Tibial-I | 214 | 96.8 |
| 7 | Greater occipital | 213 | 96.4 |
| 8 | Suprascapular-I (infraspinatus) | 212 | 95.9 |
| 9 | Lateral antebrachial cutaneous | 211 | 95.5 |
| 10 | Sural-I | 209 | 94.6 |
| 11 | Lateral or medial popliteal | 207 | 93.7 |
| 12 | Superficial radial-I | 203 | 91.9 |
| 13 | Dorsal scapular-I | 201 | 91.0 |
| 14 | Superior cluneal | 198 | 89.6 |
| 15 | Posterior cutaneous of L2 | 196 | 88.7 |
| 16 | Inferior gluteal | 195 | 88.2 |
| 17 | Lateral pectoral | 192 | 86.9 |
| 18 | Iliotibial-I | 185 | 83.7 |
| 19 | Infraorbital | 184 | 83.3 |
| 20 | Spinous process of T7 | 178 | 80.5 |
| 21 | Posterior cutaneous of T6 | 172 | 77.8 |
| 22 | Posterior cutaneous of L5 | 168 | 76.0 |
| 23 | Supraorbital | 167 | 75.6 |
| 24 | Common peroneal-I | 165 | 74.7 |

of them had deep radial-I in the passive phase. Translated into percentages, 99.5% of all patients had that acupoint in the passive phase. Taking the supraorbital point as another example, 167 patients, or 75.6%, had that acupoint in the passive phase. Only three patients, or 1.4%, had the olecranon point in the passive phase. That was the lowest ranking for any acupoint.

## 12.5 TRIGGER POINTS IN FOUR GROUPS

We decided to divide the 110 trigger points into four groups: primary, secondary, tertiary, and nonspecific. The reason for such divisions will be explained in the later chapters. For the time being, it is useful to remember the sequence in which acupoints turn from the latent to passive phase or the sequential order in which trigger points appear. One hundred and ten is not a small number to deal with. It is very difficult, if not totally impossible, to memorize all of them in correct sequence. The primary points are the most important and used in acupuncture practice all the time (there are 24 of them). It should be possible to become acquainted with their names, if not their correct sequence. For other trigger points in the secondary, tertiary, and nonspecific groups, it will be sufficient to remember a few in each group for acupuncture practice. Which of them are beneficial to remember will be suggested in the following descriptions.

Pain and Measurement

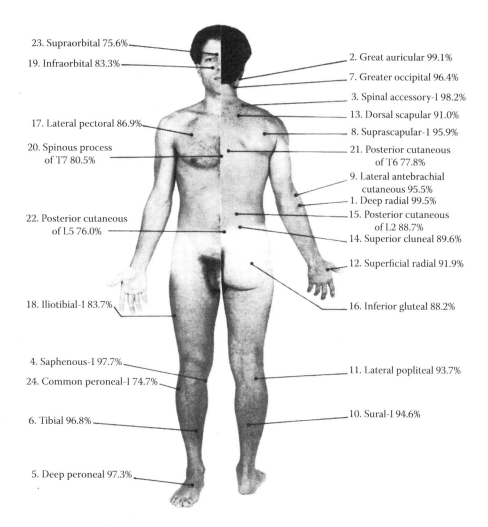

**FIGURE 12.1** Anatomic locations of 24 primary trigger points.

## 12.5.1 Primary Points

The first 24 acupoints to become trigger points are considered as the primary points. The justification for claiming a total of 24 acupoints will be offered in Chapter 13. The names of these 24 points are listed in Table 12.2, and their anatomic locations are shown in Figure 12.1.

Gradually, the author figured out one adequate and appropriate scale for rating objective pain in 12 degrees. Each degree encompasses eight trigger points. Therefore, if a patient had the first 24 trigger points detectable with painful sensitivity, that patient was estimated to have at least third-degree objective pain. The same rule will apply to the secondary, tertiary, and nonspecific trigger points.

## 12.5.2 Secondary Points

The next 28 points in sequence are grouped as the secondary points. Their names are listed in Table 12.3, and their anatomic locations are shown in Figure 12.2. We can divide 28 by three to have nine trigger points representing one degree of objective pain. We suggest keeping three of the 28

## TABLE 12.3
### Names of the Secondary Trigger Points in Sequence of Appearance

| Sequence | Acupuncture Points (Anatomical Nomenclature) | Passive Phase Frequency | (%) |
|---|---|---|---|
| 25 | Medial antebrachial cutaneous | 164 | 74.6 |
| 26 | Tibial-II | 164 | 74.6 |
| 27 | Temporomandibular | 164 | 74.6 |
| 28 | Cervical plexus | 163 | 74.2 |
| 29 | Deep radial-II | 163 | 74.2 |
| 30 | Masseter | 162 | 73.6 |
| 31 | Femoral | 161 | 72.9 |
| 32 | Xyphoid | 160 | 72.4 |
| 33 | Saphenous-II | 156 | 70.6 |
| 34 | Lesser occipital | 152 | 68.8 |
| 35 | Posterior cutaneous of T4 | 148 | 67.0 |
| 36 | Iliotibial-II | 147 | 66.5 |
| 37 | Medial pectoral | 146 | 66.1 |
| 38 | Radial | 143 | 64.7 |
| 39 | Spinous process of T5 | 142 | 64.3 |
| 40 | Axillary | 138 | 62.4 |
| 41 | Posterior cutaneous of L1 | 138 | 62.4 |
| 42 | Spinal accessory-II | 135 | 61.1 |
| 43 | Superficial peroneal | 134 | 60.6 |
| 44 | Sural-II | 132 | 59.7 |
| 45 | Posterior cutaneous of L3 | 128 | 57.9 |
| 46 | Recurrent of median | 123 | 55.7 |
| 47 | Posterior cutaneous of T8 | 122 | 55.2 |
| 48 | Common peroneal-II | 114 | 51.6 |
| 49 | Suprascapular-II (superspinatus) | 111 | 50.2 |
| 50 | Mental | 110 | 49.8 |
| 51 | Superior auricular | 108 | 49.3 |
| 52 | Acromioclavicular | 106 | 48.8 |

points in mind: the medial antebrachial cutaneous in the sequence of 25, the lesser occipital in 34, and the mental in 50. The medial antebrachial cutaneous can be used to compare with the lateral antebrachial cutaneous of the primary points in the sequence of nine. If the lateral antebrachial cutaneous point is tender and the medial antebrachial cutaneous is not, the objective pain in the patient is third degree or lower. If the medial antebrachial cutaneous begins to exhibit sensitivity but the intensity of tenderness is less than that of the lateral antebrachial cutaneous, this is an indicator that the pain is reaching the fourth degree. If tender sensitivity in both points is equal, the pain is unquestionably exceeding the fifth degree. Many more examples can be cited to explain how to use trigger points for measuring objective pain. The best way to learn this method is by using it in clinical practice. Of course, it is simple to recognize that having the lesser occipital point in the passive phase indicates pain at the fifth degree, and having the mental point in the passive phase indicates pain at the sixth degree.

# Pain and Measurement

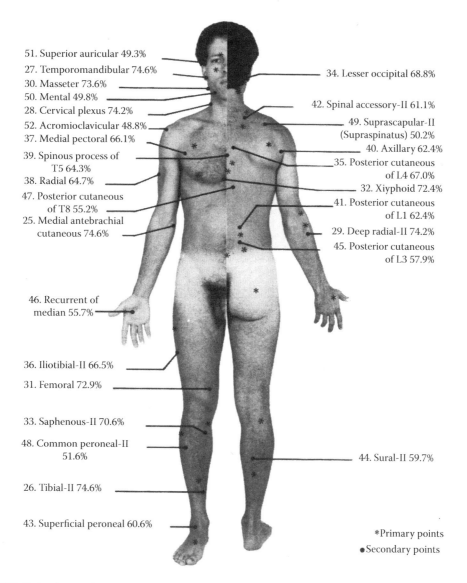

**FIGURE 12.2** Anatomic locations of 28 secondary trigger points.

## 12.5.3 TERTIARY POINTS

As listed in Table 12.4, there are 27 points in this group. Their anatomic locations are shown in Figure 12.3. Three in this group are easily accessible and convenient to use: the transverse cervical, the temporalis, and the medial brachial cutaneous. When the medial brachial cutaneous is used to compare with two other cutaneous points in the arm, the lateral antebrachial and the medial antebrachial, one will quickly realize how much objective pain the patient has. By the time the medial brachial cutaneous is passive, the pain is reaching the ninth degree. The objective pain at nine degrees makes the subjective pain rather difficult to manage.

## TABLE 12.4
### Names of the Tertiary Trigger Points in Sequence of Appearance

| Sequence | Acupuncture Points (Anatomical Nomenclature) | Passive Phase Frequency | (%) |
|---|---|---|---|
| 53 | Transverse cervical | 108 | 48.8 |
| 54 | Achilles | 107 | 48.4 |
| 55 | Upper biceps brachii | 105 | 47.5 |
| 56 | Inferolateral malleolus | 104 | 47.1 |
| 57 | Inferomedial malleolus | 104 | 47.1 |
| 58 | Intercostobrachial | 102 | 46.2 |
| 59 | Temporalis | 102 | 46.2 |
| 60 | Lateral cutaneous of T8 | 100 | 45.2 |
| 61 | Spinous process of T3 | 95 | 43.0 |
| 62 | Iliotibial-III | 93 | 42.1 |
| 63 | Obturator | 91 | 41.2 |
| 64 | Spinous process of T6 | 83 | 37.6 |
| 65 | Plantar | 81 | 36.7 |
| 66 | Ilioinguinal | 79 | 35.8 |
| 67 | Costal margin | 78 | 35.3 |
| 68 | Saphenous-III | 76 | 34.4 |
| 69 | Third metatarsal | 73 | 33.0 |
| 70 | Spinal accessory-III | 72 | 32.6 |
| 71 | Coronal suture | 71 | 32.1 |
| 72 | Pterion | 71 | 32.1 |
| 73 | Greater trochanter | 70 | 31.7 |
| 74 | Medial brachial cutaneous | 69 | 31.2 |
| 75 | Bregma | 67 | 30.3 |
| 76 | Common peroneal-III | 65 | 29.4 |
| 77 | Posterior brachial cutaneous | 63 | 28.5 |
| 78 | Deltoid | 63 | 28.5 |
| 79 | Deep radial-III | 61 | 27.7 |

### 12.5.4 Nonspecific Points

When objective pain gets to the tenth degree or higher, subjective pain becomes very difficult to manage. The degrees of the objective pain encompassed by the last 31 nonspecific points, as indicated in Table 12.5, are ranked 10, 11, and 12. Sometimes, the degree can go higher than that because other nonspecific points, which are not included in the table, can turn functionally to the passive phase. It is not necessary to remember which points are associated with tenth-, eleventh- or twelfth-degree pain because subjective pain involving nonspecific points is not only difficult to manage, but also the trigger points can be ubiquitous.

Figure 12.4 shows the anatomic locations of 31 nonspecific trigger points, although their number can be greater. Often, people with that many nonspecific trigger points will cry out in pain when a portion of their body is gripped unexpectedly.

## 12.6 TRIGGER POINTS ON THE SPINOUS PROCESSES

Trigger points can also appear on the spinous processes of some vertebrae. Figure 12.5 is taken from a drawing in a traditional acupuncture textbook [4]. The drawing shows acupoints on the spinous

Pain and Measurement

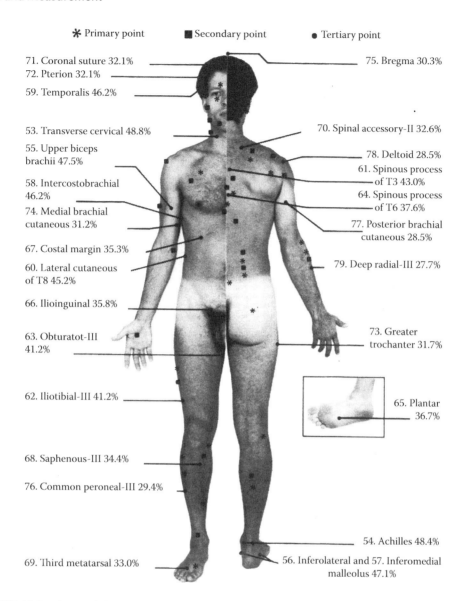

FIGURE 12.3 Anatomic locations of 27 tertiary trigger points.

processes of the seventh cervical and first, third, fifth, sixth, and seventh thoracic vertebrae. The second and fourth thoracic vertebrae have no acupoints on their processes. A study was undertaken to determine if there were no acupoints on these two processes because no trigger point was formed on them [5,6]. Here is a brief summary of this study:

First, the drawing of acupoints shown in Figure 12.5 needs to be converted into an anatomic illustration in English, as seen in Figure 12.6. Using Figure 12.6 as a guide, the anatomic location of each spinous process for the first seven thoracic vertebrae can be easily determined. The spinous process of T1 is located approximately 1 to 2 cm inferior to the vertebral prominence, which is the spinous process of the seventh cervical vertebrate. The spinous of T3 can be palpated on the midpoint of the line connecting the base of the spines of two scapulae. The spinous process between T1 above and T3 below should belong to T2. If we draw a line connecting the two inferior angles of the scapulae, the spinous process of T7 is found at the midpoint of the line. The spinous processes

## TABLE 12.5
### Names of Nonspecific Trigger Points in Sequence of Appearance

| Sequence | Acupuncture Points (Anatomical Nomenclature) | Passive Phase Frequency | (%) |
|---|---|---|---|
| 80 | Intermediate supraclavicular | 61 | 27.6 |
| 81 | Fifth metatarsal | 60 | 27.1 |
| 82 | Medial sural | 58 | 26.2 |
| 83 | Zygomaticofacial | 55 | 24.9 |
| 84 | Saphenous-N | 51 | 23.1 |
| 85 | Medial supraclavicular | 48 | 21.7 |
| 86 | Lateral supraclavicular | 44 | 19.9 |
| 87 | Common peroneal-N | 41 | 18.6 |
| 88 | Peroneus brevis | 39 | 17.6 |
| 89 | Sternal angle | 37 | 16.7 |
| 90 | Posterior auricular | 35 | 15.8 |
| 91 | Median-N | 34 | 15.4 |
| 92 | Depressor septi | 32 | 14.5 |
| 93 | Vastus medialis | 28 | 12.7 |
| 94 | Lateral cutaneous of T10 | 26 | 11.8 |
| 95 | Nasion | 24 | 10.9 |
| 96 | Occipital protuberance | 21 | 9.5 |
| 97 | Rectus femoris | 20 | 9.0 |
| 98 | Frontalis | 18 | 8.1 |
| 99 | Spinous process of T10 | 17 | 7.6 |
| 100 | Lacrimal | 16 | 7.2 |
| 101 | Mentalis | 15 | 6.8 |
| 102 | Posterior cutaneous of S3 | 14 | 6.3 |
| 103 | Anterior cutaneous of T10 | 13 | 5.9 |
| 104 | Great toe | 12 | 5.4 |
| 105 | Posterior interosseus | 11 | 5.0 |
| 106 | Third proximal interphalangeal | 9 | 4.0 |
| 107 | Anterior cutaneous of T8 | 8 | 3.6 |
| 108 | Heel | 7 | 3.2 |
| 109 | Third distal interphalangeal | 6 | 2.7 |
| 110 | Olecranon | 3 | 1.4 |

of T4, T5, and T6 can be located sequentially either from above starting at T3 or from below beginning with T7.

After becoming familiar with the anatomic locations of the thoracic spinous processes, we turn to Figure 12.7 for a more realistic view of the body's dorsal surface taken in a photograph. The model stood with the upper limbs abducted about 30 degrees. Thus, the inferior angles of the scapulae were slightly protracted upward. They are clearly visible, nevertheless, and their anatomic locations are easy to identify for recognizing the acupoints.

To test for the appearance of any trigger points in the spinous processes, patients were asked to undress from the waist up. In a prone position, they laid flat on an examination table. Their upper limbs were kept close to the body to maintain an anatomic position akin to standing. The acupoint on the spinous process of the seventh thoracic vertebra was tested first using a thumb or index finger to apply 2 lb. of pressure to determine if it had become a trigger point. The same test was repeated

# Pain and Measurement

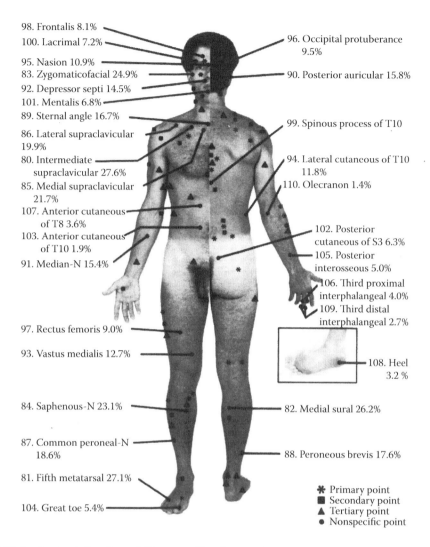

**FIGURE 12.4** Anatomic locations of 31 nonspecific trigger points.

for the spinous processes of other eight thoracic vertebrae as indicated in Table 12.6. A total of 219 patients were available for the study. As can be seen in the table, 177 (80.9%) of them had a trigger point on T7. Next, in rank to T7 is T5, with 147 patients having a trigger point on that spinous process. The lowest frequency for a trigger point was found on the spinous process of T2. Only 17 out of 219 patients (7.8%) were found to have that trigger point in T2. The sex and age distributions of the 219 patients for the study of trigger points in the spinous processes of the thoracic vertebrae are tabulated in Table 12.7.

## 12.7 RESULTS OF PAIN MEASUREMENT

In this chapter, we describe two ways to measure pain. One way is to quantify trigger points detectable throughout the body. The trigger points are divided into four groups: primary, secondary, tertiary, and nonspecific. Each group encompasses three degrees of pain, providing a scale of 12 degrees. Another way is to quantify trigger points in the spinous processes of nine thoracic

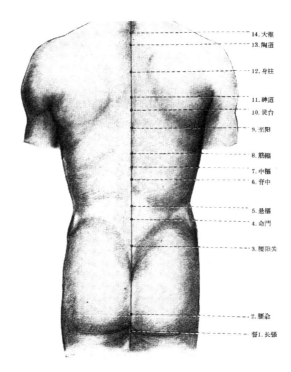

**FIGURE 12.5** Acupoints on the tips of spinous processes of some vertebrae.

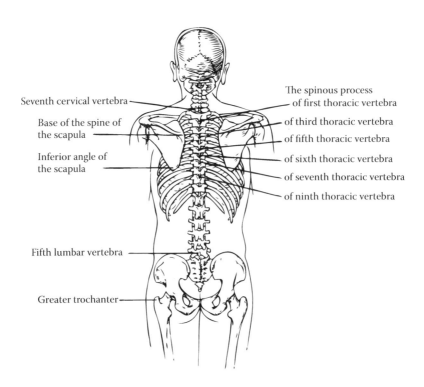

**FIGURE 12.6** A posterior view of the vertebral column.

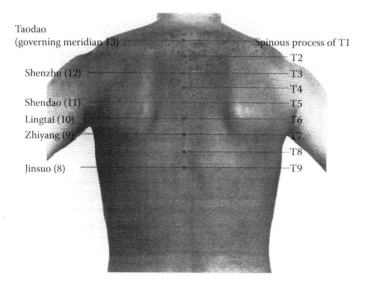

**FIGURE 12.7** A photograph of the posterior thoracic wall showing the anatomical locations of the spinous processes of the upper nine thoracic vertebrae and the names of the acupoints translated from Chinese.

**TABLE 12.6**
**Acupoints on the Spinous Processes of the Thoracic Vertebrae in the Passive Phase in Patients with Pain Symptoms**

| Spinous Process | Acupuncture Points (Traditional Chinese Terms) | In Passive Phase Frequency | (%) |
|---|---|---|---|
| T1 | Taodao | 42 | 19.2 |
| T2 | | 17 | 7.8 |
| T3 | Shenzhu | 90 | 41.1 |
| T4 | | 31 | 14.2 |
| T5 | Shendao | 147 | 67.1 |
| T6 | Lingtai | 79 | 36.1 |
| T7 | Zhiyang | 177 | 80.9 |
| T8 | | 32 | 14.6 |
| T9 | Jinsuo | 39 | 17.8 |

vertebrae. The results of pain measurement using the number of trigger points in the thoracic vertebrae will be discussed first, followed by the results of pain measurement in which the four groups of trigger points are used.

### 12.7.1 PAIN MEASUREMENT BY COUNTING TRIGGER POINTS IN THE THORACIC VERTEBRAE

For all nine thoracic spinous processes in Table 12.6, T7 is the first one to become a trigger point. T5 will be the second to convert, followed by T3, T6, and T9. Although the sequence for the last three points can vary, they always turn into trigger points after T7 and T5. In other words, T3, T6, and T9 will not become trigger points if T7 and T5 have not already done so. In turn, the spinous processes of T1, T2, T4, and T8 will not become trigger points before the other five points have already done so. More spinous processes in the thoracic vertebrae turning into trigger points seem to indicate a

### TABLE 12.7
### Sex and Age Distributions of Patients Surveyed for Passive Acupuncture Points on the Spinous Processes of the First Nine Thoracic Vertebrae

|              | Male Patients |      | Female Patients |      | Total Patients |       |
| ------------ | ------------- | ---- | --------------- | ---- | -------------- | ----- |
| Age in Years | No.           | (%)  | No.             | (%)  | No.            | (%)   |
| 10–19        | 0             | 0.0  | 1               | 0.8  | 1              | 0.5   |
| 20–29        | 6             | 6.8  | 8               | 6.1  | 14             | 6.4   |
| 30–39        | 16            | 18.2 | 24              | 18.3 | 40             | 18.3  |
| 40–49        | 15            | 17.0 | 21              | 16.0 | 36             | 16.4  |
| 50–59        | 16            | 18.2 | 28              | 21.4 | 44             | 20.1  |
| 60–69        | 21            | 23.9 | 33              | 25.2 | 54             | 24.6  |
| 70–79        | 31            | 14.8 | 14              | 10.7 | 27             | 12.3  |
| 80–89        | 1             | 1.1  | 2               | 1.5  | 3              | 1.4   |
|              | 88            | 40.2 | 131             | 58.9 | 219            | 100.0 |

longer duration of pain in the patient. We believe that T7 can be appropriately used as a primary point; T5 as a secondary; T3, T6, and T9 as tertiary; and T1, T2, T4, and T8 as nonspecific.

Patients frequently reported a discrepancy in sensitivity during the process of checking trigger points in the thoracic spinous processes. Many times when T7 was first tested, patients would respond by saying that it was painful. As the test was moved to T5, the same patients might also indicate pain, but then add that it was not as painful as the previous point. The responses clearly indicated some difference in the quantity of pain at the two trigger points. Thus, painful sensitivity in T7 could deserve a full credit and in T5 only partial credit with less perceivable pain. The same consideration should also apply to other trigger points in the thoracic spinous processes: one full credit for tenderness equal to that of T5 and partial credit for tenderness less than that of T7. The degree of pain for patients can be calculated using the formula $T \times 2 = D$, where $T$ is the number of trigger points gaining full or half credit for sensitivity. By the time T7 becomes a trigger point, the objective pain has reached the second degree. Rarely, will more than six thoracic spinous processes turn into trigger points, and even if they do, one or more of them will have only half a credit in sensitivity, making 12 the highest degree of objective pain possible.

Measuring objective pain in the patients using the method described sounds rather simple. However, some experience is required to obtain accurate measurements of objective pain efficiently. For example, if a patient has no trigger points in the thoracic spinous processes, $T$ in the formula will be considered as equal to zero, and the degree of the objective pain in the patient will also be zero. However, this zero degree doesn't mean that the patient is free of pain. The reason is that the acupoint in the spinous process of the seventh thoracic vertebrate ranks twentieth in the sequence of primary acupoints becoming trigger points. Out of all the patients we received, only 80.5% were found to have T7 in the passive phase, and for some of them, the tenderness at that point could be considered as having only partial credit because it was less sensitive compared with primary points that ranked higher in the sequence. It is also possible for patients to have third-degree objective pain measured using trigger points distributed systematically throughout the body, yet still have their T7 in the latent phase.

Another example of experience required is determining whether a trigger point should be given full credit or half credit. In general, T7 will be most sensitive among all trigger points in the same patients. Anything less sensitive than T7 should gain only half credit. Sometimes, two or more other trigger points have sensitivity equal to that of T7. Then, it will be acceptable to give all of them only half credit. A lot of clinical practice with many patients will naturally improve one's skill for measuring objective pain correctively and reliably.

Finally, although T6 becomes a trigger point much less often than T5, when it does turn, it can be as sensitive as T5.

There are many more examples that can be cited to discuss applying the trigger points in the thoracic spinous processes to measure objective pain. They will be realized after more experience is obtained in using trigger points for pain measurement.

One last comment about trigger points in the thoracic spinous processes: Why acupoints on the thoracic spinous processes turn into trigger points in such an orderly sequence is unknown. No physiological explanation is available. Anatomically, we know that the tips of the spinous processes are joined by a strong supraspinous ligament. The supraspinous ligament expands to form the ligamentum nuchae in the cervical and thoracic vertebral regions. At the attachments of the ligament to the spinous processes, there are numerous free nerve endings that are terminals of nonmyelinated and finely myelinated afferent fibers, which are nociceptive in nature. We don't know if one spinous process has more of the nociceptive afferent fibers than others. From our study, the spinous process of T2, T4, and T8 were not recognized as having acupoints in traditional acupuncture schools simply because the frequency for them to become trigger points is much lower than for other thoracic spinous processes.

### 12.7.2 Pain Measurement by Counting Trigger Points in the Body

The second method for measuring pain is by counting the number of trigger points detected in the entire body. We were able to garner 436 patients for this study. Their sex and age distributions are shown in Table 12.8. Using this number, we constructed Figures 12.8 through 12.11. Before interpreting what these four figures mean in the measurement of objective pain, it will help to make a few comments on how the results of the study were collected. First, in this study, only the first 96 acupoints in sequence were used, meaning that each degree of objective pain was encompassed by eight trigger points. The last 14 acupoints were dropped because they were so infrequently found to become passive. Second, there were some variations noticed in our testing to determine whether acupoints had indeed been converted from latent to passive phase and become trigger points. There was some subjectivity involved in testing. For example, different trigger points in a patient could exhibit different intensities of tenderness. This variation in intensity made it difficult to regard them as having full credit or half credit. Thus, no such full/half credit distinction is made for the trigger points; they are considered the same as long as they are tender upon testing. Generally speaking, trigger points ranking higher in the sequence will be more sensitive and it is easier for patients to

**TABLE 12.8**
**Sex and Age Distributions of Patients Coming in for Pain Management and Pain Quantification**

| Age in Years | Female Patients | | Male Patients | | Total Patients | |
|---|---|---|---|---|---|---|
| | No. | (%) | No. | (%) | No. | (%) |
| 10–19 | 5 | 1.98 | 2 | 1.09 | 7 | 0.61 |
| 20–29 | 22 | 8.73 | 13 | 7.07 | 35 | 8.03 |
| 30–39 | 39 | 15.47 | 36 | 19.57 | 75 | 17.20 |
| 40–49 | 49 | 19.44 | 33 | 17.93 | 82 | 18.80 |
| 50–59 | 51 | 20.24 | 38 | 20.65 | 89 | 20.42 |
| 60–69 | 42 | 16.67 | 38 | 20.65 | 80 | 18.35 |
| 70–79 | 35 | 13.89 | 21 | 11.41 | 56 | 12.84 |
| 80–89 | 9 | 3.59 | 3 | 1.63 | 12 | 2.75 |
| | 252 | 100 | 184 | 100 | 436 | 100.0 |

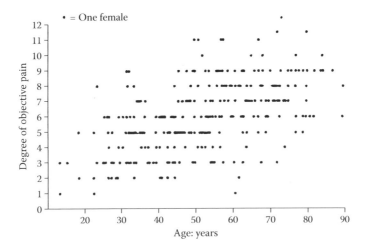

**FIGURE 12.8** Degrees of objective pain in female patients with their trigger points counted. Each degree encompasses eight trigger points.

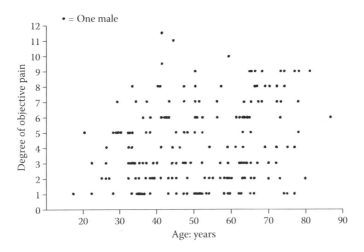

**FIGURE 12.9** Degrees of objective pain in male patients with their trigger points counted. Each degree encompasses eight trigger points.

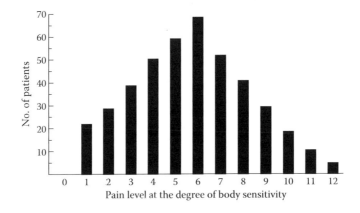

**FIGURE 12.10** Total number of patients and their pain levels and degree of sensitivity.

Pain and Measurement

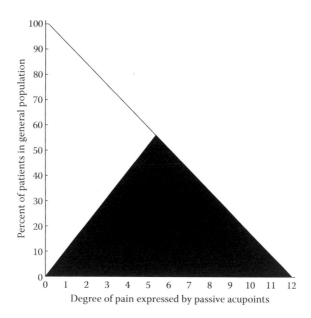

**FIGURE 12.11** Percentage of patients in the general population and their degrees of objective pain.

feel pain when they are pressed. Trigger points ranking lower in the sequence will be less sensitive and it is harder for patients to perceive pain when they are pressed. The transition for acupoints to become trigger points can be abrupt. In some cases, the point which ranks no. 26 in sequence is tender, whereas a point ranking no. 27 is not. In other instances, the point which ranks 26 is tender, and those ranking 27 to 29 are also tender but with less intensity. The possibility also exists for nos. 26 and 29 to become trigger points, but nos. 27 and 28 could stay in the latent phase, without tenderness perceived by the patients. The sequence for acupoints to change from latent to passive phase is not absolute. Their sequential order is based on statistical results, and variance is expected. The variations are most likely to appear toward the end of the sequence of the objective pain in a particular degree. For instance, if the objective pain is fifth degree, the last acupoint to become a trigger could be nos. 40, 41, or even 42.

Figures 12.8 and 12.9 are the results of the study described above. Figure 12.8 is charted from 252 female patients, whereas Figure 12.9 is from 184 male patients. Both charts summarize the distributions of objective pain in degrees from 0 to 12 for patients aged 13 to 90 years. As explained above, the degree of objective pain is obtained by counting how many trigger points the patients have. Each patient was found to have a different number of trigger points. The number varies from individual to individual, and whether each of them has the same or different kinds of pain. The number of trigger points collected can be considered as objective because patients were blind to what was going on for them. Patients knew neither the location of acupoints nor the sequence of the trigger points. It would be difficult, if not impossible, for patients to fake the results of testing trigger points. Determining the honesty of patients in testing is relatively easy. We first test an acupoint at a lower ranking of the sequence, and the patient's response to the test is positive. Then, another acupoint at a higher sequence ranking is tested, and the response is negative. We then know that patient is faking the test. The only time patients know where acupoints are located is when acupoints turn to trigger points that are in the active phase. Trigger points in the active phase are what we describe as subjective pain.

As we inspect Figures 12.8 and 12.9, we notice one difference. The distribution of objective pain in Figure 12.9 is rather random. Some young men have high degrees of objective pain, and some older male patients have low degrees of objective pain. The distribution of objective pain in

Figure 12.8 seems to have a tendency to increase with age. It seems that as female patients grow older, their objective pain tends to become higher in degree. This difference in genders may be due to functional differences in physiology. One such physiological difference is menstrual activity in female patients. A large number of female patients seen in the clinic suffered dysmenorrhea with frequent monthly menstrual cramping, which we believe is a serious source of subjective pain with endogenous origins. If a subjective pain is not or cannot be stopped, the objective pain will be increased and perpetuated. This is why the objective pain in female patients has a tendency to go higher in degree as they grow older.

Figure 12.10 is a chart constructed using both male and female patients in the study. Each degree of objective pain consists of a number of patients among the total of 436. For example, 68 patients had sixth-degree objective pain, 39 patients had third-degree pain, six patients had twelfth-degree pain, and so on.

The distribution of patients in each of the 12 degrees of objective pain forms a bell-shaped curve. The highest number is in the sixth degree, and the number decreases toward both ends of the curve. Such a distribution is unexpected. The expected distribution was a straight line, with the highest number at degree one and lowest at 12, as shown in Figure 12.11. As shown in the drawing, most patients who came for acupuncture tended to have higher degrees of objective pain. In fact, the majority were higher than the sixth degree. Fewer patients had objective pain that was less than the fifth degree. One feasible explanation was that subjective pain in patients with lower degrees of objective pain was easier to manage by conventional therapeutic approaches, such as over-the-counter painkillers, chiropractic adjustments, physical therapy, and other neuromodulation remedies. Most of us are needle-phobic. Going to acupuncturists is most likely the last thought to come to mind when people face painful distress in the early stages. Acupuncture for almost all of the patients we encountered was the last resort after other available means to cure or stop their pain failed. Of course, there may be other reasons for the way acupuncture has been received in the United States, but adequately covering all those reasons is beyond the scope of this book.

## 12.8 ACUTE VERSUS CHRONIC PAIN

One of the most commonly used criteria in clinically defining which pain is acute and which is chronic is time duration. The most often used time duration is 3 to 6 months, which is clearly arbitrary and illogical. How should a pain be classified when the duration is 1 to 3 days shorter or longer than 3 or 6 months? How about a pain that suddenly disappears 1 week before a duration of 6 months is reached, then reappears 1 month later? Should such a pain be considered as acute or a chronic? There are many more contradictions that medical doctors will face if we insist on defining acute and chronic pain based on the time element alone. The contradictions are due to one single fact: To this day, we all attempt to differentiate acute pain from chronic pain based on our comprehension of what subjective pain is. Subjective pain is capricious; it changes frequently from time to time. It cannot be fathomed. We suggest using objective pain to define acute and chronic pain.

The objective pain produced in trigger points is stable. It can and will stay in the trigger points unchanged for months to years. Yes, objective pain invariably accompanies or follows subjective pain. However, there are times when subjective pain has subsided, and objective pain has remained in the trigger points. Without preexisting objective pain in any acupoint, or in other words, without having trigger points, new injury of endogenous or exogenous origin has little or no chance to develop into a chronic state. The injury will heal on its own or will be treated medically, and the subjective pain, which is acute in nature, should subside in time. On the other hand, if patients have a number of trigger points already existing in the body before any injury of endogenous or exogenous origin, the injury may seem to be acute, yet have the potential to become chronic. How long it will take for an acute pain to develop into a chronic pain depends on how high a degree of objective pain the patient has. No favorable circumstances are available for us to conduct clinical studies, and no scientific data has been collected to prove a meaningful relationship between the degree of objective pain and the speed at which an acute pain is capable of becoming chronic. From our observations, we have reasons to believe the duration of time for acute pain to grow into the chronic stage can be stated in four simple terms. For patients with trigger points limited to the primary group of acupoints, the time duration can be many months or even years. For patients having trigger points within the secondary group, the time duration can be weeks to months. If trigger points reach the tertiary group of acupoints, an acute pain will not take long at all, an estimated period of days to weeks, to become chronic. For patients who have trigger points in the nonspecific group, any fresh injury can be considered as chronic from the time it occurs. Only time will tell whether what has been said above is correct. It is our wish that those who have interest in the study of acupuncture and pain will take time to look into the matters mentioned here. If what is said should be proven to be accurate, it will be a revolutionary way for us to understand the relationship between acute and chronic pain.

## REFERENCES

1. Melzack, R. and P.D. Wall. *The Challenge of Pain.* Basic Books, Inc., New York, 1983.
2. Bonica, J.J. *The Management of Pain*, vols. I and II, 2nd ed. Lea & Febiger, Philadelphia, 1990.
3. Bond, M.R. *Pain: Its Nature, Analysis and Treatment.* Churchill Livingstone, New York, 1979.
4. *Essentials of Chinese Acupuncture.* Foreign Languages Press, Beijing, China, 1980.
5. Dung, H.C. A simple new method for the quantification of chronic pain. *American Journal of Acupuncture* 13:59, 1985.
6. Dung, H.C. Survey of passive acupuncture points on thoracic spinous processes in individuals suffering from pain. *American Journal of Acupuncture* 14:15, 1986.

# 13 Good to Excellent Applications

## 13.1 GENERAL GUIDELINES

After learning of the possibility of measuring objective pain in patients, a study was set to determine if there might be relationships between the objective pain measured and the results of acupuncture applications. The specific relationships investigated included the percentage of patients who gained relief from acupuncture treatments, how many treatments were required to achieve noticeable relief, the probability of the same pain relapsing, and if so, the probable time lapse before its recurrence. The results of the study were tabulated in Table 13.1. The data presented in the table were collected from 436 patients.

Objective pain was rated on a scale of 1 to 12 degrees and was divided into four groups: primary, secondary, tertiary, and nonspecific, as listed in the table. The general guidelines described in this chapter were drawn from these four groups of patients as the basis for referral. Take the patients in the primary group, whose objective pain ranged from 0 to 3 degrees, for example. Twenty-three out of 100 patients were in this group. Of those 23, the manageability of their subjective pain could range from 75% to 100%, meaning that there is a 75% to 100% possibility for relief. Achieving such an outcome would most likely require four to eight treatments. The chance for the same pain to relapse was 25% at most. On the other hand, only seven out of 100 were in the nonspecific group. The possibility of totally eradicating their pain was 25% at most, but could also turn out to be a total failure without any noticeable improvement, even after many repeated acupuncture sessions. How many tests are needed before such a conclusion can be drawn? The answer is uncertain. The same guidelines listed could similarly apply to patients in the secondary and tertiary groups.

One comment about the number of treatments required to achieve total relief of pain is that it involves a personal assumption of ideal circumstances—specifically, that patients will follow recommendations. For example, patients in the tertiary group are recommended to come for 16 to 32 acupuncture treatments for a chance at total eradication of their subjective pain. After total relief, the same pain will not recur for a long time. In reality, very few patients with objective pain at the tertiary stage have come for so many treatments, for a couple of reasons. Some patients had substantial pain relief before the required number of treatments was reached, and stopped coming for further therapy. The subjective pain was noticeably reduced, but was not completely eradicated, giving the same pain a chance to return. Other patients gave up on acupuncture after four or five sessions without noticeable improvement. They might have thought that acupuncture was not helpful, but in fact, they didn't give it a sufficient chance to work.

With respect to the duration of pain relief, there is a relation between how many treatments are received and how long the relief may last before a relapse. Not all patients come for the expected and required number of treatments. If they come for a few sessions, the duration of the relief can be shorter than anticipated. The overall results will not be different because if we add the number of treatments and the duration of relief together, the end results will be very much the same. We could use any patient as an example. One patient had objective pain in the secondary group and came for four treatments. The subjective pain disappeared. Acupuncture treatment was stopped. Four months later, the same patient returned with the same subjective pain. Three more treatments were provided, and the pain subsided again. The same pain relapsed again in 4 months, making the duration of relief 8 months in total. If the same patient had come continuously for a total of seven treatments from the beginning, the relief could last for the 8 months uninterrupted. In our practice,

**TABLE 13.1**
**A Summary of Chronic Pain Measurements Using Quantified Passive Acupoints as the Caliber to Measure Degrees or Levels of Pain**

| | Levels of Pain | | | |
|---|---|---|---|---|
| | Primary | Secondary | Tertiary | Nonspecific |
| | 1st–3rd Degree | 4th–6th degree | 7th–9th degree | 10th–12th degree |
| Estimated number of every 100 new patients received | 23 | 38 | 32 | 7 |
| Percentage of estimated number effectively treatable | 100–75 | 75–50 | 50–25 | 25–0 |
| Number of treatments required to achieve total relief of pain | 4–8 | 8–16 | 16–32 | >32 |
| Percentage of probability for the same pain to relapse or recur | 0–25 | 25–50 | 50–75 | 75–100 |
| Possible time lapse before the recurrence of same pain | Years | Months to years | Weeks to months | Days to weeks |

*Note:* A summary of patients seen in the clinic. Results indicate their objective pain measured in relation to therapeutic outcome in acupuncture treatments.

once the subjective pain disappears, no more justification exists to request the patient to come and receive more needles. The number of treatments required to achieve total pain relief is more of an ideal suggestion. Very few patients need to come for the required number of treatments to achieve the goal of pain relief.

Regarding the potential time lapse before the recurrence of the same pain, the decision to use days, weeks, months, and years was made for the sake of easy memorization. Few patients with objective pain in the primary group have the same pain recur after its elimination by acupuncture. To say these patients have years of relief should be a reasonable claim. The relief, if any, for patients in the nonspecific group is only days, or at the most, weeks. If all the patients are pooled together, the average relief of subjective pain in acupuncture therapy is approximately 4 to 6 months.

In a final analysis, to be a competent acupuncturist, one needs the sophistication to answer a few questions: Can any pain in a patient be successfully managed? If yes, then how many needling sessions will be required to stop the pain? What is the possibility for the same pain to return after its eradication, and after how long an interval? Observations from clinical experiences seem to suggest that the answers for questions of this inquisitive nature can be given in a few terms. These terms need to be rather broad and inclusive. We have chosen three headings for the terms. The first heading is good to excellent applications, which is described in this chapter. The second heading is applications with mixed and limited results, which will be found in Chapter 14. The third heading is poor results and difficult patients for acupuncture, which is covered in Chapter 15.

## 13.2 SAMPLES OF PAIN FOR DEMONSTRATION

We don't know how many different kinds of pain there are medically. It is not easy to determine which among the different kinds of pain we know will be most appropriate to use in clinical demonstrations showing how acupuncture treatments can be given. There is no scientific merit to saying

## TABLE 13.2
### Different Types of Pain Described by Acupuncture Patients

|  | 1981 | | 1982 | | 1983 | | 1984 | |
| --- | --- | --- | --- | --- | --- | --- | --- | --- |
|  | No. | (%) | No. | (%) | No. | (%) | No. | (%) |
| Lower back pain | 201 | 33.9 | 220 | 34.9 | 253 | 34.6 | 229 | 35.8 |
| Arthritic pain | 81 | 13.6 | 85 | 13.5 | 94 | 12.8 | 77 | 12.1 |
| Pain in neck and shoulder | 81 | 13.6 | 84 | 13.3 | 98 | 13.4 | 84 | 13.1 |
| Pain in knee and leg | 55 | 9.3 | 64 | 10.1 | 72 | 9.8 | 68 | 10.6 |
| Headache | 50 | 8.5 | 57 | 9.0 | 53 | 7.2 | 45 | 7.0 |
| Pain in ankle and foot | 20 | 3.4 | 22 | 3.9 | 24 | 3.3 | 20 | 3.1 |
| Pain in arm and elbow | 18 | 3.0 | 16 | 2.5 | 26 | 3.6 | 25 | 3.9 |
| Pain in wrist and hand | 16 | 2.8 | 11 | 1.7 | 22 | 3.0 | 21 | 3.2 |
| Myofascial pain | 15 | 2.5 | 15 | 2.4 | 19 | 2.6 | 13 | 2.0 |
| Cramping | 13 | 2.2 | 10 | 1.5 | 14 | 1.9 | 11 | 1.7 |
| Temporomandibular pain | 6 | 1.0 | 5 | 0.8 | 3 | 0.4 | 7 | 1.1 |
| Neuritis and neuropathy | 5 | 0.8 | 7 | 1.1 | 5 | 0.7 | 6 | 0.9 |
| Herpes | 4 | 0.7 | 5 | 0.7 | 8 | 1.1 | 7 | 1.1 |
| Trigeminal neuralgia | 1 | 0.2 | 3 | 0.4 | 5 | 0.7 | 3 | 0.5 |
| All others | 27 | 4.5 | 27 | 4.2 | 36 | 4.9 | 23 | 3.6 |

*Note:* Types of pain as described by acupuncture patients.

that arthritic pain is more important than headaches, or that lower back pain is less urgent than a herpes infection. Pain is pain, regardless of where and for whatever reason it occurs. The types of pain seen in the clinic have stayed the same throughout many years. As can be seen in Table 13.2, the pain that is most commonly mentioned in writing by patients is lower back pain, followed by arthritic pain, pain in the neck and shoulder, pain in the knee and leg, headaches, and so on. There are 14 pains listed in the table. No checklists are available for all other kinds of pain, which involves only 3.6% of the total number of patients we have.

In the end, we thought it would be fair to select pain based on anatomical locations, such as headache, neck pain, pain in the upper limb, pain in the body trunk, and pain in the lower limb. Two kinds of pain from each of these five localities can serve as representatives for one area. The pains chosen are those most commonly suffered by patients arriving in the clinic. In the head, the types of pain selected are headache and temporomandibular pain. Headache can be tension, cluster, migraine, trigeminal, or postherpetic neuralgia. Pain in the neck and shoulder can be whiplash, arthritis, rotator cuff damage, or stiff neck. Pain in the upper limb can be tennis elbow, superficial radial neuropathy, carpal tunnel syndrome, and arthritic pain in the wrist or in the fingers. Pain in the body trunk can be myofascial pain, menstrual cramping, herpes infection, or lower back pain. Pain in the lower limb can be osteoarthritic knee, splinted ankle, tarsal tunnel syndrome, or plantar fasciatis. Two to three cases will be chosen from our large patient pool to represent one type of pain selected for demonstration. Demographic data of the patient pool from which the examples were chosen is summarized in Table 13.3. There were 3,669 patients, of which 1,074 (41.4%) were male and 2,595 (58.6%) were female. In all the statistics we have, there are always significantly more female patients than male patients. Only a tiny number of patients were selected for the purpose of demonstration compared with the total number of examples we have.

**TABLE 13.3**
**Sex and Age Distributions of Patients Examined for Passive Acupuncture Points**

| Age in Years | Male No. | Male (%) | Female No. | Female (%) | Total No. | Total (%) |
|---|---|---|---|---|---|---|
| Younger than 19 | 15 | 1.4 | 24 | 1.6 | 39 | 1.5 |
| 20–29 | 100 | 9.3 | 131 | 8.6 | 231 | 8.9 |
| 30–39 | 202 | 18.8 | 254 | 16.7 | 456 | 17.6 |
| 40–49 | 185 | 17.2 | 239 | 15.7 | 424 | 16.4 |
| 50–59 | 208 | 19.4 | 309 | 20.3 | 517 | 19.9 |
| 60–69 | 213 | 19.8 | 280 | 18.4 | 493 | 19.0 |
| 70–79 | 137 | 12.8 | 213 | 14.1 | 350 | 13.5 |
| Older than 80 | 14 | 1.3 | 71 | 4.7 | 85 | 3.3 |
| Total | 1,074 | 41.4 | 1,521 | 58.6 | 2,595 | 100.0 |

*Note:* Sex and age distributions of patients with pain as the main reason for seeking acupuncture treatment.

## 13.3 DEFINING GOOD TO EXCELLENT RESULTS

From the demographic profiles collected, patients who will have good to excellent results from acupuncture treatments can be summarized as follows. They are younger than 40 years of age and appear physically healthy without other illness besides the pain for which they come to seek relief. Their pain is invariably new and acute in nature. They are suffering the pain for the first time. It is in a single locality that is limited to only one area. The degree of objective pain measured is no more than fourth degree, sometimes only first or second degree, and the number of trigger points detected is 10 or less. In such patients, less than 16 needles are required to stop the pain in one or two sessions.

Therapeutically, the subjective pain in patients whose objective pain is no more than fourth degree can be effectively managed by taking nonprescription analgesic medicine of some kind. Other methods that have neuromodulation function, such as chiropractic adjustments, physical therapies, use of transcutaneous electrical nerve stimulation (TENS) units, massage, and rubbing in reflexology, can all be useful in managing pain in patients whose objective pain is fourth degree or less. Very rarely will patients in this group with objective pain between first and fourth degree ever return for the same kind of pain.

## 13.4 PAIN IN THE FACE AND HEAD

It is correct to say that all pain occurring in the face and head originates from the trigeminal nerve. The afferent fibers in this cranial nerve are ubiquitous. They are distributed throughout the entire face and head, including the facial surface and interior cavities of the head, such as the nasal sinuses, their linings, and meninges. Disturbance, irritation, infection, or inflammation of any of these afferent fibers will result in generating nociceptive sensation to produce pain.

Approximately 8% to 9% of patients can be considered as having pain in the face and head [1]. In 1995, out of 881 patients coming to visit for the first time, 74 could be considered as having pain in the face and head. Their pain can be divided into two essential kinds: headache and nonheadache. Sixty-nine of them used the word "headache" to describe their medical problem. Only five used words other than headache, even though, upon inquiry, they revealed that they were not totally free of headache. The adjectives used to describe their headache included migraine, cluster, tension, sinus, depression, premenstrual, and pressure. The headaches could be felt in the front or back of the head. The causes of headaches, in their opinion, consisted of allergies, smoking, neuralgia, brain damage, tumor, herpes, muscle spasms, and concussion. Most headache patients didn't distinguish these different kinds; all they wrote down was "headache." The five nonheadache patients indicated that they had Bell's palsy, or facial paralysis and twitching in the face. A few cases of patients with headache have been selected as examples to demonstrate how acupuncture works to stop their pain in the head. The number is small, but may serve sufficient purpose to show how acupuncture works to manage headache or other kinds of pain.

*Case 1*: Marsha O. was a 31-year-old female. On her first visit, she used the words "acute migraine" to describe her problem. She said that she had been to medical doctors, and none of them had really helped to ease her misery. She did have brief relief from a chiropractor, but had to keep going frequently. Finally, she had stopped going because she had grown tired of chiropractic manipulation. She had also tried reflexology using foot rubbing, without any appreciable result. The bad headache attacks could come as frequently as three times in a week. During bad attacks, she had been hospitalized and received injections. During migraine attacks, she had nausea, although she didn't experience vomiting. During menstrual periods, she would have severe cramping, which would exacerbate the headache. Bright light and loud noise could trigger the headaches. She felt tired all the time. Most headaches began on the left side of the head, but they could also start from the right. Regardless, each headache always ended on the left side. Her objective pain was measured to be fourth degree. Her primary acupoints in the face (supraorbital and infraorbital) and in the neck (great auricular, greater occipital, and spinal accessory) were all in passive phase with palpable tenderness. The secondary acupoints (mental, masseter, superior auricular, temporomandibular, lesser occipital, and cervical plexus) were also passive with tender sensation. Even a few tertiary acupoints, such as the bregma, pterion, and temporalis were slightly tender. Outside of the head and neck, only primary acupoints were found to be in passive phase. The appearance of passive acupoints in patients like Marsha is rather typical because the main pain is in the face and head. Therefore, more trigger points will appear in the painful region to begin with. This phenomenon is particularly prevalent in the early stages of headache development. Systematically considering the body as a whole, objective pain in Marsha can be categorized as in the range of the primary points. Because she also had trigger points in the secondary and tertiary groups, she was assigned fourth-degree objective pain. At this degree, subjective pain occurring as headaches can be effectively managed with good to excellent results. Such was the case for Marsha. The method to treat her headache, or patients with other kinds of pain within four degrees of objective pain, is relatively simple and requires few (four or fewer) in sessions. For the first treatment, Marsha was placed in a supine position. One needle was inserted into each of the trigger points listed in the primary group as shown in Figure 12.2. Additional needles were placed in three of the secondary (mental, masseter, and superior auricular) trigger points mentioned above, for a total of 34 needles used, with 17 along one side of the body from the face down to the feet. Two days later, she came for the second treatment. She was placed in the prone position. Trigger points used included all primary group points in the back (Figure 12.2) and the temporomandibular, lesser occipital, and cervical plexus in the secondary group. A total of 35 needles were used, one more than in the first session of treatments. That one needle was on the spinous process of the seventh thoracic vertebra. On her third visit, 2 days after the second treatment, she reported that she hadn't had any headaches in the previous 4 days. Patients with any kind of headache are asked to take a sitting position for the third treatment. In that position, all of the trigger points in the primary and secondary groups located in the head, face and neck regions, plus a few trigger points in the tertiary group (bregma, pterion, and temporalis) are available for needling. A total of 29 needles were used. By the time the patient came for her fourth treatment, she hadn't had a headache for a week. She did have tension in the back of her head because she had to take care of a disabled husband at home. She often didn't know what to expect after a day of work, and claimed that she had a great deal of stress and tension. For the fourth treatment, she was placed in the supine position again, repeating what had been done for her in the first treatment. Fifteen days after the first treatment, she came for a fifth visit. She reported that the headache had relapsed once in a week's time because she was under a lot of stress and pressure. She had lived under a great deal of tension the previous week. Fortunately, that headache subsided on its own without her having to take any drugs. Acupuncture treatments were repeated using the supine, prone, and sitting positions in an alternated manner. The number of needles used in each treatment was maintained the same, using very much the same trigger points described for each of them. For two consecutive months, she came in three times for one week each month, for a total of 11 treatments. One month after her last visit, she called to cancel the next appointment because she said that she already hadn't had any headache for more than a month. She indicated that she would call if her migraine attacked again. We have not received a telephone call from Marsha O. for more than 28 years. Migraine has one difference from other types of headache with respect to changes of objective pain. The objective pain in migraine can vary from as low as 1 or 2 degrees to as high as 11 or 12. This is the reason we think that some migraines are easy to manage with good to excellent results, whereas some are very difficult to treat and the results are often poor. Patients having other kinds of headaches, such as cluster, tension, or allergic, tend to have objective pain no higher than six degrees. Thus, they are relatively easy to care for. On the other hand, most patients suffering from tic douloureux and postherpetic neuralgia along the trigeminal nerve will have objective pain at the eighth degree or higher. This is why these kinds of headaches are often difficult to manage. Their management will be discussed in the next two chapters. To ensure that the same type of headache will not return, it is prudent to provide an additional series of three treatments during that interval. If the headache hadn't returned after 1 month, the chances of it coming back will be minimal.

*Case 2*: James M. was 69 years old. He was selected to represent patients with cluster headache, which is not commonly seen, often no more than one to two cases in a year. In fact, he indicated on the form he filled out that he had cluster migraine. The term did not come from diagnosis by his physician but his own opinion. How he came to conclude that his headache was cluster migraine is a mystery to us. His recollection was that he had had the headache for the last 30 years of his life. He claimed that, for all those years, he was able to ease the headache by taking medicine, although he did not elaborate on what kind. Sometimes, he would stop taking medicine for months, although he did not explain why. When he stopped taking medicine, his headache would get worse. Most times, the headache was on the left side of the face around the ocular area. His objective pain was measured to be fifth degree. During his first visit, he was placed in the supine position. The trigger points used were all in the primary group. The second and third treatments for James were similar to those for Marsha. The first three acupuncture treatments for all patients coming with a headache are the same. The sequential order of positions taken is supine, prone, and sitting. The trigger points are mostly from the primary group. A few secondary or even tertiary trigger points can be added if such an addition is helpful in patients whose objective pain can be higher than third degree. Most of the patients having cluster headaches were male. They were easy to manage. All but one acknowledged that the headache was gone after three or four acupuncture sessions. None of the patients with cluster headache, including James, ever returned with the same problem. He came for three treatments, the last of which was in March 22, 1985. He did come back on March 16, 1987, not because of the headache, but because he wanted to stop smoking. For 2 years, he was free of any headache. On January 19, 1988, he visited again because he had "left sciatic pain." At that time, his objective pain was measured to be only third degree. The procedures for treating lower back pain will be described subsequently. For James's case, all we will say here is that he was free of "left sciatic pain" after four sessions. He has not come again since February 1, 1988.

*Case 3*: Steffany T. was a 17-year-old high school student suffering temporomandibular joint syndrome (TMJ), about which we have a few preliminary comments. This term is used to include pain located in the temporomandibular joint without direct cause from dental and orofacial origins. The pain can be associated with the muscles of mastication or the TMJ itself. The pathophysiology of this pain disorder is not very well understood. Even the existence of the syndrome is controversial. Dental professionals accept the reality of the problem and treat it as such. There are medical practitioners who don't believe that there is such a disease as TMJ syndrome. Patients like Steffany are not common. She came with a rather complete medical history, presented in writing. She brought her report upon visiting the clinic on June 17, 1996. The report described her problem as "my neck, shoulders, and throat are always tight. My throat gets real tight when I sing, talk, or chew. My ears ache as if I have swimmer's ears. I always have a headache at the temples and in between my eyes. My temples and the upper right side of my jaws are tender to the touch. My left side pops at the joint, but it doesn't bother me as much as the right side does. My bottom teeth feel like they are going to fall out. When I eat soft food, talk very little and don't sing, it helps. I constantly take Ibuprofen, Tylenol, and Excedrin to relieve the pain. Ice packs and Mineral Ice are great to use while the pain killers are kicking in. It hurts when I whistle and for some unknown reason I am always crying. These symptoms have been going on for about three years. I have been to see: one oral dental surgeon who took out my wisdom teeth, thinking they were pressing on a nerve, two chiropractors who couldn't find anything wrong, one orthodontist who gave me a prescribed mouthpiece, and a regular dentist who said my problem was caused by tension." Using the method described in Chapter 12, Steffany was measured to have objective pain at the sixth degree. This is the highest degree of objective pain that would limit the manageability of symptoms described for this patient while still having good to excellent results after acupuncture treatments. Steffany was the youngest patient we have had with TMJ. Young age is a very favorable factor in acupuncture therapy. At sixth degree, TMJ would be harder to manage if her age was, say, 45 years or older. The first treatment was provided with her in the supine position. Trigger points in the primary group, plus one needle each in the auriculotemporal and TMJ points in front of one ear were used. Two days later, on June 19, she came for the second treatment. She was asked if she knew her blood pressure, and she said explicitly that it was 70 mm Hg diastolically and 93 mm Hg systolically. Having blood pressure so low is a possible reason for the symptoms she had. Another causative factor is menstrual cramping, and Steffany did suffer from monthly cramping pain during her period. She indicated that the first treatment seemed to help her feel better. The second treatment was made with her in the prone position, using all trigger points in the primary group. Her third treatment was given on June 21 with her sitting upright, using the trigger points in the primary and secondary groups accessible in the head, face, neck and upper limbs, plus the auriculotemporal and TMJ points. There was a 1-week break between two series of three treatments each. She came for the fourth visit on June 28. During her fourth visit, she reported that most of her problems were at the left ear only, and the discomfort was slight. When she came for the fifth treatment, she was asked to lay on her right side so the focus could be on the left ear. In addition to the primary group of trigger points accessible, four needles were placed around the left ear at the auriculotemporal, TMJ, superior auricular and posterior auricular points. She was told that four treatments should be able to stop her pain for at least a while, and that if for any reason the symptoms persisted, she could return for more treatments. She came back on October 21, 1996. Her TMJ symptoms had relapsed, which she attributed to her excessive gum-chewing and too much jumping exercises. She said that sweating seemed to ease pain momentarily. Over the next 5 days, three more treatments were given with the same protocol described above for the first three visits. Her last visit was on October 26, and she has not returned since. Steffany ended up coming for a total of seven treatments. It is possible that she might have needed fewer treatments if she had come in at an earlier stage of the development of her problem, as the degree of the objective pain would most likely have been lower. Nevertheless, it is still reasonable to conclude that the result of acupuncture treatments for the patient can be considered good to excellent.

## 13.5 PAIN IN THE NECK AND SHOULDERS

Anatomically, the neck and shoulder are interconnected and continuous with each other. Muscles such as the trapezius cover both areas. Pain in the region originates from the greater occipital, lesser occipital, third occipital, great auricular, transverse cervical, supraclavicular, dorsal scapular, and spinal accessory nerves. The spinal accessory is a cranial nerve. The lesser occipital, great auricular, transverse cervical, and supraclavicular are branches of the cervical plexus. The dorsal scapular and suprascapular are branches of the brachial plexus. Efferent fibers in the spinal accessory are originated in the upper cervical spinal cord. They go through the foramen magnum to enter the cranial cavity, and reemerge out of the cavity by way of the jugular foramen. These efferent fibers control the actions of the trapezius and the sternocleidomastoid muscles. However, the afferent fibers responsible for nociception to the same muscles come directly from the cervical plexus without going through the cranial cavity. The dorsal scapular and the suprascapular nerves are both muscular. Muscular nerve branches contain afferent, efferent, and postganglionic sympathetic fibers. Three muscles are innervated by the dorsal scapular nerve: the levator scapulae, and the rhomboidus minor and major muscles, which attach to the medial border of the scapula. The motor point formed between the dorsal scapular nerve and the muscles is located right at the base of the spine of the scapula where the rhomboidus minor is inserted into the bone. The suprascapular nerve innervates the supraspinatus and infraspinatus muscles. Their motor points are located right at the geometric center of each muscle. This brief review shows that anatomical arrangements for the innervations in the neck and shoulder seem to be rather haphazard. Pain in the neck and shoulder can cross from a cranial nerve cephalically to branches of cervical and brachial plexuses caudally. Occasionally, patients will describe having pain from the shoulder blade to the middle point of the shoulder bridge ending up in the back of head, as shown in Figure 13.1. It is quite easy to see how pain in the neck and shoulder can be complicated. Is pain in the upper back a headache or a neckache? It all depends on how patients present their pain to you. There are many forms of pain in the neck and shoulder. One of the most often encountered pains in the neck is whiplash. Whiplash can be due to a minor automobile accident, resulting in a fracture in the cervical vertebrae. Here is a classic case of whiplash resulting from an auto accident. It is clearly a case with acute pain, and the degree of objective pain is not too high. The result of acupuncture treatment can be confidently claimed as good to excellent.

Kuang-Hua Chang (Figure 13.2) was a 29-year-old captain in the Taiwan Air Force. We decided to use his case as an example for a few reasons: He agreed for us to use his picture and name, the duration of his pain was short, and his pain was, without any doubt, acute. The captain was a student

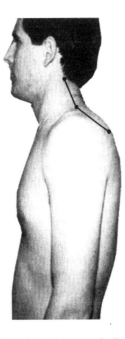

**FIGURE 13.1** The black line in the neck and shoulder area indicates the location of pain from the trigger point on the dorsal scapular below, to the spinal accessory over the trapezius muscle, ending at the greater occipital right at the hairline above. There are intercommunications between these three nerves.

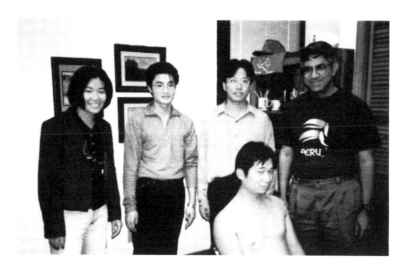

**FIGURE 13.2** Captain Kuang-Hua Chang (sitting), accompanied by three of his military comrades from Taiwan and one of his instructors.

at the Defense Language Institute on Lackland Air Force Base, San Antonio, Texas. He was brought to our clinic on October 17, 1996 by his instructor, who was an acquaintance, because of a rather severe automobile accident the previous week. He had received very good medical care after the incident. No bones were fractured, yet he had experienced terrible neck pain since. He couldn't turn his neck at all. He was told he had whiplash, from which acute pain would be expected, and that nothing could be done to speed up his recuperation. It would take time to recover from the injury, and the pain would naturally subside. However, the captain said that he was unable to sleep. Without proper sleep and rest, he had no way to learn effectively at the language school, and he had only a limited time to learn his English for the next destination in his training program. He needed to have immediate relief, without further delay. His physician at Wilford Hall USAF Hospital suggested that he come for my acupuncture, and one of his instructors, who knew me, brought him to me. After a routine examination, his objective pain in general was measured as being fourth degree. However, more trigger points were detected in the neck and shoulder areas. Therefore, he was given a fifth-degree rating for his objective pain. For the first treatment, he was asked to lie in the supine position. In addition to 24 trigger points in the primary group on the anterior side of the body, a few trigger points in the secondary and tertiary groups were also needled. These were the lesser occipital, third occipital, biceps brachii tendon, cervical plexus, and spinal accessory-II points. Two days later, on October 19, he came for the second treatment. He claimed that the pain was reduced substantially, and he was able to sleep much more comfortably. He was laid in a prone position for the second treatment, which used all trigger points in the primary group, again adding trigger points in the secondary and tertiary groups in the neck and shoulder. The day after the second treatment, the first cold front of the year arrived in San Antonio. The captain had a flare-up that was attributed to the sudden weather change. He had difficulty turning his neck for a couple of days. Four days after his first visit, he came for the third treatment, during which he was in a sitting position, as can be seen in Figure 13.2, and needles were placed in all trigger points of the primary, secondary, and tertiary groups in the neck, shoulder, and the upper limbs. His fourth visit was on October 24. The supine position was repeated from the first treatment. He described his pain as being more than 80% improved. He ended up coming for a total of six treatments. By his fifth visit, he was practically free of pain. To ensure that his pain wouldn't relapse, he was urged to come for one last time on October 28. He was advised to call and visit for more treatments if needed. The service for him was free of charge as a goodwill gesture for foreign visiting military officers, particularly as he was from my home country of Taiwan. He didn't come again.

## 13.6 PAIN IN THE UPPER LIMBS

In this context, subjective pain of the upper limbs implies any pain that is perceived in the shoulder joint and areas distal to the joint down to fingertips. Three bones participate to form the shoulder joint: the clavicle, acromion of the scapula, and humerus head. Below the shoulder is the elbow. The elbow joint is formed by the humerus, the radius, and the ulna. Between the forearm and hand is the wrist joint, which has eight carpal and 30 phalangeal or finger bones. These many bones form a number of joints that are interconnected by ligaments and tendons. To move a joint, one or more muscles are needed. There are 42 named muscles, which have attachments to the bones in the upper limbs. Everything mentioned previously receives nerve innervations from branches of the brachial plexus. The brachial plexus is everywhere in the region. Therefore, it is understandable that subjective pain can be perceived anywhere in the entire upper limb. It would be impractically time-consuming to describe every possible pain in the upper limb. There are two kinds of subjective pain most often seen in the upper limb. Medically, they are known as rotator cuff injury and carpal tunnel syndrome. One example for each of the two abnormalities is chosen to explain how acupuncture can manage these two kinds of subjective pain in the upper limb.

Elmer G. was 61 years old, in the "supply" profession. His first visit was on January 6, 1989. He said that he had a "pinched nerve" in the left shoulder. That pinched nerve gave him pain inside the left shoulder joint. He also had lower back problems that had been kept at bay through faithful exercise, which indicated that the degree of his objective pain couldn't be too high. After measurement, his objective pain was estimated to be fourth degree. He stated that the pain inside his left shoulder, meaning the shoulder joint, had been bothering him for about 5 years. During that time, he had gone to a chiropractor for adjustments and visited his medical doctor, who gave him pain pills and muscle relaxants to take. None of them provided long-lasting relief. He used his right index finger to pinpoint the left greater occipital as the origin of the pain, which would spread down inferiorly to the spinal accessory and to the dorsal scapular, as we have described previously. The pain would be felt inside the shoulder joint. He said that he had been healthy throughout his entire life. He hadn't had any surgery, and no injury had been inflicted upon his body except for a cut on the left thumb that would suffer stiffness at times. He had had low blood pressure, 110 over 70, for as long as he could remember. Low blood pressure is fairly common among patients of middle age coming with pain in the neck and shoulder. There may be a causal relationship between neck and shoulder pain and low blood pressure from an adolescent age. Elmer was 61, and his blood pressure was still low. He certainly was not unique. Many other patients of his age had similar medical backgrounds: low blood pressure from a young age with a history of neck stiffness and pain in the shoulder joints. Besides trigger points in the primary group, two more points that stood out prominently were located right over the tendon belonging to the long head of the biceps brachii muscle. The tendon is lodged in the intertubercular groove of the humerus head. He had normal motion for both shoulder joints. However, when he extended his left arm backward or abducted it upward laterally, slight pain could be perceived in the joint along the biceps tendon. The pain in his left shoulder took only two treatments to eliminate. The first treatment was given on the day he came for the first visit. It was decided to treat him in the sitting position because of his rather intense pain from the left greater occipital point down to the medial border of his left shoulder blade, where the dorsal scapular point is located. Sitting upright offers the most convenience for placing needles in these regions. In addition to the trigger points in the primary group, a total of six needles were added on the biceps tendons in both shoulder joints. Elmer came for the second treatment on January 8. He claimed that the first treatment had helped to ease his pain, and that he had slept well for the past two nights. He was placed in the supine position for the second treatment. Besides all trigger points in the primary group, another six needles were added along the biceps tendon areas. A third treatment was suggested to him, but he failed to come for the appointment. Subjective pain in the shoulder joint is relatively common—in one out of 10 patients, by our estimate. Books and other publications written about the shoulder joint are in no short supply. Their opinions are that the culprit is the rotator cuff. We have a great deal of reservation in condemning the rotator cuff. If indeed, subjective pain in the shoulder joint is caused by any damage in the cuff, acupuncture is unlikely to reduce or stop it, but the truth is that the pain can be effectively managed with good to excellent results. Most pain in the joint is possible to detect as the trigger points along the tendon of the long head of the biceps brachii muscle, as described above. The rotator cuff is a broad band of tendinous tissue extending from four large muscles: the teres minor, infraspinatus, supraspinatus, and subscapularis. This cuff covers almost the entire circumference of the humeral head. The area is rather lengthy. If there is damage or injury to the rotator cuff, a few trigger points should appear in the acromion of the scapula and the humeral head.

Another type of subjective pain we want to mention is known as carpal tunnel syndrome. As we know, there are two rows of carpal bones. The proximal row has the scaphoid (also known as the navicular), the lunate or semilunar, and two triquetral bones, one of which is also known as the pisiform. The distal row consists of the trapezium, trapezoid, capitates, and hamate bones. These bones form a tunnel in the ventral side of the wrist. Taking into consideration all the ligaments that interconnect these bones, the wrist is a very complicated structural unit in which many things can go wrong and end up causing pain here and there. One of these pains is carpal tunnel syndrome. Patients with this syndrome are fewer in number than those having pain in the shoulder. There are more females than males. They are usually middle-aged people. One thing they often blame for having symptoms of carpal tunnel is modern technology, such as repetitive stress in typing on a keyboard. Medical doctors believe carpal tunnel syndrome is caused by a compression of the median nerve inside the carpal tunnel in the wrist area. After running through the tunnel, the nerve branches out to distribute to the thumb, index, and middle fingers. Most sufferers who come to visit complain of numbness, tingling, and pain sensations. Patients with milder stages of the problem indicate that they are wakened by these symptoms in the early morning hours. Patients with severe symptoms can become so uncomfortable that they wake up in the middle of the night. Manageability of these symptoms depends very much on the degree of objective pain patients have. If the pain is fifth degree or lower, three treatments are generally sufficient to take care of the symptoms. If the pain is between the sixth and eighth degrees, carpal tunnel syndrome is still possible to manage, with the possibility of relapse in 4 to 6 months. Once the objective pain of the patients reaches the ninth degree or higher, the problem becomes difficult to manage. By then, surgery will be the only alternative that these patients have. For patients with carpal tunnel syndrome having objective pain lower than fifth degree, subjective pain is invariably limited only to the hand and fingers. Objective pain between the fifth and eighth degrees will be likely to have subjective pain in one other location, such as backache, headache, shoulder pain, etc. Once the objective pain exceeds the ninth degree, there will be multiple sites of pain in different areas of the body. That is why carpal tunnel becomes a difficult problem to manage. Treating simple carpal tunnel syndrome is easy For the first treatment, place patients in the supine position. All trigger points of the primary group, plus the median and median recurrent, are used. The median recurrent and median points belong to the secondary and tertiary groups, respectively. Their anatomical locations are shown in Figure 12.2 (for median recurrent) and Figure 12.4 (for median, which is marked with an unlabeled black triangle superior to the wrist in the right forearm). For the second treatment, patients are placed in the prone position. Again, all trigger points of the primary and the two additional points are used. The third and last treatment is given in the sitting position. Trigger points of the primary and secondary groups in the head, neck, and upper limbs are used. Patients are asked to wait for a week and return for more treatments if the symptoms persist. Most of them will just disappear without needing further acupuncture therapy.

## 13.7 PAIN IN THE BODY TRUNK

If the skin's surface is used as a guideline to gauge the frequency for pain to occur, the body trunk has a large area with less potential to have subjective pain, if the lower back is excluded. Not too many patients who come for acupuncture treatments have pain in various regions of the body trunk, which includes the thorax, abdomen, and back. We think that there are reasons for such an outcome. First, pain in these regions is very likely a referral or reflection of disease or illness from internal organs or viscera. Pain of this kind constitutes an emergency. Patients who have this kind of urgent pain will be smart enough not to come to us for emergency care. Besides, as an acupuncturist, it is wise to not deal with pain of possible internal origins. Another reason is anatomical. As explained in the previous chapters, except for the lumbar region, no nerve branches distributed throughout the body trunk are major in size. We have a total of 66 acupoints in the thoracic and abdominal regions. Most of them belong to either the tertiary or the nonspecific groups. These acupoints rarely have potential to be converted to the passive phase and become trigger points. One disease that has the ability to do so is herpes infection, which can develop to become postherpetic neuralgia. We will use this neuralgia as an example to illustrate pain in the body trunk. Skin breakouts due to herpes infection can occur anywhere in the entire body. More will be said about postherpetic neuralagia in the following chapters. Herpes infections occurring in the body trunk are characteristically dermatomic, as seen in Figures 13.3 and 13.4. The patient shown in Figure 13.3 had scars on the skin of the right scapular region. The scars were formed by a herpes infection that had broken out 19 days before

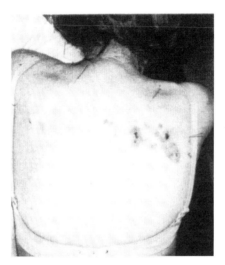

**FIGURE 13.3** A patient with herpes infection affecting dermatomes of the fourth and fifth thoracic spinal nerves.

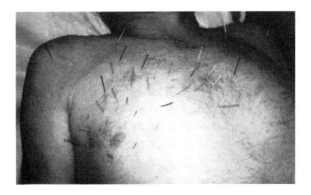

**FIGURE 13.4** A patient with herpes infection showing as many as two dozen needles placed in the affected area.

this picture was taken. The infected skin is along the dermatomes of the fourth and fifth thoracic spinal nerves. The herpes infections we saw affected two to three dermatomes. In the thorax and abdomen, the scars are linear. The skin area where the scars of the infection are located has a dozen or more trigger points, as can be seen in Figure 13.4. The purpose of this photo is to show how many needles an acupuncture treatment will take to manage the subjective pain produced by postherpetic neuralgia. The infected area in the pectoral region is densely filled with trigger points. Patients coming with subjective pain caused by postherpetic neuralgia were diagnosed by their attending physicians. With few exceptions, pain in patients with postherpetic neuralgia is difficult to manage and produces poor results (see Chapter 15). One simple reason is that they apparently have a higher degree of objective pain. The lowest objective pain measured was second degree for Clifton M. He was a 71-year-old rancher. The postherpetic neuralgia was diagnosed 3 months prior to his first visit to the clinic. His subjective pain was perceived in the skin area above the left eye extending upward to the frontal head in the territory innervated by the ophthalmic division of the left trigeminal nerve. After four treatments between August 3 and August 20, 1995, his pain disappeared. The first treatment was given with the patient in the supine position. Trigger points in the primary group, plus 18 needles belonging to the nonspecific points, were used in the manner shown in Figure 13.4. He was placed in the prone position for the second treatment using very much the same points in the primary and nonspecific groups. The third treatment was offered with the patient sitting upright. Trigger points of the primary and secondary groups accessible in the head, neck and upper limbs, plus nonspecific points were needled. He lived in Kerrville, more than an hour away from San Antonio. We suggested that he wait for 2 weeks to see if the pain would subside in that time. He did come on August 20, saying he was practically free of pain in the head region, but decided to have one more treatment to make sure that pain was eliminated forever. A few days later, we received a call from a doctor at the VA hospital in Kerrville. The physician wanted to know what we had done for Clifton to get rid of his headache. Our answer was simple: acupuncture. He was told to come to learn acupuncture, if he had such a desire. As usual, this doctor didn't accept our altruistic gesture.

As can be seen in Table 13.2, approximately one in three patients (34%) come to seek acupuncture because of lower back pain. An entire book can be written to describe acupuncture for treating lower back pain alone. As with other pain types, pain in the lower back can have good to excellent, mixed with limited and poor results, depending on the degree of objective pain that patients are measured to have. A couple of examples will be cited in this section to describe lower back pain in which patients can be treated with good to excellent results. Patients with mixed and limited results are the targets for Chapter 14. Difficult to impossible cases will be discussed in Chapter 15.

*Case 1*: It is only sensible for us to mention Woodie C. and Jim B. together, as Jim came to us because of urging from Woodie. Both of them had lower back pain, even though Jim was initially told to seek acupuncture treatment to quit dipping tobacco. Jim said that he had had a tobacco-chewing habit since high school. He had decided to stop chewing tobacco because of his six children—three sons and three daughters—who told him that they hated to see him doing so. Before coming, he had tried nicotine patches, but still seemed to have difficulty in overcoming the addiction. Someone in his home town suggested that he should try acupuncture to stop chewing tobacco, that person being Woodie. We will gloss over further detail of the tobacco chewing and focus only on the lower back pain for both of them. All we will say further on it is that Jim kicked his habit of dipping tobacco after two acupuncture treatments without having to suffer withdrawal symptoms.

Woodie came for acupuncture first on November 15, 1987, when he was 46 years old. He wrote "back" as his main problem, and "pumper" as his job. The lower back pain would sometimes run down to his right hip and thigh. This indicated that the roots of the lower lumbar and upper sacral spinal nerves were involved, as with the pinching of a herniated disc. His objective pain was measured at second to third degree. The last five acupoints in the primary group had no tender sensitivity. In other words, there were enough trigger points to qualify him for having second degree but not enough to place him at third degree. Using the prone position, needles were given at each of the trigger points in the primary group only. Needles in each of the trigger points of the primary group

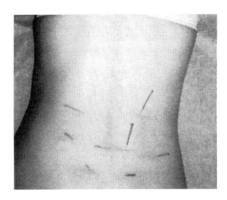

**FIGURE13.5** A photo showing primary acupoints for needles to manage lower back pain.

in the lumbar area are shown in Figure 13.5. Anatomical names for these trigger points can be found in Figure 12.1. Because of the low degree of objective pain, one treatment could be sufficient to stop his lower back pain. We suggested that he wait for 1 week and then call if the pain didn't go away. He didn't call until September 25, 1988, when he began to feel some aching in his back again. The first treatment was repeated. He came again 2 days later, not because of his lower back, but because he wanted to stop smoking. Discussing how acupuncture can help smokers kick their habits would require another dissertation. Suffice it to say that Woodie stopped smoking after four acupuncture sessions between September 25 and October 4 of 1988. On his last visit, he claimed that he had no more craving for cigarettes, and his lower back was free of pain. As a pumper for oil companies, he had to drive several hundred miles every day to check many oil pumps. Long-distance driving made his back tired, and when he happened to be in town, he would appear without appointment for one needling session in the back. For him, an acupuncture treatment was a tune-up that made him relax as well as loosened his back tension.

Because of his good and excellent results, Woodie recommended acupuncture to Jim. On March 15, 1990, Jim was 21 years old, and came as an emergency without prior appointment because his lower back was hurting "real bad." He said he had had lower backache since the age of 10, although the cause was not elaborated. In all those 11 years, he had not consulted a medical doctor, even when he sometimes suffered a great deal of pain in the lower back. That was the reason Woodie had urged him to come. Because he came as an emergency patient, there was no time to properly quantify his objective pain. It was suspected that it would not be too high. Otherwise, one treatment would not be able to clear the pain in his back. His second visit was on October 25, 1996, more than 6 years after his first. During this not-so-short period, he had not had any lower back pain. He came because he wanted to quit dipping tobacco for the sake of his six kids. If Jim does not come again, we will not know whether he had good to excellent results from acupuncture treatment.

*Case 2*: The next case of lower back pain was selected to represent that good to excellent results can occasionally be immediately visible. Mary Lou V. (Figure 13.6) is such a case. This patient arrived with her right hip slouching toward the side (left two photos of the figure). A slouching posture toward one side is always an unspoken indication that the person has lower back pain. Patients whose lower back pain is evident from a tilted body are seen now and then. Sometimes, patients with visible signs of lower back pain will have dramatic and drastic results from acupuncture treatments. Immediately after the needles were removed, Mary Lou appeared to be able to stand straighter, as can be seen from two photos on the right of the figure. The subjective pain she perceived was reduced substantially. Again, such obvious good to excellent results were possible because her objective pain was low, between third and fourth degree. Mary Lou was a 46-year-old clerk typist. At the age of 23, she was involved in an automobile accident. She ended up landing on asphalt pavement with a chipped tailbone. Pain caused by a fracture in the coccyx is not easy to

Good to Excellent Applications 163

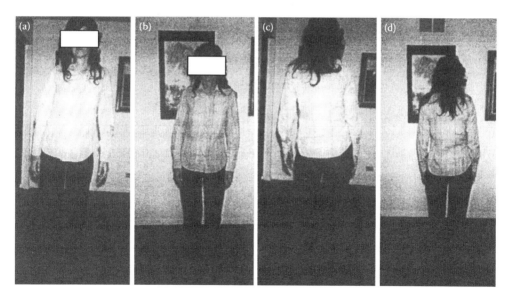

**FIGURE 13.6** Photos of Mary Lou taken before (left) and immediately after (right) the first acupuncture treatment. An improvement in her standing posture can be clearly seen.

manage. Yet, after four treatments, pain in the coccygeal area subsided because of her low degree of objective pain. The diagnosis from her doctor was "tendonitis [sic] and a chip on the coccyx," although medical dictionaries give the spelling "tendinitis." She couldn't recall precisely when her lower back started to have pain, but it had worsened about 2 years ago. The pain had become more frequent, occurring once every 2 days. She had received physical therapy, was taking hot baths three or four times a day, and was using Tylenol, Advil, and Ascriptin pills. They helped for a short period. She had had some kind of breast operation in 1973, and in 1984, she had had a hysterectomy because of endometriosis. She was told her back pain would disappear after the surgery, but that prediction failed to materialize. The lower back pain persisted. She had had some dysmenorrhea with mild cramping during menstrual periods, but there was no more cramping after the hysterectomy. Her obstetric-gynecologist also told her that the uterus had precancer cells. She said that she slept well but would wake up with pain every morning around 5:30. She also had occasional constipation. Before coming for acupuncture, she had had four cortisone injections: one in the midback, one at the coccyx, and two inside the pelvic bone. She also complained of numbness in the right thumb and index finger, particularly in the morning after a night's sleep. Her feet would become uncomfortable after standing for any period of time. For the first treatment on November 3, 1984, in the prone position, 25 needles were placed in each of the trigger points in the primary group. The relief was immediate after the needles were removed. The second treatment was given on November 5, using trigger points in the primary group on the supine position. Three additional needles were placed around the right tibial points proximal to the medial malleolus of the right ankle, because active pain was perceived in that area. Mary Lou came for two more treatments, on November 9 and November 12. On both occasions, she was asked to lie in the prone position. For these two last treatments, an additional three points of the secondary and tertiary groups in each limb were used. She reported that her pain was much reduced and that she slept very well, without any discomfort. She stopped coming after her fourth visit.

## 13.8 PAIN IN THE LOWER LIMBS

Because nerve branches in the lower limb come from the lumbar and sacral plexus, there is pain associated with each of these points. If we wanted to pick pain in just two regions in the lower limb to describe, for example, these would be knee pain and meralgia paraesthetica (which is also known as Bernhardt disease). Knee pain related to osteoarthritis is the most common complaint in the entire lower limb. Meralgic pain from the greater trochanter is not as common as knee pain. It is a pain that can lead to hip joint replacement if the problem is not effectively taken care of. The cause of meralgia paraesthetica is not clearly understood. Knee pain often is the consequence of joint degeneration.

### 13.8.1 Meralgia Paraesthetica or Bernhardt Disease

We have mentioned this pain condition in a previous chapter. The pain almost always starts in the greater trochanter, which is a bony process of the femur that can be easily and conveniently palpated on the upper end of the thigh. Laypeople often refer to the trochanter as the hip. Between the greater trochanter above and the lateral aspect of the knee below, there is a strong aponeurotic ligament known as the iliotibial tract, a thickening portion of the fascia lata covering the lateral side of the thigh. Bernhardt disease involves tingling, formication, itching, and other forms of paresthesia on the outer side of the thigh beginning at the greater trochanter and running down to the lateral epicondyle of the femur, and is a very commonly seen condition. Most patients seen in the clinic with this disease have objective pain at fifth degree or higher. Acupuncture for them will have mixed and limited results, which are presented in Chapter 14. The pain in some of the patients will be difficult to manage with poor results, and are presented in Chapter 15. In our opinion, meralgia paraesthetica is an expected extension of pain deriving from lower back pain. In other words, people who have Bernhardt disease will have had lower back pain to start with, and it could be with them for years. Some medical doctors believe that the pain originates from the trochanteric bursa, which covers the outer surface of the greater trochanter. Therefore, the disease is also known as trochanteric bursitis. However, most patients who have a biopsy done by aspirating synovial fluid from the trochanteric bursa were found to have no pathological indication of any infection. The symptoms of pain, tingling, formication, itching, and other forms of paresthesia are easy to manage if the objective pain in the patient is no higher than fourth degree. The results are always good to excellent. To treat meralgia paraesthetica or Bernhardt disease, patients are first placed in the prone position, using trigger points in the primary group. The second treatment is given in the supine position, again using the trigger points in the primary group. Patients are placed a lateral recumbent position, meaning lying on one side. If the uncomfortable sensation is more prominent on the right side, place patients on the left hip, and vice versa. Trigger points used include all primary group accessible locations, plus four trigger points of the secondary group in the available locations. Needles placed over the greater trochanter and iliotibial tract are essential for managing the disease. In the lateral recumbent position, the greater trochanter is easy to palpate and locate. There will be an obvious trigger point detectable right on the top of the trochanter. A needle must be inserted right at that locus. Approximately 1.5 in. peripherally from that needle, six additional needles are needed to circle it. Finally, trigger points along the iliotibial tract must be searched out. There are often three to five of them found along the tract. Each is inserted with one needle to complete the third treatment. The fourth treatment is repeated as described for the third on the other side of the hip. Four treatments are enough to erase symptoms of Bernhardt disease if the objective pain in the patients is fourth degree or lower. If symptoms persist for any reason after four needle sessions, the same protocol of four treatments should be repeated once more no later than 2 weeks afterwards. Very rarely are additional series of therapy required.

### 13.8.2 Pain in the Region of the Knee Joint

When we say "knee pain," some people may have a narrow concept of pain inside the knee joint only. It is more inclusive to say pain in the region of the knee joint. Anatomically, the region consists of the distal end of the femur with the lateral and medial epicondyles, the patella, and the proximal ends of fibula and tibia with their heads and the lateral and medial condyles of the tibia. In this entire region, one trigger point that often becomes the first to be detectable is formed by the saphenous nerve. This saphenous nerve point is clearly not in the knee joint. The point becomes sensitive with pain or tenderness palpable early in the sequence of acupoints turning from latent to passive phase. It ranks fourth in the sequence of all acupoints that have potential to become trigger points. In fact, pain that appears in the knee due to an injury inside or outside the joint will have the saphenous point turning to a trigger point. Injuries inside the knee joint can include tearing of the meniscus or damage to cruciate ligaments. Injuries outside the joint can include rupturing of muscles or collateral ligaments that attach to the bones of the joint. The pain caused by these types of injuries is acute in nature. The injured parties are most likely young and healthy athletes. Their pain has the potential to stay in the acute stage for years. This kind of acute pain can turn chronic only if the same injury happens repetitively over a period of many years, or if the original pain was not totally eliminated. Years later, trigger points will appear in other loci of the knee joint region. More about chronic pain in the region of the knee joint will be discussed in the next two chapters. Here, one reality concerning chronic pain in the knee is useful to point out. This chronic pain will often be mistakenly regarded as acute because the knee has suddenly begun hurting in the past few days or week when, in fact, the aching knee has been degenerating for years. Such is the case particularly for female patients who have passed the postmenopausal age. They already have numerous trigger points in the body with osteoarthritis going on inside their knee joints for a number of years without being able to perceive subjective pain in their knees. Of course, the patients themselves have no idea that the pain in their knee is already in the chronic stage when one day they become aware of it. This fact explains why degenerative osteoarthritis in the knee often is difficult to manage with poor results, whether using acupuncture or whatever other remedies. Knee pain is easy to manage with good to excellent results if the patients have an objective pain that is no higher than fourth degree and if there are no other trigger points detectable in the region of the knee joints. Here is an example.

Lila M. was a 96-year-old tour director. She is certainly unique because she is the oldest patient on our records, an old-fashioned schoolteacher, and had remained single her entire life. After retiring from teaching, she became a tour director because of her penchant for traveling. She belonged to a club whose membership requirement is to travel to at least 100 countries. At the age of 84, she was still leading tour groups to China.

Lila first came to visit on November 27, 1995. She indicated that she'd come because of a suggestion from a Dr. Richard Carraghan. No such name was found in the local telephone directory. Her main problem was "arthritis in the left knee" with pain for about 3 months. After checking her trigger points, her objective pain was measured to be fifth degree, which could be considered low for her age. This fact might explain why she had a successful total hip replacement in 1988. The hip surgery was necessary because she had Bernhardt disease in the left hip joint, which her physician told her was already "bone to bone" contact in the joint. After the surgery, the problem was completely solved. Surgery for her left knee was not justifiable because the arthritis was "minimal." Because of her relatively low degree of objective pain, it was predicted that four treatments would be able to manage her subjective pain in the knee.

To stop Lila's knee pain, she was first placed in the supine position, and needles were inserted in all trigger points of the primary group, plus an additional four needles in the saphenous area, which had more sensitivity. She came for a second treatment on November 29. Pain relief in the knee was obvious because she came without a walking cane. She reported that she was able to walk to the post office and work in the yard without using her cane. She was very happy with the results. In the prone position, needles were placed in the trigger points of the primary group with an additional four needles in the left knee. By the time she came for her third visit on December 1, she said that she was free of pain in the left knee. In a sitting position, all trigger points accessible in the primary group plus four additional in the knee were used for needling. She was advised to call if the knee became painful again. She returned for a fourth visit on January 15, 1996, because the knee had begun to bother her again. A series of three treatments was repeated, mimicking the first three sessions in the first series of four, on January 17 and January 19, 1996. In the meantime, a letter from Orthopaedic Surgery Associates of San Antonio arrived to compliment Ms. Lila M., reading: "I am absolutely delighted that you have had such an excellent response to the acupuncture therapy. I trust that it will be of lasting duration for you..." It was signed by one of the physicians at that practice.

### 13.8.3 Pain in Other Locations of the Lower Limb

Subjective pain can appear in many locations of the lower limb. Acupoints where subjective pain has been seen include the ilioinguinal, genitofemoral, and obturator at the junction of the lower body trunk and upper end of the lower limb. Subjective pain in the popliteal fossa (known as Baker's cyst), along the shaft of tibia and fibula, around the ankle, between the toes (Morton's neuroma), under the foot (tarsal tunnel syndrome), calcaneal or plantar fascitis, and bunions on either the big or little toe are just some of the pain types seen in the clinic. Some of them will be mentioned in the next two chapters.

## REFERENCES

1. Dung, H.C. Biostatistical profiles of individuals seeking acupuncture treatments in the United States. *Chinese Medical Journal* 98:835, 1985.
2. Macnab, I. and J. McCulloch. *Neck Ache and Shoulder Pain*. Williams & Wilkins, Baltimore, 1994.
3. Cailliet, R. *Shoulder Pain*, 5th ed. F.A. Davis Company, Philadelphia, 1973.

# 14 Applications with Mixed and Limited Results

Acupuncture has a tendency to be contentious. All manner of news media are filled with information that can be considered as misleading. One example is found in an issue of *Consumer Reports* [1]. The magazine describes how a patient diagnosed with systemic lupus erythematosus received acupuncture treatments. Reports that a disease of this nature can be treated with acupuncture will surely draw a great deal of skepticism from people with medical sophistication. Obviously, acupuncture is neither a panacea nor a charade. The treatments, without a doubt, can produce good to excellent results, as presented in the previous chapter. They can also be ineffective and produce poor results. Most of the results obtained from acupuncture treatments will be appropriately described as mixed and limited. Thus, we have the title for this chapter.

## 14.1 DEFINING MIXED AND LIMITED

"Mixed" is used here to mean that patients can have more than two kinds of pain at once. They may perceive any two or more of headaches, lower back pain, pain in the shoulder, knee pain, pain under the foot, and other kinds at the same time. Pain may also be mixed with other medical problems or symptoms; patients with headache or lower back pain may suffer from hot flashes, indigestion, stomach ulcers, hiatal hernia, constipation, insomnia, depression, dysmenorrhea, menstrual cramping, hypoglycemia, low blood pressure (hypotension), anemia, and so on. Acupuncture may be useful for solving one or more of these diseases or symptoms, but not all of them at one time. Thus, the results are best described as mixed. Subjective pain in some patients is perceived in many locations. This pain can be managed with good and excellent results in some locations, but not in others. Such results are best categorized as mixed.

Clinically, patients commonly express that their pain is better, but they are not completely well or totally free of the pain subjectively perceived. The relief is clearly limited. Mixed relief in pain also consists of limited relief in pain. Mixed and limited can be best explained by using the three terms below.

### 14.1.1 IN TERMS OF PATIENT PROFILES

Most patients are of middle age or older. They often consume multiple prescription drugs simultaneously. Adverse reactions to medicines taken are rather common. Most medicines taken for pain are not helpful, or if they are, the relief of pain is short—lasting only hours, not days—unless the medicines contain narcotics. Other medical modalities, including physical therapy, prescribed analgesics, antiinflammatories, muscle relaxants, and steroid injections have all been tried without lasting relief. One thing they want to avoid is the need to undergo surgery to solve their painful problems. Surgery can be beneficial for managing the pain of some patients in this group. Their pain can be considered as being chronic in nature. The objective pain measured for these patients is from sixth to ninth degree. Nonprescription drugs are a waste of money because they are useless. Chiropractic adjustments are not of much help, and have the potential to generate more pain after the adjustments. Massage, TENS units, or any other counterirritants are all similar wastes of time and money.

### 14.1.2 IN TERMS OF NUMBER OF TREATMENTS

It will require a minimum of four sessions to administer a proper number of acupuncture treatments to see mixed and limited results. Most of the time, six sessions are needed to see subjective relief. Substantial relief may not be achieved until as many as 16 treatments are given. In the long term, patients in this group come hundreds of times because their subjective pain can relapse from time to time. Patients in this group constitute the majority of our acupuncture clientele. Our estimate is that 63% of all patients belong to this group with mixed and limited results. The greatest appreciation of acupuncture is found among them, and they are the most enthusiastic in urging others to try acupuncture for the relief of chronic pain.

### 14.1.3 IN TERMS OF PAIN RELIEF AND RELAPSE

We don't collect statistical data to say for sure how many treatments are required before subjective pain in a patient shows noticeable improvement. We do know that after as few as four treatments, some patients report being better. Only a small number of patients are fortunate enough to have such a quick outcome. Some patients will take six or more treatments to see an improvement. As many as 12 treatments to see relief of subjective pain is not unusual at all. The number of treatments required to conclude with a desirable result also varies from patient to patient. Some of them have satisfactory relief after four sessions, and no more will be required until the same pain relapses. Some may need as many as 16 treatments. The duration of pain relief ordinarily lasts from 4 to 6 months. Of course, the period can be shorter or longer for a small percentage of patients. The time until relapse of the same subjective pain will increase as the patients return for more series of treatments.

## 14.2 IRRELEVANT TO PAIN

By now, it has to be clearly understood that the main purpose for using acupuncture is for managing pain. The matter may not be that simple because not all people seeking acupuncture do so due to pain. Among the patients received, some want acupuncture to help them quit smoking, stop dipping tobacco, or kick other addictive habits. There are women who cannot get pregnant and want to have babies. Overweight individuals hope placing needles in their ears will help them to reduce weight. Wrinkles come with age, and some women expect acupuncture to smooth their facial skin, or give them a face-lift. Patients with nasal congestion due to allergic sinusitis may not experience any pain. Even without any subjective pain perceived, these people have to be included in the acupuncture clientele. Acupuncture is known to be useful in offering solutions for their problems. The solutions are not complete. Some will be helped, and some will not have fruitful results. Therefore, the results of treating these patients can be suitably described as mixed and limited. Some of these patients, of course, can have pain of one kind or another. If they don't have any subjective pain perceived at the time of their first visit, they can be appropriately placed into the group of patients who are irrelevant to pain. Describing how to take care of patients who are irrelevant to pain would involve a great deal of space. We have no intention of undertaking such a big task. Nevertheless, two examples can be provided for demonstrating what mixed and limited results are in the acupuncture practice. These are weight reduction and infertility.

### 14.2.1 WEIGHT REDUCTION

The popularity of using acupuncture to reduce body weight has faded to some extent in America. In the early 1980s, overweight patrons knocked on the clinic's door every day to seek acupuncture's help in solving their problem of excessive caloric intake. The phenomenon speaks of a social problem in an affluent nation. Americans simply eat more than they need. The unutilized energy is then converted into fat for storage in the stomach and elsewhere. One can fairly say that obesity is one of the unique dilemmas of the United States. This social peculiarity became an expectation that was unheard of in the history of acupuncture. No mention of using acupuncture to reduce body weight was found in any of the writings or publications available prior to 1970. The real story behind how acupuncture became popular for weight reduction is fascinating, but we have neither the time nor the need to repeat it in this book. The acupuncturist who started the practice of acupuncture face-lifting was a personal friend. He resided in Hollywood, where the abundance of movie stars is a well-known fact. They don't mind spending cash to keep themselves young. Such a reality explains why acupuncture for face-lifting became popular in California and throughout the country at one time. The results of face-lifting are also mixed and limited, with a tendency to be on the very poor side. We have no desire to explain why. We do want to have a rational anatomical explanation for understanding why placing three or four press needles, known as auriculopuncture, in the ears will be able to help some people to reduce a few pounds of their body weight in a few weeks. This rational explanation was reported in two publications [2,3]. Briefly, the principal scheme relies on the distribution of the vagus nerve to the ears, as shown in Figure 14.1. The anatomic mechanism for suppressing appetite by inserting very small press needles in the ear concha is the auricular branch, a small nerve branching from the vagus. Nerve signals generated in the concha by the press needles will interfere with hunger signals coming from digestive organs carrying the vagus nerve. This interference must be able to confuse the central nervous system's desire for food intake. When food intake is reduced over a period of time, body weight will have a chance to decrease. Overall, such a reduction only occurs in approximately 23% of people who tried it and were able to drop 2 or 3 pounds during a 2- to 3-week period. Therefore, we say the results are mixed and limited. Mixed because some people had the expected results of shedding a few pounds of their weight, and some

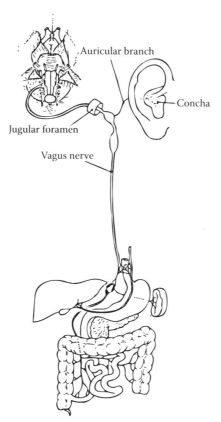

**FIGURE 14.1** A diagrammatic drawing to depict distribution of the vagus nerve and its branches. (Modified from K.L. Moore, *Clinically Oriented Anatomy*, 1st ed. Williams & Wilkins, Baltimore, 1980.)

didn't. Limited because body weight reduced was limited to just a few pounds, and for only a small number of people who tried the method.

### 14.2.2 Infertile Pregnancy

Describing a pregnancy as infertile is an oxymoron. A total of 67 females came for acupuncture procedures with the hope of becoming pregnant. Slightly more than 50% of them achieved pregnancy, with 35 of them reported as having a baby. Among these, one mother had twins, as shown in Figure 14.2. Her name is Pamela Sadler (her name is used with permission). She was 29 years of age, and taught at an elementary school in San Marcos. Her mother, Kathie P., received a total of 55 acupuncture treatments between January 18, 1992 and December 2, 1995 because of back pain after an unsuccessful lumbar fusion. Kathie is considered as having mixed and limited results. The treatments helped to ease the back pain, which relapsed repeatedly during 4 to 6 months after receiving two to four needling sessions per series. In early 1996, Kathie inquired into the possibility of using acupuncture to improve her daughter Pam's infertility. Pam came on February 10, 1996. She indicated her "failure to conceive is due to ovulation disorder." More knowledge of this ovulation disorder would have been helpful to determine whether acupuncture was able to make her infertility into pregnancy. The diagnosis of the disorder was given by her fertility doctor in Austin. Her doctor had tried every means in his arsenal to overcome her infertility, without success. Pam said that she had already spent a lot of money trying to have a baby, but that she would not mind spending more, if anything could help her become a mother. We told her we would try to make her pregnant free of charge. Our only request for reciprocation was that she show us a picture of her baby after his or her arrival in the world. Pam kept her promise, and that is the reason we have the photo for this book. To be able to conceive, the father has to have a sufficient sperm count, and the mother must have normal menstrual cycles with ovulation occurring. The best time to have acupuncture is about 1 week prior to expected ovulation. Three to four sessions will constitute a series of treatments in promoting fertility. The sequence of treatments is supine first, then prone. Both times, only acupoints in the primary group are used. The third treatment is done in a sitting position using the primary and the secondary points accessible. The fourth treatment, if such a chance is available, is repeated in the supine position using only the primary points. After four series and a total of 13 treatments by May 13, Kathie called on June 6. Her excitement was beyond words, because her daughter Pam had been confirmed as pregnant. Her happiness was painfully brief. An unexpected spontaneous abortion occurred, just a couple of weeks after the pregnancy. Pam returned for two more series in July and

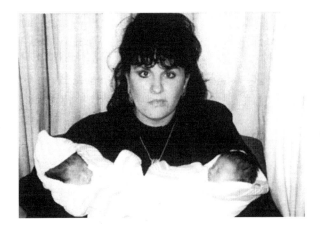

**FIGURE 14.2** Pamela Sadler with her twin sons, Wesley and John. Residual symptoms of facial paralysis due to Bell's palsy are still visible on her face.

Applications with Mixed and Limited Results 171

August. A second pregnancy was confirmed on August 16. By then, 18 treatments had been provided. On December 17, 1996, Kathie informed us that Pam was expecting twin boys on April 24, 1997. The twins arrived more than 1 month early. A week before the childbirth, Pam developed Bell's palsy with paralysis on the right side of her face. She was assured not to worry. Most facial paralysis would improve by itself without medical intervention. She did take steroids as prescribed. No initial attempt was made to see if acupuncture would improve her condition. The symptoms of facial paralysis on the right side of Pam's face persisted, and she came for six treatments to get rid of her Bell's palsy, which can be treated with good to excellent results in the early stages of the disease. The treatment procedures are given using the primary points and trigger points in the face and head.

Another case of infertility pregnancy is that of Norma G., a 31-year-old wife of a district judge in Brownsville. She came to the clinic on January 17, 1983, through a referral by her nephew, Dr. Joe Zayas, a graduate of UTHSC's dental school. Without this connection, it would be difficult for someone more than 300 miles away to become aware of our clinic's existence. Because of the distance, Norma could come and stay for no more than three treatments, and then only when she and her entire family came to San Antonio for various reasons and activities. She had "severe headache" of the migraine and tension type. The headaches often landed her in the hospital, where she would receive Demerol injections to ease her suffering. In reply to our inquiry, she indicated that her menarche occurred when she was 11 years of age. Thereafter, she would have severe cramping every month, and her periods would last 6 days. At the time of her first visit, she had one child, who was mentally disabled, as can be seen from Figure 14.3. The family picture was mailed as a Christmas greeting years later. The boy in the chair is their first son. Because of their first son's disability, she and her husband decided to wait before having a second child. When they decided to have another child 3 years later, she was unable to become pregnant. She consulted every medical

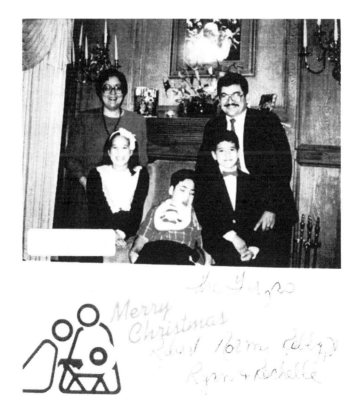

**FIGURE 14.3** A Christmas greeting from Norma with her husband, Robert, second son Ryan, daughter, Rochelle, and first son, Robby, Jr., in the chair.

resource available to her, but still could not conceive. She blamed the stress and anxiety of taking care of a brain-damaged son and becoming infertile as the reasons for her headache. This is a typical patient attributing subjective pain to psychological factors. We do agree that Norma's psychology might have played a role in creating "severe" headaches as she described them. The degree of her objective pain was only between five and six. At such a degree, headaches should not be severe all the time, unless one is regularly under a great deal of psychological stress. The family stayed in San Antonio for 3 days. She came once a day during that time for three acupuncture treatments, using the supine, prone, and sitting positions. The number of trigger points used has been given in the previous descriptions of headache treatments.

It was almost 11 months later, December 10, 1983, when Norma returned again. On that day, she reported that a few weeks after the acupuncture received in January, she became pregnant. She adamantly insisted that her pregnancy was the result of the acupuncture treatments, because she had tried very hard for several years without any luck. She jokingly said that after her pregnancy was confirmed, she paid a visit to her fertility doctor's office, and was told that the reason she couldn't conceive was because she was not ovulating. She then told the receptionist at the fertility clinic that she had already become pregnant because of acupuncture treatments received in San Antonio. She was so thrilled that the first thing she did when she stepped into the clinic was to give this author a hug. She said that she was very happy to have had a healthy boy, Ryan, the week before coming to San Antonio. He was a big baby, 10 pounds in weight at birth. She said this author was a miracle-worker because her headache had gone away after the three treatments and remained at bay until the birth of her second son. She received two treatments for her second series at the clinic, once a day for 2 days. A year later, she had her daughter, Rochelle. During her pregnancy with Rochelle, her headache got better. However, it kept relapsing, and she came about once every 6 to 8 months through July 9, 1996. By then, she had been given a total of 38 acupuncture treatments not only for headache but also for lower back pain, neck pain, and shoulder and knee pain. Her whole family has grown so enamored of acupuncture that all, but one, have become patients at the clinic in time. Each of them has two to three acupuncture treatments when they come to San Antonio.

## 14.3 SUBJECTIVE PAIN PERCEIVED

Acupuncture is used to control and manage perceivable pain, which is subjective. Subjective pain gives all of us uncomfortable sensations. Uncomfortable sensations are not restricted to pain. They can include numbness, itching, burning, prickling, stabbing, and many more. Acupuncture needles can eliminate some of these unpleasant sensations sooner and more easily than others. The intention of using "mixed" and "limited" is to imply such results. The treatments improve some of these problems, but not all of them. The improvement for some of them is more profound and longer-lasting than for others. Quantitatively, pain can be described as being somewhat relieved but not eradicated. It is not uncommon for patients to say that they feel somewhat better, but are still hurting. Such comments lead to an understanding that pain relief can have a quantitative aspect. "Limited improvement" would suitably describe such a quantitative change. "Limited" can also be used to define the duration of pain relief. In Chapter 13, good to excellent results are used to define patients who don't return for the same pain after four or fewer treatments. In this chapter, it will be found that most patients return for the same pain after some time. In most cases, this period is 4 to 6 months. Norma is an example. This period of 4 to 6 months of relief can also be viewed as a limit. Most acupuncture patients will have a limited time of relief. Except for those patients whose objective pain is fourth degree or lower, anyone expecting permanent relief could be disappointed.

With respect to age, patients with good to excellent results tend to be younger. Older patients with good to excellent results are fewer in number. Mixed and limited results are more often observed for patients who are older than 20 years and can be as old as 90. A reasonable explanation is that latent acupoints can be converted to passive at any age. Young patients with objective pain of sixth to ninth degree are less common. Older patients provide the possibility for having a higher degree of objective pain. If, indeed, pain can be acute and chronic, all of the patients who will have mixed and limited results must have chronic pain. Our reasoning is that their objective pain is almost always at sixth degree or higher, and anyone at this level of pain can be viewed as having subjective pain in the chronic stage.

In determining whether the results will be mixed and limited, we must discuss the number of treatments involved. The answer is six to 12 for 85% of the patients treated. The other 15% can take fewer or more treatments to obtain the same results. The duration of relief for subjective pain can be from weeks to years but, as already mentioned, 4 to 6 months is most likely.

One of the reasons that patients have mixed and limited results is subjective pain in multiple locations. Usually, a subjective pain is described as appearing first in one location. Another subjective pain can then appear later in a second location, and so will a third or fourth pain. Take, for example, patients with lower back pain, who can eventually have pain in the groin or lateral surface of the thigh. Some of these pains can have anatomical relations, and others may not. Let us examine the two example secondary pains mentioned. Pain in the groin always occurs at the ilioinguinal point, the nerve of which is a branch of first lumbar spinal nerve. Chronic lower back pain most often begins from the fifth lumbar. In time, the pain will involve the first lumbar. Pain in the lateral surface of the thigh is Bernhardt's syndrome, which is part of sciatica. Patients who have lower back pain can also suffer from chronic headache. Subjective pain in one location is almost always easier to manage than in multiple locations.

With very few exceptions, the overwhelming majority of patients who have had mixed and limited results after treatment had consulted at least one medical doctor before coming for acupuncture. It is obvious that when pain is perceived, acupuncture was most likely the last remedy to come to their minds. If acupuncture becomes popularly accepted as a legitimate therapy, people suffering from pain will go to acupuncture as the first choice, at which point their problems can be easily and quickly solved. One patient had seen at least 14 doctors before trying acupuncture, the highest number seen by any given patient prior to coming to us for treatment. None of them had given him good relief. Before acupuncture, therapeutic regimens given by their physicians consisted most commonly of pain pills (prescribed or nonprescribed), injections of one substance or another (most often steroids), and surgical interventions (for the elimination of pain or other pathologic reasons). Of the regimens mentioned, the number who had received surgery was relatively small. Nevertheless, saying that they were not regularly seen is not an overstatement.

Other forms of treatment received and mentioned by the patients include physical therapy, chiropractic adjustments, reflexology, and massage. Of these, chiropractic adjustments seem to provide temporary relief for some time. One reason that they decided to try acupuncture was because chiropractors became ineffective in providing even momentary relief. It was not infrequent for some patients to confess having their pain aggravated by their chiropractors. In the beginning of their pain, nonprescription pills might have helped for a short while. In time, the pain pills would become useless. Then, drugs prescribed by their physicians would follow. The three types of drugs most commonly prescribed medically were pills for pain, muscle relaxation, and counterinflammation. Individual drugs must come in and out of fashion because their names have changed rather often in just a few short years. Drug treatments provide relief at the beginning of their consumption, but after a while, they become of little use for the purpose of relieving pain.

Next to drugs, another often-mentioned treatment is the injection of steroids. The first injection often worked beautifully for patients who had mixed to limited results from acupuncture treatments. The relief usually lasted for as long as 6 months, but was much shorter after the second injection. Very few patients received more than three injections, at which point they were likely to have minimal or no relief. At that juncture, acupuncture would come to mind.

We suspect that patients who have mixed and limited results have a poorer homeostatic state than normal, as manifested in a number of conditions. They complain of easily becoming fatigued, of having difficulty sleeping at night, and of a tendency for indigestion and constipation, and are more likely to be stressed, become depressed, and be sensitive to environmental changes during the arrival of rain or a cold front. These patients have a higher incidence of allergies to chemicals and toxic substances, and have low tolerances for medications. It is not uncommon for them to describe how one pill could turn their stomachs upside down.

Pathologically, subjective pain originates more from endogenous causes in females, and more from exogenous causes (e.g., sports and work injuries) in males. One main source of pathological changes, which have endogenous origins, is menstrual malfunction. A large proportion of females with chronic pain seemed to have a medical history related to dysmenorrhea. Many of them had had a hysterectomy by the time of they reached the age of menopause. Other pathologic conditions that were mentioned by patients, and which produced mixed and limited results, included hiatal hernia, gastritis associated with excessive gastric acids, colitis, and diverticulitis. With improvements in the quality of drugs for pain, such as better buffering against indigestion, illness in the digestive system seems to be more seldom seen among patients. The availability of medicines such as cimetidine, packaged as Tagamet, may be another reason for the substantial decrease in gastrointestinal problems among patients with chronic pain. We suspect that there is a causal relationship between the irritation of the digestive tract and the consumption of pain pills that is observed so frequently among patients coming with chronic pain. It may be a simple coincidence but we wonder why the three most frequently advertised medicines on commercial TV during the 1980s and the 1990s seemed to be for pain, excessive stomach acids, and constipation. Subjective pain in patients who have some kind of gastrointestinal abnormality can be anticipated to be harder to manage. Again, we come to the purpose for this chapter's title.

Managing subjective pain with mixed and limited results will be described following the approach used in a previous chapter. The body is divided into five regions: face and head, neck and shoulder, upper limb, body trunk, and lower limb. Two or three kinds of subjective pain are chosen to represent each of the five regions. Some of the pain types chosen can be identical in one region, and some may be different. The reasons for such discrepancies will be explained whenever the circumstance is appropriate.

## 14.4 PAIN IN THE FACE AND HEAD

The three kinds of subjective pain in the face and head region chosen as examples are migraine, tic douloureux, and postherpetic neuralgia. Two cases for each of these three sicknesses are used to illustrate how subjective pain in the face and head can be managed.

### 14.4.1 MIGRAINE

Over more than 20 years, we have had several hundred patients come to us with migraine headaches. A few dozen of them have good to excellent results after four or fewer acupuncture treatments, and practically no patient in this first group was known to return for further migraine treatment. Clinically, most migraines have mixed and limited results. Migraine headache can certainly be managed, although with more frustration than satisfaction. Before we explain why migraines are not easy to manage, a short review of the medical literature will be helpful.

Essays in the form of books [5–8], periodicals [9–11], reviews [12,13], and others [14,15] about migraines constitute a greater volume than any person can possibly digest. The number of reports published by different investigators regarding headaches is astronomical. Medical experts must know a great deal about migraines. To this author, after dealing with the problem for so many years and in so many patients, migraines are still an enigma. To say that no two migraines are alike is altogether reasonable. The first conspicuous discrepancy is in gender. There are far more female migraine sufferers than males. Three out of every four cases of migraine are in women. This type of headache can assault victims as young as 10 years or as old as 60 years. Individuals older than 65 years seem to be immune to migraines. We have seen only two migraine patients older than 70 years. By the time the patients arrive in the clinic, the duration of their headaches can be from 1 year to more than 30 years. The interval between headaches can vary from days to years. Some migraines can relapse after years of remission. The severity of the headaches can be extreme, ranging from mild discomfort to paroxysmal sensations resulting in fainting and vomiting. Some patients didn't have to depend on too much medication to subdue their headaches. Others had a long history of consuming different types of drugs for combating tenacious migraines. The symptoms, their intensity, and characteristic sensitivity can change with age for many patients. Clinical variables in migraines are almost unlimited. Because of the possibility of such wide variations, the predictability for acupuncture managing migraines is less reliable than for other kinds of pain. "Mixed and limited" is unquestionably more appropriate for describing the results in managing migraine headaches than for any other kind of pain. Two patients are selected to serve as examples for migraine management.

*Case 1*: Lois C. was 26 years old. She didn't mention what her job was. She was literally brought to the clinic by Joyce Mauk, a senior-year student of the medical school who was taking the Anatomical Acupuncture elective for which I was the instructor. Lois used "common migraine" to describe her main problem. She gave us a written report in which she said, "headache since 9 or 10 (prepubescent). Head x-rays done around that time ruled out tumor. Headaches usually unilateral accompanied by nausea and vomiting. Over-the-counter medication (aspirin, Tylenol, etc.) didn't work. Usually slept the headaches off by going to a dark room and sleeping through the night. Headaches have always started around midday and reached their peak around 6 to 7 pm. Nothing in particular ever seemed to trigger them. Never occurred at any particular time during the month, and frequency was around once a week. As I have gotten older, nausea less of a problem. The only time headache-free was when I was pregnant (once). Now headaches are one-sided (right). They occur almost weekly and last for 2 to 3 days running (even sleeping didn't help). In November of 1982, went to a neurologist in San Antonio who did a CT scan to rule out tumor and was prescribed 50 mg Endep nightly and Midrin at the start of any headache. When headaches persisted, he prescribed Cafergot at the start of the headaches. On December 15 of the same year, started to take Inderal (60 mg) daily. It prevented any headaches for about 1 month. When I did get a headache, he increased the Inderal to 120 mg daily, and this was successful in relieving the headaches. Diagnosis was common migraines." Lois couldn't relate the headaches to menstrual function; the headaches came once a week, whereas menstruation naturally occurred once a month. Her periods were regular; she was taking contraceptive pills. During her periods, she would feel puffy and swollen, but no other discomfort or pain. Her objective pain was estimated as sixth degree. However, some trigger points in the tertiary group were detected in the head region, making her to be between sixth and seventh degree.

The first acupuncture treatment given to Lois was on February 26, 1983, the day she came to visit. Using the supine position, all trigger points in the primary group from the supraorbital in the head down to the deep peroneal in the feet were used for needling. When she came for the second treatment 2 days later, she indicated that she had cut down her Inderal intake to 60 mg daily. In the prone position, trigger points in the primary group were used. Additional trigger points in the secondary group, including the lesser occipital and third occipital, were also used. The third treatment was given on March 2, using the sitting position. Trigger points of the primary and secondary groups in the head, neck, shoulder, arms, forearms and hands, plus tertiary points on the scalp, including the bregma, coronal, pterion, and temporalis, were also needled. The first three treatments were repeated after a 1-week break. By March 24, when she came for her ninth treatment, she claimed that she had had no headache for a week. She felt elated because she was free from migraines. The author suggested that she keep coming for a few more treatments to prevent relapse. The treatments were free of charge because she was willing to be used as a teaching case for my Anatomical Acupuncture elective. Six days after her ninth visit, the headache relapsed, but subsided on its own within the day. She returned on March 30 for the tenth time. She said that a headache seemed to be building up, and upon her arrival, she was suffering. It was also at that time she began her new menstrual period. This coincidence led to the reasonable suspicion that the migraine and menstrual activity were related. Lois was advised to return after 2 days instead of waiting for a week, so that migraine could be suppressed without having a chance to rebound. The eleventh treatment was on April 1. She reported that the headache went away after the last treatment she received. The remainder of her visits were on April 6, 11, and 25. The modus operandi was the same, using the supine, prone, and sitting positions. The trigger points used were the primary, secondary, and tertiary in combinations. Lois's next menstrual period was on April 26. She came on April 27 for the fifteenth treatment. She again had a headache, which was not as bad as the ones she used to have. She was asked to come again on April 29 for her sixteenth treatment. Her seventeeth visit was on May 21 because she was expecting a new menstrual period and wanted to make sure that the headache would not relapse. Lois received two more treatments on May 23 and May 25. She returned again beginning June 11 for another series of four treatments (June 11, 15, 19, and 22), for which, as with all subsequent services she received, she was charged as a regular patient. Her headaches kept bouncing back every so often. They were mild headaches, without any severity to speak of. She had come for a total of 38 treatments by October 20, 1983. She returned for her thirty-ninth treatment on March 2, 1984, because she'd begun to have headaches after almost 4 months of freedom from suffering. The headaches seemed to coincide with the arrival of menstrual periods again. Migraines and acupuncture became a seesaw for the next 8 months, through October 6, 1984. By then, she had come for a total of 57 treatments. We have not seen Lois since. We hope that she is free of migraines after all these years.

*Case 2*: Bill G. was a 75-year-old retired rancher. He was our oldest patient to have migraines, and one of only two who were older than 70. He couldn't remember for how many years the headaches had been with him, or when he was diagnosed as having migraines. Most of the headaches were in the temporal area on both sides. The headache attacks were infrequent and impossible to anticipate. He had a headache upon arrival at the clinic, although not a severe one. Severe headaches appeared only very occasionally. He had not taken prescription or nonprescription medicine for headaches in years. His headaches were more a nuisance than a threat to his life. Most of the time, he just ignored the discomfort and carried on with whatever he had to do. He decided to try acupuncture because so many good friends in his town of Uvalde had urged him to come. He arrived on March 3, 1995 for the first visit. After giving him an examination to check the number of trigger points he had, his objective pain was measured as being fourth degree. He was assured that his headache could definitely be managed. Because of the pain's relatively long duration, the possibility for his headaches to relapse would be high. To us, pain is like a tree; it will grow in time. A small tree is easy to pull up at the roots. If a tree grows to 100 feet tall, the trunk can be cut down, but digging out all the branches of the roots can be difficult. He understood the analogy and decided to take the chance. The first treatment was in the supine position. The trigger points used were all in the primary group. Three extra needles were added to each temporal region. On his second visit (March 5, 1995), he described how his headache had subsided a few hours after his first visit, but then rebounded a day later. He came, more or less, as an emergency case because of his relapsed headache. He now felt pain around the rims of his eyes. The second treatment was again given in the supine position. In addition to the primary group trigger points, three needles were placed in the temporal areas and three were placed around the orbital margins, including the lacrimal, the lateral angle of the eyes, and the zygomaticofacial points. He came back for the third time on March 7, still suffering from headaches. The treatment was provided on the prone position. Trigger points used were all in the primary group. Two days later, on March 9, he came for the fourth treatment, which was made with him sitting. Needles used included six on each half of the scalp, and trigger points in the primary and secondary groups in the neck, shoulder, and upper limbs. The fifth treatment was given on March 11 and repeated the same needles as the first time in the supine position, adding secondary-group trigger points in the head, face, and neck. A total of 48 needles were used. He came for the sixth treatment on March 15 and reported that he hadn't had a headache for the last 3 days. Needles were given with him in the prone position. This time, only trigger points of the primary group were used. He was advised to wait for a week, unless the headache rebounded. He came for the seventh visit on March 22, 1995 because he felt as though a headache was impending, although it didn't materialize. The fourth treatment given on March 9 was repeated for this seventh visit with him sitting on a chair. He waited for 5 more days and returned for the eighth visit on March 27. He said that unmaterialized headaches could still be apprehended. The inconclusive battle to conquer his headaches would go on for the next 5 months, until August 29, 1995. By then, Bill had come for 21 treatments. During this time, he mentioned that he also had pain in the shoulder, neck, and lower back, as well as indications of tinnitus. He stopped coming until February 26 1996, which was the date for his 22nd treatment. Briefly, he hadn't had many headaches for about 5 months. The headaches then gradually began to sneak back. To combat his migraines, he returned on May 31, 1996. He received a total of 44 acupuncture treatments before he decided not to come again. The results of acupuncture therapy for Bill can be properly categorized as having mixed and limited outcome. The treatments helped to ease some of his migraine, but did not totally stop the headaches. The relief from the headaches was only for a limited period.

### 14.4.2 Trigeminal Neuralgia or Tic Douloureux

Our patients have a tendency to express opinions about their problems. Upon close scrutiny, they will confess that the conclusions they have are derived without prior medical diagnosis. One exception for this tendency is the disease clinically known as trigeminal neuralgia, also known as tic douloureux. The tic is not a very commonly seen illness in the acupuncture clinic. As recorded in Table 14.1, in 7 years' time, a total of 16 patients were seen with the tic, ranging from none in one year (1991) to four at the most in another (1994), with an average of 2.3 of these cases per year. All of them positively indicated that they suffered from trigeminal neuralgia or tic douloureux (even though most of them couldn't spell the words correctly), as diagnosed by their physicians. Because of their rarity, tic patients were not commercially significant. Nevertheless, from a clinical point of view, the tic is a very important problem for the patients. It is one of the worst sufferings a living soul can possibly have. Descriptions of the condition include terms like "excruciating pain" and "lancing, stabbing, burning sensations." The severe pain will attack suddenly with slight or even no provocation. The pain can last briefly, disappearing in seconds, or can endure minutes or longer. The pain can be so sharp as to collapse its victim. It must be merciful to experience relief from such a pain. For that reason, we have always had a strong compassion for patients with the tic, even though in our hearts, we know that the chance of helping these patients is not very good. Most tic cases have a poor prognosis and are difficult to manage with acupuncture treatments. Only a small percentage of them will have mixed and limited results. Here is an example.

Linda H. was a 12-year-old student. She and her case are unique for the following reasons: at 12 years old, she was the youngest among the patients seen suffering from the tic, which is a disease of the elderly, but does occur very uncommonly among the young [16]. There are more female than male patients with the disease. Among the tic patients received, 87% were women. No scientific evidence is available to explain why more females than males should suffer from the tic. Our own speculation is that, after middle age, there are more female then male patients with the tendency to have a higher degree of objective pain measured [17]. We were surprised to find out that Linda had seventh-degree objective pain at only 12 years of age. Subjective pain with seventh-degree objective pain is, indeed, not easy to manage. Linda's tic had been treated by several dentists and medical doctors. None of them were able to help her. She ended up in our acupuncture clinic through the referral of a pediatric neurologist, Dr. Sheldon Gross.

A few words about Dr. Sheldon Gross, MD, PA, FAAP: He was a graduate of the medical school in the Health Science Center in the mid-1970s. He was a very friendly and courteous student. We developed a good camaraderie during his student years. He had been our guest for dinner a number of times during his school years, because he had been tutoring piano lessons for our son. After his postgraduate training, he set up his practice of pediatric neurology in an office across the street from his alma mater. It is just a short walk to drop by his clinic to pay him a visit whenever we desired. We went to visit Dr. Gross unannounced on March 4, 1997 to inquire about Linda. After checking her file, Dr. Gross told me that the acupuncture had cured her tic. This is possibly the only time a

## TABLE 14.1
## Biostatistical Data for Patients with Trigeminal Neuralgia

| Year | Case No. | Name | Patient's Code No. | Sex and Age | Etiology | Side and Division of Trigeminal | Duration | Degree of Pain | No. of Treatments | Results |
|---|---|---|---|---|---|---|---|---|---|---|
| 1990 | 1 | Linda H. | 90208H551 | F12 | Didn't mention | R-Maxillary | 2 months | 7 | 7 | Good |
|  | 2 | Allen M. | 90326M533 | M63 | Postherpetic neuralgia | R-Maxillary | 10 years | 5 | 9 | Pain reduced |
| 1991 | 0 |  |  |  |  |  |  |  |  |  |
| 1992 | 1 | Anna M. | 92160M656 | F44 | Extensive dental drilling | L-Maxillary | 5 years | 9 | 2 | Needles were too painful |
|  | 2 | Francis V. | 92640V146 | F71 | Unknown | R-Maxillary | 5 years | 8 | 7 | Didn't call for appointment again |
| 1993 | 1 | Eva G. | 93047G595 | F73 | Didn't remember | L-Maxillary | 10 years | 10 | 12 | Feeling better |
|  | 2 | Maria R. | 93141R553 | F84 | Dental treatments | R-Maxillary | 6 months | 8 | 7 | Less pain but still hurting |
|  | 3 | J.C.B. | 93651B874 | M53 | Dentist | R-Maxillary | 2 years | 3 | 3 | Good |
| 1994 | 1 | Cathy S. | 94005S078 | F55 | Not sure | L-Maxillary | 2 years | 5 | 5 | No improvement |
|  | 2 | Elsie Mc. | 94020Mc155 | F73 | Unknown | L-Maxillary | Couldn't remember | 12 | 4 | No improvement |
|  | 3 | Geraldine M. | 94039M750 | F63 | Dental implantation | R-Mandibular | 6 months | 8 | 4 | Pain reduced |
|  | 4 | Mildred B. | 94666B927 | F80 | Dental care | R-Maxillary | 20 years | 9 | 28 | Limited improvement |
| 1995 | 1 | Janine V. | 95726V172 | F46 | Due to automobile wreck | R-Mandibular | 11 years | 4 | 3 | No improvement |
|  | 2 | Jane B. | 95726B992 | F74 | Unknown | L-Mandibular | 5 years | 7 | 17 | Still has attacks |
|  | 3 | Ruby Mc. | 95759Mc174 | F51 | Dental filling | R-Maxillary | 7 years | 5 | 26 | Substantially improved |
| 1996 | 1 | Jean A. | 96746A422 | F75 | Blaming her dentist | L-Mandibular | 3 months | 5 | 3 | Excellent |
|  | 2 | Alice M. | 96768M969 | F64 | Unknown | L-Maxillary | 3 years | 8 | 10 | Still hurting the same |

result of acupuncture treatment was able to be verified by a medical doctor. Linda was lucky. Her tic took seven treatments to stop because she had had it for only 2 months. It definitely would have been different had the duration of the tic been much longer.

The protocol for treating the tic is very similar to that for migraines, with emphasis around the maxillary and mandibular regions. The tic seems to involve only the maxillary and mandibular divisions of the trigeminal nerve. We do not profess knowledge as to why it skips the ophthalmic division. Seven out of 16 tic patients, as shown in Table 14.1, indicated that before having headaches, they received rather extensive dental drilling. Because of their high degree of objective pain, injury to the nerve inside the tooth pulp provoked general pain in the face and head. If this turns out to be accurate, people who have a high degree of objective pain need to watch out before undergoing dental drilling.

### 14.4.3 POSTHERPETIC NEURALGIA IN THE FACE AND HEAD

Postherpetic neuralgia in the face and head is another kind of trigeminal neuralgia. Both of them are headaches. One difference is that trigeminal neuralgia seems to involve the maxillary and mandibular divisions, whereas postherpetic neuralgia involves the ophthalmic and maxillary divisions. The reason the mandibular division is not involved is unknown. Both neuralgias are due to damage in the same nerve. Yet, by talking to the victims, it becomes obvious that the tic hurts more than herpetic infection. There is an anatomical difference. Nerve fibers that produce tic pain are in the tooth pulp. The herpes virus destroys ordinary afferent fibers distributed to the skin. Both kinds of pain are not easy to overcome. Nevertheless, postherpetic neuralgia has a better chance of being managed than tic douloureux. A few cases of postherpetic neuralgia have had good to excellent results. Approximately 60% of the patients can expect to have mixed and limited results, whereas 40% end up being difficult to manage with poor to impossible results. The manageability of the pain very much depends on the degree of the objective pain the patients have and the duration since the skin outbreak caused by the infection. Within 2 months after the skin infection, chances for good to excellent results are high. As this period is prolonged, the manageability will decrease, and the results will turn to mixed and limited. After 1 year, it is reasonable to expect poor and difficult results. The reason is that, scientifically, we know the herpes virus can erode and dissolve myelin sheaths wrapped around the nerve fibers after about a year's time, from the terminal end of nociceptors to the dorsal root ganglia. The procedures to manage pain generated by herpetic infection are very much the same as for other kinds of headaches. The positions used, in order, are supine, prone, and sitting.

Figure 14.4 is provided to visualize where the needles are placed for managing headache perceived in postherpetic neuralgia. The picture was taken as the patient was sitting to receive his third acupuncture treatment. His headache was perceived in the area where needles were inserted. As can be noticed, needles over the scalp were inserted in the primary, secondary, tertiary, and even a couple of nonspecific points. Needles in the mandible and shoulder were placed in the primary points only. The number of needles will increase after the first series of four treatments if improvement is not noticeable. If the improvement is perceived after any series of three treatments, then the same protocol can be repeated. This patient came with pain from a shingles infection affecting the scalp area innervated by the left ophthalmic division on March 25, 1996. He said that the skin infection happened more than 5 months ago, in October of 1995. He had been treated immediately by military doctors in an Air Force hospital in San Antonio. The skin healed quickly in a couple of weeks, but the pain over his head lingered. His doctors told him that sometimes it took months for the pain to subside. After waiting for 5 months, he was told that nothing more could be done for him medically. None of the medicines taken were useful in reducing his headache. Besides postherpetic neuralgia, the patient was also hard of hearing. His objective pain was measured to be sixth degree. The first treatment was given with the patient in the supine position. In addition to the trigger points in the primary group distributed throughout the entire body, trigger points in the secondary and

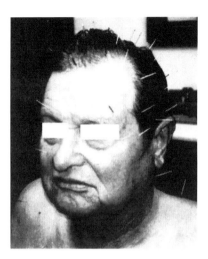

**FIGURE 14.4** Patient with postherpetic neuralgia over the scalp where needles can be seen.

tertiary groups, as shown in Figure 14.4, were also used. A total of five treatments were given as a series, one session every 2 days over 10 days. He was advised to wait for 1 week. Then, the second series of three treatments was provided. By that time, his pain began to show signs of diminishing in both the frequency of attacks and their intensity. The third and last series of three treatments was repeated after 1 more week of waiting. The eleventh and last treatment was given on April 25, 1996. The patient happily informed us that he had been free of pain for almost a week.

There are other kinds of pain in the face and head. They are known as atypical facial pain, that is, pain associated with Bell's palsy, as shown in Figures 14.5 and 14.6. Most cases of Bell's palsy are painless, but these two patients did perceive pain in the face. Acupuncture treatments for these patients had mixed and limited results. Their pain showed obvious relief, but not their facial paralysis, as can be seen from the pictures. One of the headache patients was also unusual in that she is the only patient we have had who came for treatment after a tumor was removed from her left internal acoustic meatus. Figure 14.7 includes two pictures taken before acupuncture on January 18, 1994 (top) and one taken in December of 1996 (bottom). From these pictures, we believe that she had mixed and limited results. Her face became more normal-looking, but paralysis due to damage to her facial nerve persisted. Treating symptoms associated with these problems is not any more complicated than treating other kinds of headaches.

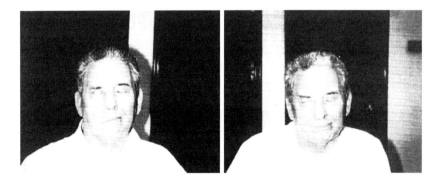

**FIGURE 14.5** Two photos taken of the same patient, one taken on April 24, 1995 before acupuncture (left), the other on June 6 of the same year after 26 treatments (right). His right eye could close better, but he still felt some paralysis in his right face.

Applications with Mixed and Limited Results 181

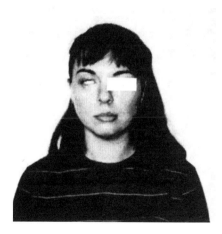

**FIGURE 14.6** A patient with Bell's palsy after eight acupuncture treatments. She still had problems closing her right eye, and the paralysis on the right face persisted.

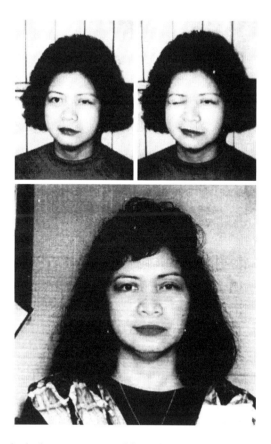

**FIGURE 14.7** A patient who had a tumor removed from the left internal acoustic meatus. The top two pictures were taken at the time of her first visit to the clinic. Due to the paralysis, her left eye was barely able to close normally because her left facial nerve was damaged in the surgery. Her face in the bottom picture, taken almost 3 years later, appears more normal.

## 14.5 PAIN IN THE NECK AND SHOULDER

We often say "pain in the neck," possibly because neck pain is rather common. Anatomically, the neck is the thinnest portion of the entire body trunk; it may also be the weakest. Yet, it has to carry the relatively heavier head on the top. It has a great degree of mobility, which inherently must compromise its stability. The form and shape in which the neck is constructed anatomically makes the region vulnerable to many possible forms of injury. If an accidental force of exogenous origins is applied to the body, the neck would have to be one of most likely regions to suffer impact. Just take automobile accidents as an example. How many of them happen every minute in the United States? The number can be a reasonable explanation of why so many people complain of whiplash. In time, whiplash will eventually become arthritis in the neck. We will use one patient as an example for each of these two kinds of pain to show how acupuncture could have mixed and limited results.

### 14.5.1 Whiplash

Many patients used whiplash as a substitute term for neck pain. Yet, whiplash is not even listed in the 21st edition of *Stedman's Medical Dictionary* (1966), as an official medical term. The dictionary does include "whiplash injury" under the heading of "injury," but not whiplash. Whiplash injury is defined there as "a popular term for hyperextension–hyperflexion of the neck. The term should not be used to imply any specific resultant pathologic condition or syndrome." In the context of this writing, whiplash means neck pain, with some exceptions, as a consequence of the automobile accidents. We understand that the force of impact in an accident will vary because of differences in the driving speeds and in the size of cars. It is a simple principle of physics: force is equal to the rate of change in speed multiplied by the factor of mass. In reality, the result might not always be as physics suggests. There are cases of whiplash with severe neck pain from low-speed collisions. There must be multiple factors involved in determining how much neck pain the injured persons will have after suffering whiplash. From our clinical experience, one general principle applies in many cases of whiplash neck pain: the degree of objective pain measured in the victims seems to be a reliable way for predicting the manageability of neck pain from whiplash. We have had many patients come with whiplash injuries for which the neck pain was totally eradicated in four or fewer treatments, and the patients were not seen to return for the same pain. In other words, we have treated neck pain from whiplash with good to excellent results. These patients invariably have objective pain at no higher than fourth degree. If the degree of the objective pain is five or higher, the results are often mixed and limited. Here is an example.

Sylvia C. was a 71-year-old retiree. Her whiplash was diagnosed by her doctor. She said a drunk driver ran into her car while she was in a funeral motorcade in 1954. She had a chiropractor adjust her neck for 3 months until she was almost killed during a manipulation. She admitted that she had occasional cramping during menstrual periods with pain in the back. She also bled a lot during her periods. Her symptoms indicated that she had dysmenorrhea. Sylvia had a hysterectomy in 1955 because her uterus was prolapsed. By the time she came in December 16, 1983, she had additional pain besides that in the neck. She had a palpable knot of muscle mass over the trapezius at the location of the spinal accessory point. Having a palpable knot of muscle mass at that location can be taken as a sign of a long chronicity of muscle tension in the region. Her objective pain was measured to be ninth degree. That is the upper limit of the manageability of subjective pain, and the manageability is often low and poor. Because of possible poor results, we decided to use more needles than normal from the beginning. For the first three sessions, in the sequence of supine, prone, and sitting, we stimulated trigger points in the primary group and a few in the secondary, including the lesser occipital, third occipital, and cervical plexus. After three treatments as a series in a week, she came for the fourth time on December 26, the day after Christmas. She believed that her neck was less painful. Three more treatments were repeated to constitute a second series. The number of needles used in the neck region was increased to cover the trigger points in the tertiary group, such as the transverse cervical and a few supraclavicular points. After the sixth treatment was given on January 6, 1983, she didn't come for more than 3 years, until March 9, 1987. She returned because she couldn't abduct her right arm without pain in the shoulder joint. She also had some pain in the left ankle when walking. The neck pain only bothered her very occasionally, and it was tolerable. What was wrong in her right shoulder was not determined medically because she came to the clinic directly without going to see a licensed physician. Her pain in the shoulder joint and the arm area is a common problem for patients seeking relief via acupuncture. To us, the problem is related to biceps tendinitis and rotator cuff damage, which are discussed in the next section. The pain in the right shoulder and left ankle Sylvia complained of was reduced after only two visits. She didn't even bother to come for the third appointment, which was suggested for March 17, 1987. On April 19, 1988, more than a year later, she came as an emergency case because she'd been kicked by a horse in her right knee, and she had difficulty walking. The pain was also felt over the left hip along the greater trochanter, which is familiar to us as meralgia paraesthetica or Bernhardt disease. Pain in both areas was taken care of in a single treatment. Her next emergency visit was on June 7, 1989, when the medial plantar surface of her left foot became painful. The pain was stopped in one visit with needles given on the primary trigger points, adding six extra needles along the medial side of the foot. On November 16, 1989, she became dizzy, a condition known medically as vertigo. Her vertigo was taken care of in two treatments using trigger points in the primary group with an additional two needles in front of each ear, at the auriculotemporal and temporomandibular joint points each time. By July 28, 1994, she had come for a total of 22 treatments. During this period, besides recurrent neck pain, she was treated for other kinds of pain, including burning sensation in the toes, loss of tactile sensation in the left hand, signs of carpal tunnel syndrome, etc. We are sure that she will keep returning for years to come, because acupuncture can only provide mixed and limited results for her. Her problem is like a brush fire. When the fire burns over only a couple of square feet, the flame is easy to put out. Fire over an area of thousands upon thousands of acres of brush and forest lands will be hard to stop. Fire in one site is eliminated, but another spot can be ignited, and it will begin to burn again.

### 14.5.2 Arthritic Neck

Many patients we have describe themselves as suffering from arthritis in the neck. The descriptions and opinions can be either their own or given by their doctors. We have no knowledge of what constitutes arthritis in the neck. Is the pain from whiplash and in an arthritic neck the same or different? Our suspicion is that when pain lasts for a long time in the neck, arthritis possibly will set in the neck between the cervical vertebrae. The following is an example.

Jean J. was a 63-year-old retiree. Her doctors at the Air Force Hospital at Lackland told her that she had arthritis in her fourth, fifth, and sixth cervical vertebrae. The pain was so bad that she had only limited motion in the neck. Her objective pain was measured as seventh degree. After four treatments with a protocol similar to that for Sylvia in the previous subsection, she was able to move her neck slightly better. Her neck pain was concentrated in the occipital region over the nuchal line, extending medially from the occipital protuberance to the insertions of the trapezius and sternocleidomastoid muscle laterally on both sides of the shoulder bridges. For the next two treatments on February 1, 1987 (fifth) and February 3, 1987 (sixth), six extra needles were placed in the occipital along the nuchal line with Jean in an upright sitting position. She received 12 treatments between January 12 and February 19 of that year. At that time, she said the pain had reduced and she could turn her neck more easily, as when backing up her car. It was suggested that she come for more sessions after a week of intermission, but she ignored the suggestion and hasn't called to request more acupuncture service since. Our prediction is that she will call sometime in the future, because we know that the results of the treatments for her are mixed and limited. The same neck pain will return sooner or later.

## 14.6 PAIN IN THE UPPER LIMB

Subjective pain in the upper limb, from shoulder joint to fingertips, is a good example to demonstrate that it can appear anywhere, particularly in the wrist and hands. Several photos in Figure 14.8 show the different deformities that can occur in the wrist and fingers. The pain can be located over the radial side of the wrist, in the interphalangeal joints, at the basal joint in the base of the thumb, and so on.

We have selected pain in two areas, the shoulder joint and the carpal tunnel, for the purpose of illuminating how the results of acupuncture treatments can be mixed and limited for managing pain in the upper limb. The anatomical term for the shoulder joint is the glenohumeral; it is the joint formed between the glenoid cavity of the scapula and the humeral head. Our clinical observations seem to indicate that the pain in the shoulder is not from diseases or pathological changes inside the joint. In most patients, the pain is produced by biceps tendinitis, as we have mentioned in Chapter 13. This kind of pain will have good to excellent results with acupuncture treatments, when patients have objective pain of fourth degree or lower. After objective pain reaches the fifth degree or higher, the results will be mixed and limited, as in the case of Tom B. described in Section 14.6.1. Shoulder pain can have poor results and could be difficult to manage once the objective pain reaches the ninth degree or higher, which will be discussed in the next chapter.

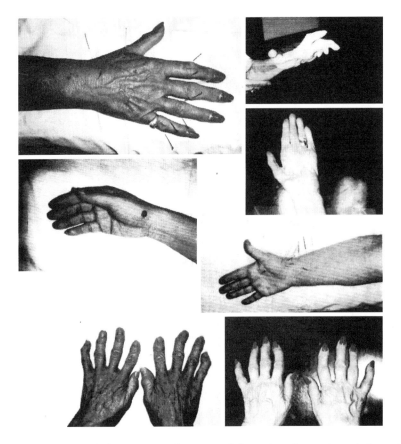

**FIGURE 14.8** In this group of pictures, some fingers are deformed, and some interphalangeal joints have needles inserted. These are the loci where the trigger points are detected.

Applications with Mixed and Limited Results 185

### 14.6.1 BICEPS TENDINITIS

The subject was Tom B., 75 years old and self-employed. We need to begin with a quote from the medical report he brought to us. A portion of the report described that "I saw Mr. B. on the morning of January 7, 1997, for an evaluation of the right shoulder. He gave a history of having trouble back in May 1995, and had x-rays made by Dr. Schoch. I think there was concern at that time the patient had a problem with his rotator cuff. He had a shot of cortisone at that point, and he said that gave him nice relief of symptoms until September 1995. Between May and September, he was able to play golf and do some hunting. He stated that in 1996, he did some fishing, maybe only two or three times, but slowed down because of right shoulder pain. He pretty much stopped playing golf altogether in October 1996. He said that since September or October of 1996, he's had a heck of a lot of trouble with his right shoulder, a lot of pain, a decrease in function and particularly has trouble sleeping at night, and his wife states that he has to get up and walk the floor or even go to sleep in a chair. She also mentioned that she has to help him get dressed because he has trouble moving the right arm. Tom has been a diabetic since the age of 40 and currently is taking four units of Humulin R and 28 units of Humulin N each morning, as well as four units of Humulin R and four units of Humulin N each night. He has not had any trouble with neuropathy in the upper extremities and his only real problem with the upper extremities has been this right shoulder. Dr. Blevins is his current endocrinologist and is managing his diabetes as well as his neuropathy. The family seems to be greatly concerned over the neuropathy problems and asked if I might suggest another person to give an opinion, and I recommend that they might want to contact Dr. Green. In summary, I believe Mr. B. suffers from pretty severe rotator cuff deficiency and muscle weakness in the right shoulder..." The report was signed by Charles A. Rockwood, Jr., MD, who ruled out surgery for Tom to rectify his shoulder problem. With such a medical history on hand, it was no surprise to find out that Tom had ninth-degree objective pain. He came on February 26, 1997, more than a month after consulting with Dr. Rockwood, having been referred to try acupuncture by one of his physicians. Acupoints around his right shoulder joint were palpated to check if Tom had any indication of damage in the rotator cuff. Many of the acupoints in his shoulder were passive with tenderness. The most sensitive acupoints in his shoulder were along the long head of the biceps brachii tendon situated inside the intertubercular sulcus. This was to be expected, because passive acupoints, which by then had already converted to become trigger points, would invariably appear at that location for all patients with shoulder pain. These trigger points are shown in Figure 14.9. Usually, one or two needles are

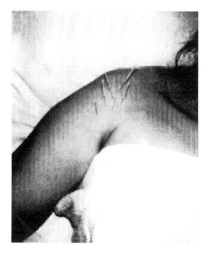

**FIGURE 14.9** A picture showing six needles inserted along the biceps brachii tendon in the intertubercular sulcus. One needle further back is in the acromioclavicular point.

used in this location. For Tom, six needles were given because his objective pain had been measured as ninth degree. Once trigger points begin to appear outside the region where the long head of the biceps brachii is located, such as the acromioclavicular and deltoid points, some diseases in the rotator cuff may be indicated, as in the case of Tom's shoulder. We predicted that it would not be possible to eradicate pain totally in Tom's shoulder. However, there could be a chance to ease some of his pain because ninth degree is the upper limit for having mixed and limited results. He came for five treatments. On his last visit on March 7, 1997, he still had pain in his right shoulder, although he believed there was a slight relief. His diabetic neuropathy seemed to be more serious than his physicians realized. The neuropathy in the lower limbs was already up to the knees. Once the neuropathy reaches the knees, acupuncture will not be very useful. Tom's case should belong to the next chapter, covering treatments with poor results and difficult manageability. He is mentioned here because he only came to the clinic five times. He might have had better results if he had tried a few more treatments. Thus, it is appropriate to include him in the category of mixed and limited results. Patients like Tom are not uncommon. They don't understand the relationship between objective pain and the outcome of treatments. As should be clear by now, the outcome of the treatments depends on how many sessions they need to receive to have substantial relief for their pain. For Tom, the projected number of treatments for the right shoulder pain to be effectively managed could be as many as 36.

### 14.6.2 CARPAL TUNNEL SYNDROME

The proper nomenclature for the carpal tunnel should be "radiocarpal joint." It is the joint formed between the distal radius and the proximal row of the carpal bones. The area of this joint is commonly referred to as the wrist. Pain in the wrist can be carpal tunnel syndrome, superficial radial neuropathy, or arthritis in the wrist. Our attention is placed on carpal tunnel syndrome.

Carpal tunnel syndrome is a clinically and medically well-defined disease. Very rarely will patients with this disease arrive without diagnosis from their doctors. We would not describe the condition as common in our practice. Only one or two cases are seen each month. Most cases (90% or more) are female. Cases seen in males are most often injury-related. In females, carpal tunnel syndrome seems to associate with having low blood pressure during premenopausal years and a history of enduring dysmenorrhea. Unless objective pain is graded to be higher than ninth degree, carpal tunnel syndrome can be adequately and effectively managed with good to excellent results. The exception is after surgery to reduce pressure on the median nerve. The median nerve runs inside the carpal tunnel. The syndrome is attributed to the fact that pressure inside the tunnel increases to compress on the nerve. This is the reason that the thumb and index finger become painful, numb, and tingling, and sometimes can have burning sensations. Larry R. is a typical example for whom acupuncture treatments provide mixed and limited results.

Larry R. was a 34-year-old railroad car repairman. Although he first came on October 27, 1980, at which time he had only carpal tunnel problem in the right hand, it would perhaps be best to begin discussion of this case by quoting a medical report later prepared by Dr. David P. Green, a very well known surgeon and coauthor with Dr. Charles A. Rockwood for their famous book about the shoulder. Larry was referred to Dr. Green by Dr. Robert Stevens. The report that we received was written by Dr. Green. Dr. Green wrote "[...]I have none of the previous medical records, but the patient relates the following history. He has had symptoms of carpal tunnel syndrome bilaterally for 3.5 to 4 years, for which he has been treated by Dr. Dung with acupuncture every 6 to 9 months with good relief of his symptoms." The story that Larry told was that of a few months before coming for acupuncture, in an attempt to catch an accidentally falling railroad tie, his right hand was injured. When he caught the tie, one of the wood block's corners hit squarely at the center of his wrist. The pain he had at that moment was beyond description. The best he could do was to say it was like going through hell. The severe pain lasted for a while. Eventually, the severity subsided to some degree, but there was always some pain in his hand. Sometime later, the pain gradually became exacerbated. By the time of his arrival, the suffering had grown intermittent. At worst, his hand would have numbness, tingling, and a hot sensation like burning fire. He even attempted to immerse his hand into a bucket of ice water, although this did nothing to alleviate the sensation. Larry was young, muscular, and tall, and a strong and handsome man. He had the appearance of a well-trained athlete. Such a person couldn't possibly have a high degree of objective pain. In 1980, we hadn't yet perfected the system to measure objective pain, so there is no record of what degree of objective pain Larry had. The protocol of treatments for him was similar to what has described many times before. First, he was laid in the supine position. Trigger points in the primary group were used. Two additional points are very important for managing the pain of carpal tunnel syndrome, the median and recurrent median, the locations for which can be seen in Chapter 12. They are located at the ventral side of the distal forearm and in the thenar compartment of the palm. These two points must be used for pain related to the median nerve. In the early stages of carpal tunnel syndrome, one of these two will become a trigger point first, although which is difficult to predict. At this stage, the objective pain is already in the secondary category. In time, both of them will turn into trigger points, and the objective pain will enter into the tertiary category. The subjective pain in the carpal tunnel will be harder to manage. Both points in Larry were tender when they were pressed during testing. Each time when Larry received treatment, these two points were used. Less than 3 min after needle insertion was completed, he began to feel nauseated, with an urge to vomit or throw up. This is one of the immediate needle reactions sometimes observed in patients who suffer from acute pain for relatively a long time, such as several months. Physiologically, the reaction is known as syncope. The syncope indicated that Larry's autonomic nervous system was becoming unstable. In time, when acute pain transforms to become chronic, the pain will have the potential to develop into reflex sympathetic dystrophy. Once syncope is observed, needles have to be removed. After a few minutes of resting, signs of syncope clear away. Having syncope is a positive indication that acute pain will show improvement soon after the treatment. When Larry returned for the second time on October 31, he was very exuberant because his pain was much reduced. What made him happy was that he had had his first two good nights of sleep since the injury to his right median nerve on the wrist. He received only three treatments to stop pain in the arm, forearm, hand, and fingers. Of course, his story was not that simple. Over the next 17 years, until March 5, 1997, he came for a total of 67 treatments. During these years, the intervals between his returns for old and new symptoms varied from 3 months to 3 years, depending on what he did in daily life. A few years later, he was given a disability retirement. There is no way for a person of his age and energy to stay idle. There were occasions when he would appear without an appointment because he was in pain after working strenuously for days to build his new home. The old pain and symptoms would take only a couple of treatments to amend. As the years passed, new problems began to appear. Some of them were beyond needle treatments, such as "losing strength in the hands." That was why he was referred to Dr. Green. Dr. Green reported "examination of both hands reveals very thick, heavy, large, working man's hands with callus formation primary over IV and V bilaterally. There is well localized tenderness over A1 pulley in right III, and active motion in this digit lacks the final few degrees. There is no triggering. Phalen's, Tinel's, and direct compression of the median nerve are all somewhat equivocal bilaterally, but definitely suggestive of median nerve compression. Two-point discrimination is 5 mm in all digits with no subjective diminution in any digit. There is excellent thenar muscle tone bilaterally, and key pinch strength is 23# right and 27# left. Grip strength is 55# right and 110# left. All intrinsic and extrinsic muscles appear to be intact." The final impression and recommendations were, "I agree that this patient appears to have bilateral carpal tunnel syndrome, although I believe that his major symptoms at the present time are due to an early trigger finger in right III. Therefore, the right carpal tunnel and the flexor tendon sheath right III were each injected with 8 mg of dexamethasone acetate. He will return in 1 month for reevaluation." One important reason for quoting this report is to show that pain can grow. When Larry first came for acupuncture, his left hand was free of any problem. Six years later, the left hand was diagnosed to have the same condition as that of the right. Thus far, neither hand has required surgical intervention for the carpal tunnel syndrome. On his latest visit, he said that both hands were doing fine. He had come instead because of a pain on his right dorsal scapular point extending to the right greater occipital point. The pain had bothered him so much that he hadn't slept well for a few nights. One treatment was sufficient to stop that pain, and he didn't return for another treatment, which we suggested if the pain persisted.

## 14.7 PAIN IN THE BODY TRUNK

The two kinds of body trunk pain we have picked to discuss are postherpetic neuralgia and lower back pain. Both of them have been mentioned in the previous chapter. We want to use them as examples again to compare and contrast good to excellent results from acupuncture treatments with mixed and limited results. To manage subjective pain perceived in the body trunk, just like pain in other parts of the body, trigger points of the primary group are essential in treatments. However, many points in the tertiary and nonspecific groups will be needed in managing pain located in this region.

### 14.7.1 Postherpetic Neuralgia

We have offered a case of headache caused by herpes infection in the previous chapter. That patient, whose headaches resulting from postherpetic neuralgia turned out to have good to excellent results, was not an exception. Postherpetic neuralgia in other regions can have good to excellent results as well, if treated with acupuncture within an appropriate period after the infection. Regretfully, such ideal circumstances are not commonly encountered. Very few patients with postherpetic neuralgia come with objective pain at fourth degree or lower. As can be seen from Table 14.2, most of them were measured to have objective pain at fifth degree or higher, placing the expected outcome of their treatments in the mixed and limited results group. Some of them will have poor results or even turn out to be impossible to manage, as explained in the next chapter. The duration of subjective pain after infection is obviously critical in managing postherpetic neuralgia. If the neuralgia is less than 3 months in duration, acupuncture will produce good to excellent results. The pain will still be manageable up to 6 months. Between 6 months to 1 year, the neuralgic pain will become obstinate, and the results of the treatments will be mixed and limited at best. After 1 year, postherpetic neuralgia

### TABLE 14.2
### Cases of Postherpetic Neuralgia Seen Over a Period of 3 Years

| Patient | Sex | Age (Years) | Pain Code | Duration | Degree of Pain | No. of Treatments |
|---|---|---|---|---|---|---|
| 1. RD (84958D094) | F | 86 | 403.X2b | 3 weeks | 4 | 6 |
| 2. CK (83006K075) | M | 66 | 203.X2a | 1 day | 5 | 7 |
| 3. SB (82902B100) | F | 46 | 303.X2b | 1 month | 6 | 6 |
| 4. HC (83437C122) | M | 65 | 303.X2b | 4 months | 7 | 10 |
| 5. MO (84472O020) | F | 49 | 303.X2b | 1 week | 10 | 5 |
| 6. FS (84579S309) | M | 65 | 203.X2b | 2 months | 3 | 3 |
| 7. TR (85199R151) | F | 34 | 403.X2b | 2 years | 4 | 3 |
| 8. JP (86009P156) | F | 72 | 203.X2b | 3 months | 7 | 9 |
| 9. BB (85124B281) | M | 61 | 203.X2b | 6 weeks | 7 | 5 |
| 10. RS (86297S443) | M | 66 | 203.X2b | 5 months | 4 | 12 |
| 11. RP (86177P169) | F | 28 | 403.X2b | 1 month | 5 | 2 |
| 12. MA (85120A084) | M | 69 | 003.X2b | 6 weeks | 2 | 9 |

*Note:* A few of these cases have good to excellent results. More have mixed and limited results. Note the Duration column, which indicates that a shorter duration of pain seems to produce better results.

becomes difficult to manage, and the results are often poor to nonexistent. The following are case reports for two patients with postherpetic neuralgia.

*Case 1*: Clifton M. was a 71-year-old rancher. His herpes could still be clearly seen (Figure 14.10) on the skin when he arrived on August 3, 1994. The infection had occurred 3 months prior to his first visit. The dermatomes involved were the third to fifth thoracic spinal nerves, because the infected area extended to the right nipple in front. His objective pain was measured to be only second degree, the lowest of all patients seen with postherpetic neuralgia. This may explain why his subjective pain diminished a little on its own during the previous 3 months, although he was still hurting, which was the reason he decided to come for acupuncture. For the first treatment, he was in the prone position, as shown in the figure. The needles were inserted into the trigger points of the primary group, plus nonspecific points seen in the picture (Figure 14.10). Two days later, he came for the second treatment, which used the supine position to needle the trigger points in the primary group and nonspecific points, approximately 24 in number, over the infected skin in the ventral thorax. He reported that the pain had been reduced by more than 50%. His third treatment was given on August 9, with him lying on the left side of his body. In addition to all the trigger points in the primary group accessible, another 50 needles were placed around the three dermatomes in the right side of the body. He returned for the fourth and last treatment on August 20. He said that he felt better that morning than at any other time in the last 4 months. He came because he felt so good that he wanted to have one more needle treatment. The second treatment was repeated for his last visit. In retrospect, the results for Clifton can be considered as good to excellent. His case is included here for the purpose of showing how needles are used in the skin area where herpes infection occurred.

The protocols for treating postherpetic neuralgia are basically the same regardless of the differences in the degree of objective pain that patients have. In the beginning, trigger points of the primary group are used. If the treatments work, then that is all we need to do. If not, trigger points of the secondary, or even tertiary and nonspecific groups can be used in increments until pain relief is obtained. In Clifton's case, his pain was totally gone after four treatments, after needling only the trigger points in the primary group and the points as seen in the figure.

*Case 2*: Norman A. was a 51-year-old gardener. He was chosen because we also have a picture to show where his herpes was (Figure 14.11). He said that he "worked hard to keep customers having a good-looking yard." His first visit was on March 23, 1988. He described his conditions as being "tinnitus, allergy, and ringing in the ears because of nerve deafening." He also had pain in both elbows, as with tennis elbow, but he didn't play tennis at all. Pain was also perceived in the deep radial point area. He had had back pain for some time and had been operated on, as can be seen in the figure. He said that his doctor told him it was a fusion. The surgery was not totally successful for Norman because he still had lower back pain. He attributed his allergy to long hours of exposure, working outdoors among all kinds of pollens. The outdoor environments were often much more noisy than they normally should be, which was why he believed his ear nerves were dying and why he heard ringing all the time. His main reason for coming was because he couldn't work due to severe pain in his right arm. He took a lot of aspirin, but still had so much pain that he couldn't

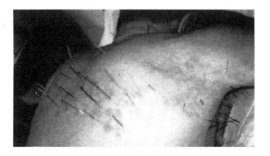

**FIGURE 14.10** Visible herpes infection in Clifton M.

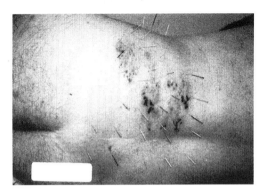

**FIGURE 14.11** A photo of Norman A. showing skin infected with herpes and needles placed over the infected area.

have a good night's sleep. At his first visit, his objective pain was measured to be seventh degree. At this level, some of the problems mentioned were better after a number of treatments, but the same problems kept coming back, and we kept giving him treatments. To save space and time, we need to jump back to discussing Norman's postherpetic neuralgia.

The picture shown in Figure 14.11 was taken 10 days after the skin broke out, which occurred on August 10, 1996. Because of its short duration of only 10 days, the condition may not qualify as postherpetic neuralgia. Clinically, pain produced by the herpes virus is known to be self-limited. For most patients, subjective pain will subside automatically once the skin lesions are healed. The irony is that no reliable prognosis is available to predict whether a herpes infection will develop into the postherpetic neuralgia. He still had seventh-degree objective pain. At this level, the possibility for his herpes infection to turn into postherpetic neuralgia was definitely there. He indicated that his pain had stayed the same for the last 10 days without noticeable diminishment. Figure 14.11 shows the needles placed in the infected skin area for the first visit, plus the trigger points in the primary group. After two more sessions, one in the supine position and another on his right side, we waited for 1 week. He returned on December 20. Pain caused by the herpes infection was gone, except for some itching in the right hip where rashes were seen. He thought the skin rashes were an indication of herpes. We told him that couldn't happen because we had never seen a herpes infection occur bilaterally. Another three treatments over a week's time stopped the herpetic pain totally.

Pain related to postherpetic neuralgia is unique; once the pain is gone, it is gone forever. We never see patients come back because of relapsed postherpetic neuralgia. Lower back pain is different. Pain in the lumbar region will keep coming back to haunt the victims faithfully in time. This interval is 4 to 6 months for most patients whose objective pain is between the fifth and eighth degrees, and thus have mixed and limited results from acupuncture.

### 14.7.2 LOWER BACK PAIN

Patients with lower back pain are all too numerous. Their records alone would be sufficient to write a big book. By regretful necessity, we will use only one example to represent all of them. There are theories to explain why *Homo sapiens* should be so vulnerable to lower back problem. One explanation is that we are upright creatures. When we stand, our center of gravity is between the fourth and fifth lumbar vertebrae, which is the location where back pain will start first. Once the pain is in the lower back, it will keep recurring for the rest of one's life. That is why there are so many cases of this pain seen in clinics. The sequence for treating lower back pain is fairly similar—practically identical, in fact—for most patients. The first treatment is always given using the prone position. The trigger points used are limited to the primary group. The most essential points are the four found on each side of the lumbar. These are shown in the anatomical charts found in Chapter 12.

Each of them must be accurately located for needle stimulation. All the needles have to be inserted in such a manner that a sensation is generated and felt by the patients. Catching the superior cluneal points can be tricky. Only a millimeter away, the needle can hit the iliac crest below, or generate no sensation if it is too far above. Individuals who have had lower back pain for years can have very tight tissues in the superior cluneal points. The tightness will be testable by needle insertion at the localities. It can be so tight that the needle becomes hard to pull out once it is placed in deep. During the 1930s, many biopsy investigations were performed by taking tissue from this area in patients who had long-term chronic pain in the lower back. The studies were not conclusive because of the variables observed in the tissues taken from different patients.

The second treatment is routinely given 48 h after the first one, if time and circumstances permit. The treatment is provided with patients in the supine position if the lower back shows substantial relief. The definition of "substantial" is subjective. However, when patients are asked how much relief they have after the first treatment, and their answer is 50% or more, that certainly can be taken as an indication of having substantial relief. Trigger points used for the second treatment in the supine position include the primary group only.

If, on their second visit, patients indicate that the lower back is still hurting, the protocol of the first treatment, inserting needles in the back using the prone position, will be repeated once more. An additional three needles are used on each side of the lumbar at the posterior cutaneous of the first lumbar spinal nerves. Occasionally, three treatments in the lumbar may have to be repeated for patients with a great deal of pain in the lower back. For us, three is the limit. At the third treatment, lumbar spinous process points have to be examined to see if any of them have already turned passive as trigger points. If so, they have to be stimulated with needles. As many as 20 needles (Figure 14.12) can be used in the entire lumbar region. The fourth treatment has to be on the supine position. After that, one or two more treatments using the prone position will be repeated for patients with lower back pain. Four or five sessions constitute a series of treatments. To give six consecutive treatments, once every 2 days, is rare. There's always a week's break between the two series of treatments. If the second series is called for, the same sequence described above will be repeated, usually with no more than four treatment sessions. Patients coming for three or more series consecutively are the minority. Most patients don't need more than eight treatments to either see the benefit of acupuncture or to give up in disappointment and stop coming. Mario is the only example given here for patients who have lower back pain.

Mario Q. was a 57-year-old tile salesman. He had a particularly good memory regarding the history of the start of his lower back pain 40 years ago. He was a teenager working for his father in a grocery store. One day, while holding a piece of ice in one arm, he slipped and fell to the ground. His back hurt ever since. Whenever he had lower back pain, he would go to a chiropractor for adjustments or take Tylenol. Either remedy would take care of his pain. He had had an inguinal

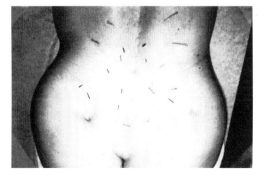

**FIGURE 14.12** A photo showing a total of 20 needles placed in the lumbar region for a patient receiving a third treatment after not receiving much relief from the first two sessions.

hernia that ruptured when he was younger, and his gall bladder was removed in 1973. Yet, he never went for medical consultation about his back because his doctor was not interested in an innocuous problem such as lower back pain. When he first appeared at our clinic on January 17, 1985, he looked as shown in Figure 14.13a and c. His posture alone was enough to indicate that he had acute pain in his lower back. He had been in this shape since the New Year. He said that he hadn't done anything but raise his hands to change a light bulb. His back pain had relapsed more frequently as he grew older. Sometimes merely turning the wrong way could make his back hurt. Chiropractic adjustments and nonprescription pain pills had reached the point of uselessness. In fact, he blamed his chiropractor for making him crooked with his last adjustment. His cousin Manuel, who was one of our patients, suggested that he should try acupuncture, because Manuel had had good to excellent results from the needle treatments. Mario explained that he had waited for more than 2 weeks to come because he was hoping that his back would get better. Besides, the drive between his home in Houston and San Antonio took 6 h for a round trip. Finally, he settled for a week at his cousin's place at Gonzales, which is about an hour's drive from the clinic. One week is long enough to have three treatments. This is a case in which improvement could be seen immediately after the first treatment, as seen in Figure 14.13. He stood straighter as compared with his appearance before needling. He claimed that he had less pain in getting up from the bed after the treatment. His objective pain was measured at seven degrees. After three treatments in prone, supine, then prone again using trigger points of the primary and some in the secondary group, his lower back pain disappeared. He was advised that the pain would relapse in 4 to 6 months. Ultimately, the pain stayed away for 11 months, until December 14, 1985. On his fourth visit, he said that he had been free of back pain the whole time, until 1 week before returning. Two treatments were given as a series, prone and supine. The back pain was under control for another 10 months until October 23, 1986. On his sixth visit, he said he had fallen again on July 4 in his front yard while mowing the lawn, and been caught by the blade of the lawnmower. His shirt had been torn and his ribs fractured. Yet he had no pain at all until the end of September. He began to have headaches on the right side, as well as right neck and

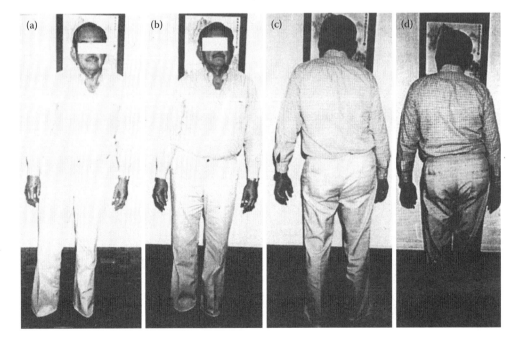

**FIGURE 14.13** Pictures taken of Mario Q. on the day of his first visit: a and c are before treatment, b and d are after treatment.

## Applications with Mixed and Limited Results

shoulder pain. The headache and neck pain were managed effectively by taking Tylenol and muscle relaxants. He started by taking a dose of one pill. By the time he came one and a half months later, even three pills were not enough to ease his pain. For a couple of weeks, pain would develop on his right shoulder (at the dorsal scapular point) at around 5 to 8 a.m. The pain then extended to the right greater occipital point.

With Mario on his left side, needles were placed in the trigger points of the primary and secondary groups located in his right upper limb, from the dorsal scapular to the greater occipital points down to the points in the hands. For the rest of the body, only the trigger points of the primary group were used. He came for two more treatments on October 24 and October 25, on the prone position using the trigger points of the primary group and an additional four needles in the secondary and tertiary groups in the scapular shoulder and occipital regions, then the supine with a similar protocol. His ninth visit was on December 29, 1986. It was an emergency call, because his back pain hit him suddenly as he attempted to pick up a heavy gas tank. This time, besides the usual trigger points in the primary group, three in the secondary group were added for a total of 14 needles in the lumbar region. He had a flare-up and came with a crutch the next day. He said that he had difficulty walking. The tenth treatment was given prone, with four needles added in the lumbar instead of three. He didn't return for his eleventh treatment the next day, which was at the end of the year. Instead, he made his eleventh visit on March 1, 1990, and received a series of three treatments, with the thirteenth on March 3. Mario is a case for acupuncture treatments having mixed and limited results. The relief lasts only for a period of several months, and the pain will relapse. He will need to come back repeatedly for an expected period. The lower back pain has the potential to go away forever after a number of repeated series of treatments, but how many times they must be repeated and over how long a period is unknown.

### 14.8 PAIN IN THE LOWER LIMB

It is not easy for us to estimate how many different kinds of pain are possible in the lower limb. One type we have seen is hip pain or trochanteric bursitis, also known as meralgia paraesthetica (Bernhardt disease). Figure 14.14 shows two patients with the disease. One of the treatments for pain

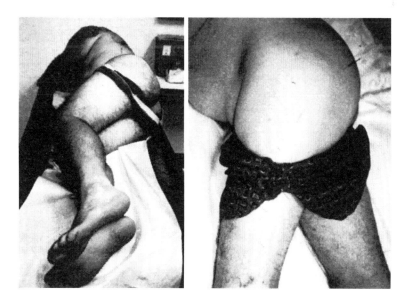

**FIGURE 14.14** Two patients having hip pain under treatment in which needles are placed over the greater trochanter area. One of them (right) had surgery to the hip without much success.

in the hip is to have patients lie on their side, as seen in the figure. The pertinent medical history and acupuncture treatments for meralgia paraesthetica or Bernhardt disease are covered in Chapter 13, and so we will omit them here.

Another known example of pain in the lower limb is caused by a Baker cyst (Figure 14.15) in the popliteal fossa. However, although it is worth mentioning, it is not a common enough case for us to spend time describing this kind of pain and how to treat it.

Ankle pain is relatively common. Causes of pain in the ankle vary, from endogenous to exogenous origins. We have two photos included in Figure 14.16. One picture shows swollen ankles due to edema without any previous injury known to the patient. Another picture shows the right ankle has been injured, as evident from the swelling. Ankle pain is easy to manage, often with positive results, which can be mixed and limited in nature.

Patients with different kinds of skin diseases are also occasionally seen. Some diseases we know, such as psoriatic arthritis (Figure 14.17). We have no idea what many others are (Figure 14.18).

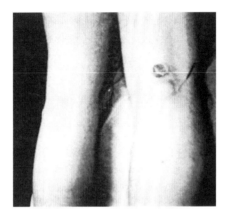

**FIGURE 14.15** A Baker cyst the size of a nickel is seen in the popliteal fossa.

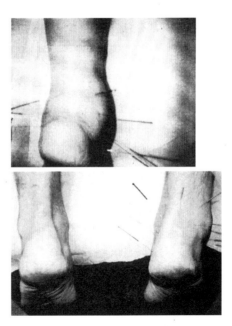

**FIGURE 14.16** The trigger points used to treat pain in the ankles are mostly nonspecific.

Applications with Mixed and Limited Results 195

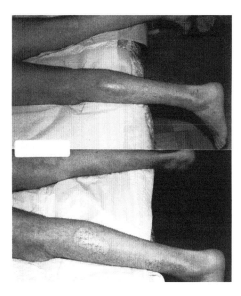

**FIGURE 14.17** A patient with psoriatic arthritis. The upper picture was taken before acupuncture, when the color of the infected skin areas was a hot red. The lower picture was taken 3 days later, and the color of the same skin areas appeared whitish. Pain in this patient was reduced, but his skin lesions remained unhealed.

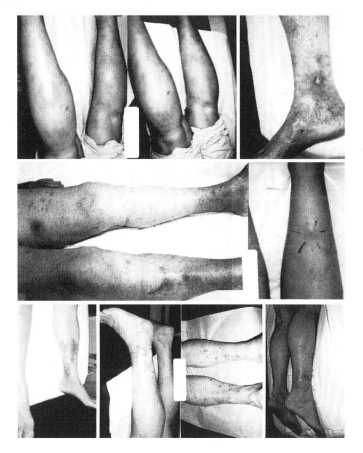

**FIGURE 14.18** Photos of patients with skin lesions that produced subjective pain in the lower limbs. The names of these dermatological diseases are unknown to us.

**196**  Acupuncture: An Anatomical Approach

Their pain is rather complicated to describe clearly. All that can be said is that acupuncture treatments have mixed and limited results for many of these patients. We still recommend trying acupuncture, if you so desire.

For us, two kinds of pain in the lower limbs have certain significance that deserves mention. They are knee pain and pain in the foot.

### 14.8.1 KNEE PAIN

Addressing pain in the knees is a daunting proposition. This conclusion is drawn from seeing a large number of patients with knee pain. But the task can be simplified into two categories: knee pain with organic diseases and those without. "Organic" in this instance means structural damage or injury in the knee joints. The most likely damaged or injured structures in the knee are the meniscus and cruciate ligaments. There are a number of ways these structures can be damaged and injured, such as sports activities and arthritic degeneration due to aging. Conditions and diseases of this nature in the knees are usually not difficult for doctors to detect and diagnose. Sophisticated medical equipment, such as the arthroscope, is available for both diagnostic and therapeutic purposes. Patients with pain of an organic nature seldom turn to acupuncture for help, and acupuncture won't be much help for patients with this kind of knee pain. Our only requirement for differentiating knee pain with organic diseases or without them is the knowledge of acupoints. If the locations of acupoints as shown in Figure 14.19 can be recognized in the knee, and one knows the sequence of their turning into trigger points, it is possible to judge whether knee pain involves organic damage and injury or not.

We name the acupoints on each side of the patellar ligament as the eyes of knee or knee eyes. The two acupoints superior to the knee eyes (Figure 14.19) are the insertion of the vastus medialis and vastus lateralis muscles, making four of them all over the kneecap region. We suspect that knee pain starts in most patients from the saphenous point. If the saphenous point is the only locus with pain in the entire knee region, that pain will be very easy to eliminate with good to excellent results. Once tenderness is detected in one of the two knee eye points, managing pain in the knee begins to become difficult. This difficulty will increase when both knee eyes become trigger points. If either acupoint formed by the vastus medialis or lateralis turns into a trigger point, such knee pain becomes quite difficult to manage. The manageability of pain in the knee is almost impossible when trigger points for both muscles are detectable. By this time, lesions inside the knee joint will be discernible and organic damage will be detected. By then, knee surgery or replacement may be inevitable to take care of the pain. If there is still hope in using acupuncture, all acupoints indicated in Figure 14.19 are beneficial to use for managing the pain. The protocol for managing knee pain is very much the same as for treating other kinds of pain. Start on the supine position by using trigger

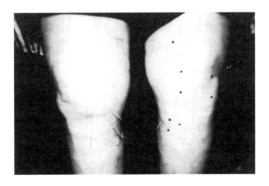

**FIGURE 14.19** A patient with knee pain. The 11 dark points marked over the knee region are used to treat knee pain.

points of the primary group, plus the points in the knee region as shown in Figure 14.19. The second treatment is on the prone position using the trigger points in the primary group, plus the accessible points around the knee. The third treatment is on the sitting position with focus on the knee region. The trigger points can be increased if more treatments are needed to produce pain relief in the knees. No case examples will be offered to show the exact manner for managing knee pain.

The knee pain in the patient seen in Figure 14.19 had mixed results. Her pain in the knee was reduced, but not completely dispelled. The same pain returned a few months later.

### 14.8.2 Pain in the Foot

We have seen patients with several kinds of pain in the feet. Specific examples include Morton neuroma between the third and fourth toes, bunions over the big toe (Figure 14.20), and on the dorsal surface of the feet (Figure 14.21), for which the name of the skin disease is not known. Again, we will not spend time here studying these pain types. Instead, the last pain in the foot we shall mention is clinically known as diabetic peripheral neuropathy.

Peripheral neuropathy is well-known medically. There exists a two-volume book, more than 2,300 pages long, with this title by Dyck et al. [18]. Yet, when we want to find out the symptoms of peripheral neuropathy, the answer simply includes pricking pain, numb sensation, burning, tightness, and cold. The symptoms can start unilaterally or bilaterally from either foot to hand, or both of them simultaneously. The symptoms will then spread proximally toward the ankle, leg, knee and thigh

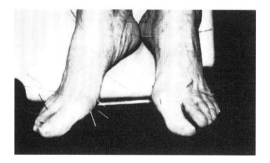

**FIGURE 14.20** Two bunions on the proximal end of each big toe surrounded by a number of needles.

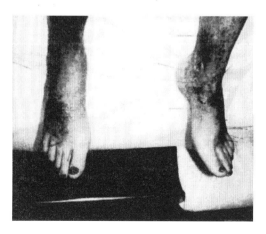

**FIGURE 14.21** Skin disease in a patient. We don't know the name of this disease, only that the patient complained that her feet hurt. Acupuncture eased her pain in the feet, but didn't heal the skin lesions during the time she came for the treatments.

in the lower limb, and the wrist, forearm, arm, and shoulder in the upper limb. The spreading of neuropathy is generally slow in speed. It can take years for the symptoms to reach the leg or forearm. Peripheral neuropathy can be associated with several disease entities, such as causalgia, reflex sympathetic dystrophy, and diabetes. Our attention is focused here on diabetic peripheral neuropathy.

Diabetes is a common illness in southern Texas. Nevertheless, diabetic peripheral neuropathy is not commonly seen among the patients we have. Only one such patient is received each month. It would be preposterous to claim that acupuncture benefits them all. However, we have no reservations about stating that acupuncture indeed helps to reduce some symptoms for some patients for a certain period. Because of our curiosity for a scientific answer as to whether acupuncture really has any use in managing diabetic peripheral neuropathy, it was an exciting thrill for us to receive a memo from a diabetic research consortium in San Antonio, soliciting a proposal for a study in diabetes. With undying naiveté, we accepted the invitation and mailed the consortium an outline of our research proposal to see if acupuncture would be able to improve the symptoms of diabetic peripheral neuropathy. To date, we have received no reply, even as a minimum of courtesy, to indicate whether our proposal had been received by the consortium. Clearly, the solicitations were delivered to us for three consecutive years before our response to the third time, purely because we were a faculty member at the health science center. Surely, people in the consortium didn't expect someone to be so crazy as to suggest acupuncture for diabetic research.

Management of diabetic peripheral neuropathy can have good to excellent results, if the symptoms are limited to the feet only. Once symptoms reach the ankle, management starts to have mixed and limited results. When neuropathologic symptoms are in the knee, they will be difficult to manage. Once above the knee, there is no hope of taking care of the symptoms.

Diabetic peripheral neuropathy is rarely seen in the upper limb, and thus we have not similarly described its occurrence there. Our example for diabetic peripheral neuropathy is among the far more typical lower limb cases.

Charles R. was a 70-year-old retiree. He described his problem as "shooting pain in the back of legs, very painful." That was on February 23, 1995. He didn't reveal how long he had suffered from diabetes, when the symptoms of pain first appeared, or when the peripheral neuropathy was first diagnosed. He didn't even mention the name of his disease, but admitted upon questioning that he had been diagnosed by his doctor to have diabetic peripheral neuropathy. He brought six pill bottles, the contents of which were perphenazine (for anxiety), Propoxy (Darvon containing narcotics), Zantac (for stomach), and Dilantin and Sulindac (for arthritis). He complained that he couldn't sleep because his muscles twitched with fibrillation (author's term) at night in bed. We thought that with the symptoms Charles had, he would have a high degree of objective pain, but it turned out to be only sixth degree. After two treatments, one supine and one prone, using only trigger points in the primary group each time, he came for a third visit on February 27. He said that he still had same symptoms: muscle jumping and jerking. He had been sleepless for the last two nights. Two more treatments were repeated, one supine and one prone, and used primary trigger points and an additional four needles in the secondary trigger points on each leg. A week later, he came for a fifth and last visit on March 10, 1995. He was pleased because the jumping muscles in the legs had been somewhat calmed down, and he had had good nights' sleep since. We urged him to come for few more sessions, but he failed to show up. Charles' feet didn't have the typical neuropathy described by diabetic patients. We were not sure that he could be classified as a patient with diabetic peripheral neuropathy even though he had been so diagnosed. Whatever his disease was, because he had diabetes and pain in his legs, we will just assume for practical purposes that he is a patient with neuropathy that was helped by acupuncture. The results, most likely, will be mixed and limited.

## 14.9 DIFFUSE PAIN

Some pain is confined to only a limited area. Headache, neck pain, and lower back pain are typical examples. Some pain is diffuse, spreading over several areas in the body. Examples include rheumatoid arthritis, osteoarthritis, Still's disease, Reiter's syndrome, reflex sympathetic dystrophy, causalgia, myofascitis, and fibromyalgia. A couple of these diseases will be mentioned in the next chapter. One of them is selected for discussion here.

Fibromyalgia was chosen to represent a pain that is diffuse in nature, and is perceived all over the body. Medically, fibromyalgia is thought to be a disease in the connective tissue. Connective tissue, just like afferent nerve fibers, is found everywhere in the body. Therefore, illness in the connective tissue can generate pain in multiple locations of the body. Is this concept scientifically valid? Medical terms found in scientific literature to describe fibromyalgia include myalgic spots, myalgia, myofascitis, myositis, fibrositis, muscular rheumatism, fibromyositis, muscular strain, and myofascial pain syndrome. Which of them is most accurate and acceptable? There may even be more terms, but if so, the matter is unimportant because all we need is an agreeable name, and there is none. Fibromyalgia is the name most often mentioned in medical reports and commonly used by the patients we have.

First, we have a brief background of our experience with fibromyalgia. Publications about fibromyalgia began to inundate us by the 1980s. We have decided to not cite any of them because after reading so many of these publications, we still had no clear understanding of what fibromyalgia is. The reason is simple: all these authoritative experts, pundits, scholars, scientists, and clinicians cannot even agree among themselves as to the definition of fibromyalgia. To this date, there are still medical professionals who seek to discredit the identity of fibromyalgia. To them, it is a fake disease, a medical fantasy or chimera. Can they be condemned for having such a stance? Not really. Fibromyalgia can be any case of pain manifesting in multiple locations, from headache on the crown of the head to fascial pain on the bottom of the feet, and all those in between. Do we believe there is such a disease as fibromyalgia? The answer is yes. That is what we will discuss next.

We begin this discussion by mentioning Dr. I. John Russell, a colleague of ours in the medical school. We knew who he was, although it is doubtful he knows who we were. He was an important faculty member heading the division of rheumatology, and we were but a minor faculty member in the same institute. He was outspoken on the issue of fibromyalgia, going to the nation's capital to speak in front of the U.S. House of Representatives' Appropriation Subcommittee on Labor, Health and Human Services to ask for more funding to study the disease. According to Dr. Russell, having tenderness in a total of 16 points in the body can be taken as an indication of suffering fibromyalgia. The 16 points he described corresponded to the trigger points in the primary group described in Chapter 12 of this book. If his criteria are used to diagnose this disease, more than 96% of our patients would be qualified as having fibromyalgia. Patients who arrived bearing their doctors' diagnosis of having the disease invariably were found to have seventh-degree objective pain or higher. That translates into 65 or more trigger points on one side of the body. This fact tells us that most pain produced by fibromyalgia can definitely be managed by acupuncture with mixed and limited results. Patients with the objective pain lower than fifth degree will certainly have good to excellent results, whereas in those with objective pain at ninth degree or higher will have poor results and will be difficult to manage. The protocol for treating fibromyalgia is similar to that used in treating other kinds of pain. The supine position is used first if the pain is mainly located in front, or in the prone position first if the back is hurting. Then, alternate positions of need are selected depending on the location of pain requiring attention. Trigger points to use begin from the primary group for the first three treatments. This gradually increases to use trigger points in the secondary group for the next three treatments, and the tertiary group eventually, if such is required.

## REFERENCES

1. Landau, I. Acupuncture: A report in three parts. *Consumer Reports,* January, 1984.
2. Dung, H.C. Role of the vagus nerve in weight reduction through auricular acupuncture. *American Journal of Acupuncture* 14:249, 1986.
3. Dung, H.C. Attempts to reduce body weight through auricular acupuncture. *American Journal of Acupuncture* 14:117, 1986.

4. Moore, K.L. *Clinically Oriented Anatomy*, 1st ed. Williams & Wilkins, Baltimore, 1980.
5. Perce, J. *Migraine: Clinical Features, Mechanisms and Management*. Charles C. Thomas, Springfield, IL, 1969.
6. Rose, F.C. and M. Gawel. *Migraine: The Facts*. Oxford University Press, New York, 1979.
7. Diamond, S. *Migraine Headache Prevention and Management*. Marcel Dekker, Inc., New York, 1990.
8. Spierings, E.L. *Management of Migraine*. Butterworth-Heinemann, Boston, 1996.
9. Solomon, S. et al. Common migraine: Criteria for diagnosis. *Headache* 28:124, 1988.
10. Mackenzie, E. et al. Functional bases for a central seratonergic involvement in classic migraine: A speculative view. *Cephalalgia* 5:69, 1985.
11. Graham, J.R. and H.G. Wolff. Mechanism of migraine headache and action of ergotamine tartrate. *Archives of Neurology and Psychiatry* 39:737, 1938.
12. Primary headaches: Migraine, cluster headache, tension-type headache. Review of world literature 1990 and 1991. *Headache* 33(suppl. 1):1, 1993.
13. Antonaci, F. et al. Chronic paroxysmal hemicrania (CPH): A review of the clinical manifestations. *Headache* 29:648, 1989.
14. Committee on Classification of Headache of the National Institute of Neurological Diseases and Blindness. Classification of Headache. *Journal of the American Medical Association* 179:717, 1962.
15. Headache Classification Committee of the International Headache Society. Classification and Diagnostic Criteria for Headache Disorders, Cranial Neuralgias, and Facial Pain. *Cephalalgia* 8(suppl. 1):1, 1988.
16. Loeser, J.D. Cranial neuralgias. In *The Management of Pain,* edited by J.J. Bonica, Lea and Febiger, Philadelphia, 1990.
17. Dung, H.C. Age and sex in relation to pain expressed through passive acupuncture points. *American Journal of Acupuncture* 13:235, 1985.
18. Dyck, P.J. et al. *Peripheral Neuropathy*, vols. I and II, 2nd ed. W. B. Saunders Company, Philadelphia, 1984.

# 15 Difficult Patients with Poor Results

## 15.1 CONNECTING DIFFICULT AND POOR

We connect the terms "difficult" and "poor" together because patients in this group have pain that is difficult take care of, and the results, after using acupuncture on them, often turn out to be poor. They are difficult to take care of because, by the time of their arrival, they already have multiple medical conditions or problems. All these conditions and problems are the consequences of failures due to previous attempts to stop their pain. For example, they may have undergone surgery that failed to manage their pain. They may have taken strong, addictive drugs that were ineffective in stopping their pain, yet it is these drugs that could have their made acupuncture treatments less effective. They may have physically perceived their subjective pain in multiple locations due to the chronic nature of their pain. Their pain may have begun when they were young, so it has been enduring for years. The patients may have passed retirement age, have limited resources, be overmedicated, or suffer other clinical complications. Combining any or all of these conditions and problems together leads us to conclude that these patients are difficult for us to deal with. Unless acupuncture can be incorporated into a more comprehensive medical practice, it is unrealistic to expect a sole practitioner to take care of multiple medical problems alone.

Nevertheless, we face difficult patients frequently. It is medically unethical and humanly immoral to refuse difficult patients from our practice. There is one advantage in caring for the difficult patients: we learn from taking care of them what poor results are in performing acupuncture. Why are the results poor? Because the patients always have higher degrees of objective pain. Their objective pain is invariably measured at seventh degree or higher, most of them being between the ninth and 12th degrees. Statistically, approximately 7% to 8% of all the patients we have examined have measurable objective pain between the 10th and 12th degrees. In other words, out of 100 patients, seven or eight of them will have objective pain at the 10th degree or higher. In proportion, they are a small minority of our clientele. Therefore, it became our policy to either charge a mere token fee or treat free of charge patients whom we considered to be difficult and have poor results from treatment. Such a policy enables us to have a sufficient opportunity to observe the outcome of acupuncture treatments. The data used in this chapter is essentially derived from this approach.

## 15.2 PROFILES OF DIFFICULT PATIENTS

Table 15.1 contains the biomedical profiles of 25 patients who were considered as difficult. The results of their acupuncture treatments were categorized as being poor. These 25 difficult patients were selected from registered records collected between 1980 and 1997. Twenty of them were female, the remaining five were male. Their subjective pain was very diversified, and pain in every location of the body was represented. Their objective pain ranged from seventh to 12th degrees. More of them were at eighth degree or higher. The total number of treatments each of these difficult patients received ranged from 100 to 392 sessions at the time the first edition of this book was written. The numbers definitely increased later on. We have had difficult patients come for more than 1000 treatments. Even though the results were poor, acupuncture was the only relief some difficult patients would have in their life. They had no alternative relief to choose from for their suffering.

## TABLE 15.1
## Biomedical Profiles of 25 Difficult-to-Treat Patients

| Name | Code No. | Age and Sex | Proclaimed Condition | Degree of Pain | Dates of First and Last Treatments | Total No. of Treatments |
|---|---|---|---|---|---|---|
| 1. Rosaline A. | 85121A085 | F65 | Arthritis | 9 | 03/04/1985 11/01/1995 | 111 |
| 2. Tony A. | 86422A129 | F56 | Swelling of right arm and shoulder | 9 | 06/12/1986 05/31/1993 | 104 |
| 3. Wendy B. | 81009B017 | F65 | Bell's Palsy | 8 | 01/14/1981 10/19/1996 | 272 |
| 4. Elizabeth B. | 88412B521 | F37 | Lower back and hip pain after surgery | 8 | 06/01/1988 02/08/1997 | 162 |
| 5. Rachel C. | 83671C135 | F43 | External ear pain | 7 | 07/24/1983 07/29/1984 | 124 |
| 6. Arlene C. | 90432C568 | F69 | Three bulging discs in the spine | 10 | 07/27/1990 12/03/1992 | 103 |
| 7. Ava D. | 84206D096 | F31 | Lower back pain | 7 | 03/28/1984 06/06/1992 | 153 |
| 8. Robert F. | 84034F081 | M42 | Nerves | 5 | 01/18/1984 03/01/1997 | 108 |
| 9. Casey F. | 85672F144 | M29 | Chronic sciatica | 10 | 12/13/1985 09/16/1996 | 132 |
| 10. Herbert J. | 80456H021 | M48 | Neck spurs | 9 | 12/17/1980 05/10/1996 | 344 |
| 11. Lucille J. | 84326J067 | F79 | Feet, back, and knees | 9 | 05/09/1984 07/20/1991 | 101 |
| 12. Villet J. | 88318J157 | F66 | Arthritis, lower back, headache, neckache | 12 | 05/03/1988 11/29/1996 | 209 |
| 13. Evelyn K. | 84391K087 | F62 | Lower back, shoulder, colon | 9 | 06/07/1984 09/17/1992 | 148 |
| 14. Kay K. | 87914K087 | F48 | Neck, head, back, leg, feet | 7 | 11/09/1987 10/08/1996 | 205 |
| 15. Doris L. | 88672L283 | F63 | Bone spurs | 8 | 09/06/1988 08/14/1996 | 153 |
| 16. Paul M. | 81396M010 | M52 | Back pain | 8 | 11/19/1981 06/10/1996 | 392 |
| 17. Betty M. | 83571M125 | F51 | Myofascial syndrome | 11 | 06/23/1983 09/09/1995 | 256 |
| 18. Lyria M. | 84742M163 | F53 | Arm, shoulder, and knees | 11 | 02/03/1984 03/30/1997 | 100 |
| 19. Ernistine M. | 93058M703 | F72 | Lower back herniated disc, hand numbness | 9 | 02/19/1993 02/20/1997 | 177 |
| 20. Carol M. | 95034M827 | F50 | Connective tissue disease | 12 | 06/18/1995 03/25/1997 | 102 |
| 21. Jeane P. | 95486P556 | F51 | Ruptured disc, fibromyalgia | 9 | 07/29/1995 02/26/1997 | 116 |
| 22. Peggy S. | 82258S060 | F51 | Allergy, tension, neck and back pain | 7 | 04/14/1982 08/19/1996 | 105 |
| 23. Robert S. | 82496S097 | M39 | Lower back pain due to disc herniation | 7 | 07/27/1988 12/02/1996 | 122 |
| 24. Virginia S. | 88625S644 | F56 | Separated lumbar fusion cervical disc | 7 | 08/20/1988 10/19/1996 | 101 |
| 25. Patsy W. | 88569W397 | F?? | Migraine headache | 7 | 07/26/1988 09/14/1996 | 118 |

The treatment protocol for difficult patients is not that critical because the results will be poor anyway. Expecting good to excellent results is sheer optimistic exuberance, as those are not possible. Mixed and limited results sometimes happen, but very rarely. The longest relief these patients can hope for is days or weeks. Occasionally, they receive a pleasant surprise of 1 or 2 months of exoneration. To achieve any beneficial results, the first treatment position can be supine, prone, sitting, or on one side of the body, depending on where the focal point of pain is located. Thereafter, the treatments will alternate through previously unused positions. The number of needles used can appropriately start at 24, then increase by three to four needles each time by using trigger points in the secondary group first, followed by the tertiary, and finally the nonspecific group. It should take six to eight consecutive sessions to reach a maximum of 50 needles. Using more than 50 needles each time is unnecessary because exceeding that number will not proportionally enhance the efficacy of acupuncture.

The best way to learn how to take care of difficult patients is to have the chance to practice. Each difficult patient is different. However, describing a large number of examples to explain what needs to be done for each kind of pain would still lead to some redundancies, along with taking up excessive space. We have therefore chosen only one or two different kinds of pain in each of the five major regions of the body as examples for our discussion below.

## 15.3 PAIN IN THE FACE AND HEAD

As described in the previous two chapters, the most difficult pains in the face and head region to take care of are migraine, postherpetic neuralgia, and tic douloureux. Only the first two will be repeated in our discussion because they are more commonly seen among our patients.

### 15.3.1 MIGRAINE

*Case 1*: Annette C. was a 31-year-old RN. After checking her objective pain, we knew that her headache would not be easy to manage. Annette stated that she had had headaches since she was 4 years old. For 4 weeks before she came to us, the headache had been bothering her day and night. She had had seizures due to overmedication with Demerol this time, so she was taking Dilantin for her seizures. None of the drugs she had taken had been very helpful, and she continued to have headaches. Her objective pain was measured at the eighth degree. At this level, with her taking the narcotic Demerol, this made her headache very difficult to manage. Poor results were expected. After our explanation, she still decided to try. A total of 22 treatments were provided in the early part of 1995. She called on March 17, 1995, and said that she would not come for any more treatments because they were not helping.

*Case 2*: Mary G. was a 46-year-old retiree. This patient first visited in June of 1996. She indicated that she had "chronic headaches" for the last 20 years. The headaches had been with her all the time, except during sleep. She stated that her headaches could be migraine, but she was without the classical symptoms of proximity. She also suffered from occasional dizzy spells, which were not severe. The headache could be on either side of the head or encompassing the entire head and would intensify after menstrual periods. She was taking multiple drugs. One would ease her suffering for a short time, and then she would have to take a different drug. Her headache always returned. Her objective pain was measured at only the sixth degree, which, of course, was in her favor. If not for her long history of headaches, we might have had a chance to reduce or stop the pain. Between June and December, she received a total of 24 treatments. After a series of three or four treatments, she would have 1 week's relief, after which the headache returned to plague her. She wrote to inform us that "my husband wants to try a different approach for my headache. I want to thank you for your gentle, professional care and your unreserving support and encouragement."

We are sorry to say that too many difficult patients with migraines like Mary's wait too long to come for acupuncture. We feel that their migraines could have been manageable if they had chosen acupuncture to stop their headaches a few years earlier. We hope that the physicians of this world are willing to refer or suggest to their patients with migraine to seek acupuncture treatments as soon as possible after they find that addictive drugs are unable to stop the headaches. This generous attitude can save a great deal of suffering for patients with migraine headaches.

### 15.3.2 POSTHERPETIC NEURALGIA

Like migraines, the manageability of headaches produced by this neuralgia is determined by the degree of objective pain and how long the subjective pain has been perceived by the patient. Twelve difficult patients with postherpetic neuralgia are listed in Table 15.2. These 12 patients were seen

## TABLE 15.2
## Pain in Patients with Postherpetic Neuralgia without Improvement after a Number of Acupuncture Treatments

| Patient | Sex | Age | Pain Code | Duration of Pain | Degree of Pain | No. of Treatments |
|---|---|---|---|---|---|---|
| 1. MR (83482R070) | F | 79 | 003.X2b | 4 years | 10 | 8 |
| 2. JJ (84618J075) | F | 75 | 303.X2b | 6 years | 5 | 5 |
| 3. CW (84773W202) | F | 78 | 003.X2b | 2 years | 5 | 4 |
| 4. EK (84742K202) | F | 81 | 403.X2b | 2 years | 5 | 5 |
| 5. GR (85211R153) | F | 75 | 303.X2b | 2.5 years | 6 | 8 |
| 6. JB (84764B256) | F | 81 | 003.X2b | 8.5 years | 11 | 8 |
| 7. MH (85461H268) | M | 77 | 003.X2b | 5 months | 6 | 8 |
| 8. LN (85526W241) | F | 75 | 303.X2b | 5 months | 11 | 8 |
| 9. LH (86179H299) | F | 66 | 303.X2b | 1.5 years | 12 | 21 |
| 10. FV (86424V063) | M | 52 | 303.X2b | 10 months | 5 | 7 |
| 11. VH (86460H321) | F | 65 | 403.X2b | 2 years | 8 | 5 |
| 12. CE (86535E102) | F | 76 | 303.X2b | 7 months | 8 | 12 |

over a period of 3 years [1]. None of them benefited from acupuncture treatments. In all but three, the duration of the subjective pain had lasted for longer than 1 year by the time of their arrival. These statistics seem to indicate that once the pain of postherpetic neuralgia has existed for longer than a year, it becomes relatively difficult to eradicate. However, we did have patients whose objective pain was fourth degree or lower and who had suffered postherpetic neuralgic pain for 6 to 12 months, and yet reported having relief. No patients obtained relief if their objective pain was ninth degree or higher. At that level, the neuralgic pain definitely would not respond to acupuncture treatments.

Childhood infection by the chickenpox virus, medically known as varicella, is the cause of herpes zoster in adults [2]. After the infection has subdued, the virus migrates to hide in the sensory ganglia, such as the trigeminal and dorsal roots. The virus remains latent and stays dormant in the ganglia until an appropriate opportunity for attack, such as when the immune system of the host is weakened by other factors. One of these factors is aging. As we age, the body's defenses decrease because of our weakened immune systems. This explains why herpes infections victimize seniors more often than younger adults. Not only are fewer young adults known to have herpes zoster but also, after the infection, they have less potential for it to develop into postherpetic neuralgia. Our thoughts are that younger people are more likely to have lower degrees of objective pain. Finding whether our speculation has any medical basis could be an important topic for scientific research with respect to understanding why only a small percentage of herpes infections become postherpetic neuralgia.

Josephine B. was an 81-year-old retired school teacher. When we first met in September 1984, she seemed to be unhappy, as can be seen in her picture (Figure 15.1). She was brought to San Antonio after a 4-h drive from San Angelo. She was very frail, requiring assistance for almost any activity. Her subjective pain in the forehead had lasted as for long as she could remember, which was the cause of her unhappiness. Her doctor told her that it was herpes neuritis, which is another name used clinically for postherpetic neuralgia. The skin area on the right forehead where the infection occurred was visibly lighter, with fine lines. She said that the pain attacked her head all the time, even when she tried to sleep. Narcotic opiates prescribed for her provided no relief at all. After carefully examining her trigger points, we measured her objective pain to be 11th degree. With the long duration of subjective pain, consumption of addictive drugs, and high degree of objective pain, acupuncture was doomed to fail. We knew treatment results for her postherpetic neuralgia could be expected to be poor before we even made the attempt. However, she was desperate, and thus still

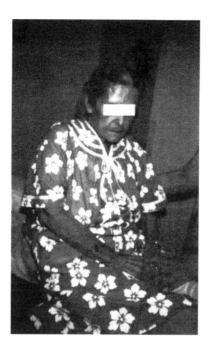

**FIGURE 15.1** Josephine B. on the day of her first visit to the clinic.

wanted to try, even with our forewarning of failure. Naturally, our services were provided free of charge. She stayed in San Antonio for 20 days and received a total of eight treatments. She became no better, and finally decided to go back home. Could more sessions improve the pain in her head? There is no way to know because more chances are not available. We would certainly be more than willing to try more. Until we reach 32 sessions, we will not give up the hope of making Josephine's pain more tolerable.

After years of taking care of difficult patients with postherpetic neuralgia pain, we still have a few questions that remain unanswered despite some effort to research the medical literature. One of the questions is why pain from this neuralgia is only perceived in the ophthalmic and maxillary divisions, and not the mandibular. The manifestation of postherpetic pain is different from that of tic douloureux, which is often perceived in the maxillary and mandibular divisions, but not in the ophthalmic. Why does the herpes virus, or varicella, only infect the trigeminal nerve in the head unilaterally and not bilaterally? Why is the infection only involved in three of the spinal nerves and not more?

The herpes virus can remain in the sensory ganglia for a long time. When physiological circumstances become favorable, the virus emerges to attack its host. The virus propagates down the axons of the spinal nerves and their branches. However, the mechanism for the reactivation of viral movement to the peripheral nerve fibers remains unknown [2]. The destination of the virus is likewise unknown. What happens once the virus reaches the cutaneous ends of the nociceptive fibers? These have to be nociceptors in the skin, so does the virus come out of the nociceptors? If so, can it damage or destroy sensory nerves? In what manner would it damage or destroy? Although none of these questions can be answered, it is logical to speculate that nociceptors and nociceptive fibers can be damaged or destroyed to generate nociception. The most likely way to damage or destroy the nerve fibers is to dissolve their myelin sheaths. This is comparable to having insulation stripped from electrical wires, which can result in electrocution. Pain felt in postherpetic neuralgia is analogous to a nerve fiber acting like an electrical wire. The destruction of myelin sheaths around nociceptive fibers must be retroactive, beginning at the terminal and peripheral ends of the nociceptors. Gradually, the myelin sheaths are dissolved toward the sensory nerve cells in the sensory ganglia. After a time, the entire nerve fibers are stripped of myelin, all the way to the bodies of the sensory neurons, and regeneration of the myelin becomes impossible. This is why after a sufficient time of a year or longer, acupuncture treatments will become unable to heal the damage incurred on the nociceptive fibers, making pain management useless. This is a field with abundant research potential for better understanding of postherpetic neuralgia and its relationship to the actions of acupuncture therapy.

## 15.4 DIFFICULT PAIN FROM THE NECK TO THE FINGERS

We all have too many difficult patients with subjective pain perceivable from the neck to the hands and fingers. A number of these patients can be selected as useful examples to show how poor results are possible in managing their pain. Four of them are chosen to represent pain in the neck, shoulder joint region, and hands and fingers. We start with an example for neck pain.

### 15.4.1 Torticollis in Perpetual Motion

Depending on the duration after the injury, torticollis has different forms. The necks of certain torticollis patients seem normal, whereas some have rigid neck muscles. Mary's torticollis was in perpetual motion.

Mary G. was 75 years old. It would be appropriate to use the term "perpetual motion" to describe her torticollis. As seen in Figure 15.2, either she or someone else had to push her head upright. Otherwise, her head would turn toward the right shoulder. The condition had originated 18 years earlier in an automobile accident. At the impact of the accident, she turned her head backward and suddenly noticed a stiffness in her neck. There was no pain at the time. A few months later, while she was under tremendous emotional strain, her neck began deviating to one side without any apparent outward cause. She was driving her car home when she noticed a pain in her neck, which worsened over time. She said that she had seen several physicians without much help until she visited an acupuncturist in 1973. After 15 treatments, the pain "completely" subsided for 6 months, which was more than 10 years prior to her coming to us. Thereafter, the pain gradually reappeared. The acupuncture clinic she patronized was closed for illegal practice of medicine, and she was then referred to our clinic. Her objective pain was estimated to be between the ninth and 10th degrees. For the first two treatments, she had a latent flare-up reaction after each session. She also complained of sinus congestion and excessive stomach acid with indigestion. After 23 treatments, she said that her neck was almost free of pain.

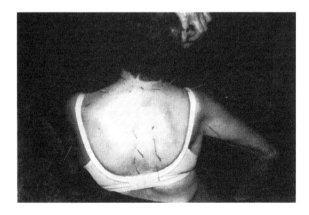

**FIGURE 15.2** Mary's head had to be pushed upward from the right side because of torticollis, which would pull her neck toward the right.

Mary returned 5 years later with pain in her right shoulder and lower back. She attributed the shoulder pain to a fall, and the lower back pain to a fracture in her ilium. She still had some pain in the neck, which was expected, because her torticollis seemed to be the same. She still used her right hand to push and support her head upward all the time. We measured her objective pain for the second time, and it was 10th degree. She came for two more treatments, and did not return thereafter.

### 15.4.2 Severe Arthritis inside the Shoulder Joint

In previous chapters, we have stated that pain in the shoulder joint area can have good to excellent results when treated with acupuncture if the trigger points are detected only on the tendon of the long head of the biceps brachii muscle. Keep in mind that, if the pain inside the joint is not properly managed and if the damage or disease is prolonged, arthritic conditions can set in the joint cavity. The subjective pain becomes very difficult to eradicate. We have no way to know how commonly such developments can occur in the shoulder. We do have one example to prove that it has the possibility of occurring in some patients.

Philip C. was a 71-year-old retiree. The patient visited in July 1993 and described having pain in the right shoulder for 2 years. He was barely able to move either shoulder joint, which we suspect indicated that the problem had existed for longer than 2 years. When both of his shoulder regions were examined for trigger points, practically every place palpated was tender. His overall objective pain was measured to be only eighth degree, despite so many nonspecific group trigger points being located around the shoulder joint regions. If we take those nonspecific trigger points into consideration, he may have qualified to be at the ninth or 10th degree. From our experience, we know that his shoulders were most likely affected by severe arthritis. He was urged to go to the Physical Medicine and Rehabilitation clinic at the university hospital for further examination. The hospital gave him x-rays for both shoulder regions. He brought the images (Figure 15.3) to show us how his shoulders looked. From the radiograms, we had no problem recognizing extensive and severe degenerative arthritis in the joint cavities of both shoulders. We pointed out to him that he ought to have had shoulder pain for more than 2 years. Philip then confessed that he had injured his right shoulder during his high school years when he slipped and fell. Thereafter, he had suffered pain in the right shoulder for the last 60 years. He ended up having more than 12 acupuncture treatments without any noticeable improvement, and stopped coming after September of 1993.

### 15.4.3 Carpal Tunnel Syndrome

This disease was first described about 70 years ago, and it has been well documented in the medical literature [3]. Anatomically, the main malefactor for the symptoms of this syndrome is the median nerve. The median nerve is very long. Medical opinion is that along its long course, a compression on the nerve will produce numbing pain in the three fingers on the radial side of the hand—the

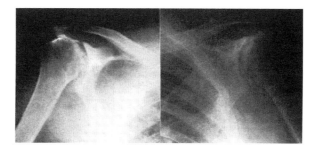

**FIGURE 15.3** Both of Philip's shoulder regions, showing extensive and severe arthritis inside the joint cavities.

thumb, index, and middle. Clinically, the most vulnerable site where the compression can occur is under the flexor retinaculum, the location known as the carpal tunnel. When the median nerve is compressed in the tunnel, it can cause numbing pain with itching and severe burning sensations. In the early phase of the disease, the pain typically begins to present on only one hand toward the end of the night. Gradually, the patients will be awakened in the middle of the night, but the pain usually subsides in the morning.

As the symptoms are prolonged, the syndrome will eventually involve both hands. A small number of patients are seen to have muscular atrophy in the thenar compartment. Once muscular atrophy sets in, acupuncture will not be of much use. Flexing and extending the diseased wrists can aggravate pain. It is a concern for industrialized societies, particularly in the computer age, due to loss of working time after symptoms of carpal tunnel syndrome begin to appear and become more serious. Many reasons, including pregnancy, kidney dialysis, diabetes, hypothyroidism, and acromegaly, are given as the causes of carpal tunnel syndrome [4]. One common indicator among our patients with the syndrome is low blood pressure beginning from the teen years. One obvious reason for having low blood pressure is protracted and excessive bleeding associated with monthly menstruation. We believe that having low blood pressure during premenopause is one of the causes of having carpal tunnel syndrome in the menopausal stage. Our female patients with carpal tunnel syndrome invariably are found to have had dysmenorrhea with menstrual cramping during their premenopausal years.

It is not that difficult to realize if a person has carpal tunnel syndrome. Patients having the syndrome are not commonly seen in our clinic. Of those seen, if the symptoms are confined to only one hand, the pain is relatively easy to eliminate. We have had many patients with good to excellent results after three to four treatments. Once both hands are involved, the pain in the fingers becomes harder to manage. Still, most patients with an objective pain lower than seventh degree will have relief. Patients with objective pain at ninth or higher degree, or pain that has persisted after hand surgery, are the exceptions. Margaret E. is one example.

Margaret E. was a 76-year-old retiree. She was diagnosed with carpal tunnel syndrome by her doctor 8 months before coming to us to ask for help. Not too long after the diagnosis, the symptoms disappeared on their own, but reappeared later. She waited for 3 months after the recurrence before coming to us. Her right hand was the first to have symptoms. After a brief intermission, both hands were affected the second time around. The left hand hurt more after the second episode. She then perceived pain in the forearms and the shoulder joints. She had difficulty abducting her right shoulder by more than 15 degrees. Her past medical history included hypothyroidism, which had been treated with synthyroid for the last 40 years. Her parathyroid glands had been removed. She had herpetic infection. Both of her index fingers were visibly deformed. She used Motrin and Tylenol to overcome her pain. Her objective pain was measured at ninth degree. After a total of 14 treatments, she said her pain was still hurting. She stopped coming thereafter.

### 15.4.4 Deformities and Pain

If a patient has deformities in the hands or feet (Figure 15.4), they will be easy to see. We don't see them very often. Almost all of them occur in patients who have been diagnosed with rheumatoid arthritis (RA). The deformities do not form in a short time, but take years to develop. We don't know if all deformities are accompanied by pain. We do know our patients with deformities come because of pain. After the fingers or feet become crooked as shown in the figure, we cannot expect acupuncture to restore their normality. Pain in patients with deformities is also not easy to manage. Because the deformities we see come from RA, and not all patients with RA have deformities, but they all have pain when they come for acupuncture, some comments regarding RA are justified. RA is a chronic disease that can last for many years throughout life. For most patients we see with RA, very few of them consult a rheumatologist within 6 months of the onset of the disease. By the time the illness is firmly and positively diagnosed, the condition could have existed in the patient's body for

Difficult Patients with Poor Results

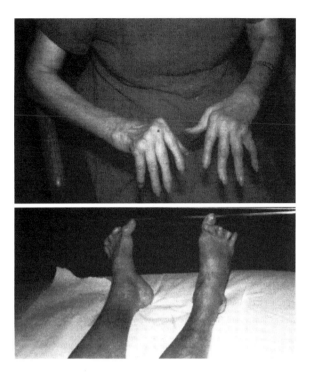

**FIGURE 15.4** Deformed extremities in patients with RA: hands and fingers (top), and feet and toes (bottom).

a year or longer. Acupuncture for subjective pain in RA patients can have good to excellent results, if they are treated within 1 year after having the disease. Mixed and limited results are reasonable to expect if the patients have objective pain at the seventh degree or lower. Once deformities appear, they become difficult patients for acupuncture to treat, and poor results are inevitable. Growth of objective pain in RA is not easy to foresee. We have patients whose objective pain increased to trigger points of the tertiary group within a year or so. We also have patients who have had RA for more than 10 years, and the objective pain stays at no more than the fifth degree. There is an unfortunate degree of uncertainty in having an accurate and reliable diagnosis for RA, even given by a physician who is not a rheumatologist. Patients may say that they have RA, but their diagnosis can be false or inaccurate if given by their general practitioners or family doctors. Vanita A. is an example of a difficult patient with poor results.

Vanita A. was a 45-year-old housewife. This patient developed RA after her first pregnancy and has had the disease for the last 20 years. She had had cortisone and gold injections. Her fingers and feet had already become deformed, but were surgically corrected. We measured her objective pain as ninth degree. After the second treatment, she had a latent flare-up reaction, and the pain increased. To ease her pain, she took Trilisate 750 for 2 days. After coming for 15 treatments, her subjective pain was reduced enough for her to be able to ride a bicycle. Unfortunately, she fell from her bicycle and broke her left ankle, with a 2-in.-long hematoma and ecchymosis visible inferiorly to the medial malleolus in the foot injured. Her RA continued to be problematic. We have not seen her for years.

## 15.5 PAIN AFTER SURGERY

Surgical remedies to stop pain are not always successful. We have received patients who were still in pain after their surgeries. The pain that surgeries attempt to manage can be at numerous different locations. Here, we pick two of the most commonly seen examples to explain how they make patients difficult to treat: lower back and hip surgeries. They become difficult patients in a different sense after unsuccessful surgeries. The difference is that it becomes difficult to predict the outcomes of the treatments. What has been described in this book for pain management is not always applicable for pain after surgery. These difficult patients may have low degrees of objective pain, and the results can still be poor. Certainly, poor results are expected if the degree of their objective pain is higher than the eighth degree. A few patients are chosen here as examples.

### 15.5.1 Lower Back Pain after Surgery

Lower back pain after surgery is commonly seen. We have received at least one such patient every 2 to 3 weeks. The surgical marks were the visible indicators. Figure 15.5 contains just four samples observed among hundreds. Some of these patients still had good to excellent results if the degree of their objective pain was not too high. Surgical procedures disturb anatomical normalcy, and the scar tissue could be dense, making needle penetration difficult, if not impossible.

*Case 1*: Paul M. was a 52-year-old disabled postal office worker. Paul is listed in Table 15.1 as patient no. 16. From the table, one can see that he is the record-holder for having the most acupuncture treatments at our clinic. He came for a total of 392 treatments from November 1981 to June 1996. That number went up to more than 1200 during 2006. We checked his objective pain intermittently. On his 79th visit, it was still at the 10th degree, although it had been higher when he came for the first visit 3 years earlier.

Paul's lower back pain began during the Korean War, where he was in hand-to-hand combat on numerous occasions. At night, he had to sleep on the snow-covered ground. Soon after that, he would occasionally experience nagging backache. He noticed that when he was tense and under

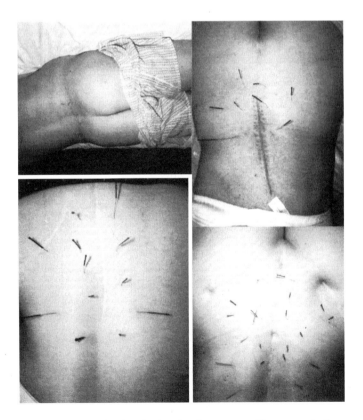

**FIGURE 15.5** Four patients still having low back pain after surgery. The one at the bottom right had undergone surgery only recently, whereas the others were from years earlier.

stress, the back would bother him more. Five years ago, he was under a great deal of emotional stress, and his back really began to hurt him. Eventually, he underwent two back surgeries in 2 years' time. The pain never completely went away. At the time of his arrival, he was in a great deal of pain. He also had neck pain, which his physicians blamed on arthritis.

His other concern was "dizziness and fear of falling." His dizziness was most likely attributable to the medications he was taking for his pain. He showed a newspaper clipping of an advice column that described another patient with similar problems. The answer given by the physician who wrote that column was "you fall into the category of what is called 'dizzy patient.' There are increasing numbers of people who have faintness, dizziness and related problems. Some are caused by ear problems, which is particularly likely in patients below the age of 50. Many of these patients have true vertigo, meaning a sensation of the body moving when it is not, or the surrounding objects moving when they are not." But, what then is true vertigo? Is there a false vertigo?

Paul's pain was not totally eliminated, but it was reduced to such a degree that he could stop taking drugs for a few months. During that time, his dizziness disappeared. His physicians disagreed, insisting his dizziness had nothing to do with the drugs prescribed. Did Paul have the "false vertigo" to which that newspaper columnist alluded? He hasn't mentioned the dizziness in the last 20 years.

Difficult patients with medical histories and physical profiles similar to Paul's often have the potential to have dispersed pain. Through the years, Paul would come complaining of pain in the shoulder, in the temporomandibular joints, from trochanteric bursitis, along the erector spinae muscle in the back of the thorax, and in the calves of the legs. These kinds of pain were relatively easy for us to manage because he'd had them for only a short duration. None of his pain can be considered as cured, because it all has the potential to come back to hurt him. That is why he keeps coming back after all these years. He said that acupuncture is the only thing saving his life from more pain. He was 83 years old in 2012 and still going strong, evidence that protracted pain can hurt but not kill.

*Case 2*: Another difficult patient was Jay N., a 50-year-old dentist (Figure 15.6) who still suffered lower back pain after four surgeries. He received 27 treatments from February 1997 to June of the same year. He will have to come for more because, as he indicated, acupuncture is his last hope to ease his lower back pain. Jay said that all his physicians would do is give him more pills. Our opinion is that his lower back pain is developing into symptoms of Bernhardt disease with paresthesia on the lateral surface of both thighs. He had seventh-degree objective pain. At that degree, without surgery, we might be willing to predict that 5 to 10 acupuncture treatments would effectively get rid of his pain, both in the lower back and thighs. After 27 treatments, his pain was essentially unchanged. How many more treatments he will need to have his pain under control is uncertain.

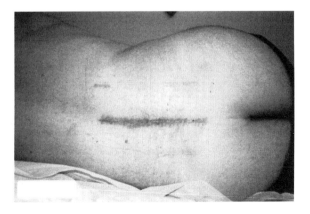

**FIGURE 15.6** The state of Jay's lower back after four surgeries.

### 15.5.2 PAIN AFTER HIP REPLACEMENT

Prosthetic surgery to replace the hip joint is only occasionally seen in our clinic. When pain remains after the surgery, patients become difficult to treat. Here are two examples.

*Case 1*: Judith M. was a 53-year-old housewife. This patient came with a walker. She claimed that surgeries to her hips crippled her legs. Thereafter, she could only walk using a walker. She had had numerous surgeries, enough that she could not remember the exact number. Years ago, she was diagnosed with RA. Her visit to us was not for her pain in the legs but because of severe pain in her chest, which was diagnosed as "pericarditis" by her physicians. We have no intention of nitpicking in defiance of medical opinion, but it is most likely that her chest pain was not solely due to pericarditis. Pain of such a pathological nature involving the pericardium will be out of reach of any acupuncture treatment, yet the patient claimed that, after four treatments, she had no more pain in the chest. The pain she felt most was in the left pectoral region, where the pectoralis major and minor muscles are innervated by the medial and lateral pectoral nerves. Anatomically, it is possible for cardiac pain to be referred to these two nerves, manifesting in the upper chest. The difficulty we faced was in explaining the pain this patient had above the clavicle, reaching as far superior as the occipital area. Cardiac innervation is from the seventh cervical and first and second thoracic spinal nerves. Nerve innervation to the occipital area is from the first and second cervical spinal nerves. They are six dermatomes apart. Of course, Judith also had pain in other locations, including the shoulder and scapular regions, lower back, hips, thighs, legs, and so on. Pain in multiple locations can be expected if the patients have objective pain of the eighth degree or higher. Judith's objective pain was eighth degree. The pain over her two hip areas was typical of trochanteric bursitis or meralgia paresthetica. Surgery was not beneficial for her, but instead aggravated the pain in the hips and the thighs. Her thighs were so sensitive that she didn't want to have needles placed in these areas. A year after the first series of four treatments, her chest pain returned. The second series of three treatments was in April of 1996. Then, she decided to take care of the pain in her hips and thighs. Three treatments were given for that purpose. Again, her chest pain was relieved, but her hip pain persisted. Judith proved to be a difficult patient for whom acupuncture treatments often have poor results. Such pain after surgery is difficult, if not impossible, to manage.

*Case 2*: Lars W. was a 68-year-old retiree from the U.S. Army. This patient had had four surgeries, with results seen in Figure 15.7. Lars was chosen as an example to show that even after surgery, acupuncture sometimes can be still useful to manage pain. His objective pain was measured at only the fifth degree. It was a pity to see a nice, gentle, and healthy man suffering so much from pain that left him looking so depressed. He was taking antidepressants when we first met. He said that he had played hockey for many years and was very athletic until an injury to his left hip in 1989.

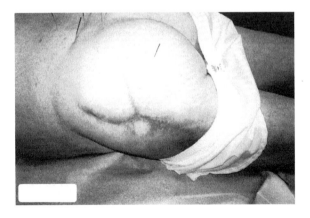

**FIGURE 15.7** Scars seen on Lars' left hip from hip joint replacement surgery.

After multiple surgeries, he had no other recourse but to pursue acupuncture. His physicians in the military had all but given up on him totally, and he was still in so much pain that he could not walk normally. It turned out that our acupuncture treatments were able to reduce his pain after 14 treatments. Ordinarily, without surgery, four or five treatments might have done the job. When he came for his 14th treatment, he told us that he felt so good that he had decided to go back to Sweden to visit his relatives.

## 15.6 PHANTOM LIMB PAIN

We do not know how many people in this world have their arms or legs amputated, willingly or unwillingly, every day. After the amputation, how many of these victims are known to suffer from relentless postoperative pain? The answer will depend on which statistics one believes [5–7]. The incidence of pain after amputation or phantom limb pain has been reported to be 10% to 25%. Postamputation or postsurgical pain is also known among patients who have lost their nose, tongue, breast, fingers, teeth, testes, penis, bladder, and anus [8–11]. An extensive damage to tissues, either accidentally or performed for medical reasons, can potentiate patients to perceive pain of a phantom nature. Physicians are still in total darkness when it comes to predicting who will be the next victim to have postamputative or postsurgical pain. There is a need for surgeons to know if the development of phantom pain can be predicted. The principles of acupuncture discussed in this book may offer a useful answer. This is the reason phantom limb pain is included here for our discussion. Patients seen with phantom limb pain were found to have objective pain at relatively high degrees. This observation leads us to speculate that patients with phantom limb pain could have some kinds of pain for a long duration before amputation. Our thinking is in agreement with that of Roberts et al. [12], who reported that "the role of preamputation pain in the genesis of phantom limb pain is unclear. Some have suggested that pain prior to amputation increases the likelihood of severe phantom limb pain. Others have not found this association." At the time the first edition of this book was in print, only eight cases of phantom limb pain had been seen in the clinic. All of them involved lower limb amputation, and only one of the patients was female. Their objective pain was seventh degree or higher, with a specific objective pain distribution of one at the seventh degree, three at the eighth degree, two at the ninth degree, and two at the tenth degree. Four of these eight difficult patients are briefly mentioned here as examples to show their poor results. Their medical histories are condensed but otherwise the descriptions are quite lengthy, and thus will be omitted.

Ruth S. was 45 years old, and did not tell us what her profession was. Her right leg was amputated, as shown in Figure 15.8. The reason for the amputation was an automobile accident in 1969, 15 years before her first visit to us. She had seventh-degree objective pain, the lowest level among the eight patients with phantom limb pain. From March 24 to April 17, 1983, she came for eight treatments. Two years later, on April 13, 1985, she returned because of recurring lower back pain. That is how we found out that acupuncture treatments stopped her phantom limb pain.

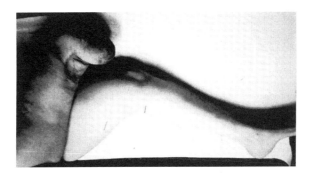

**FIGURE 15.8** Ruth's right leg after the amputation.

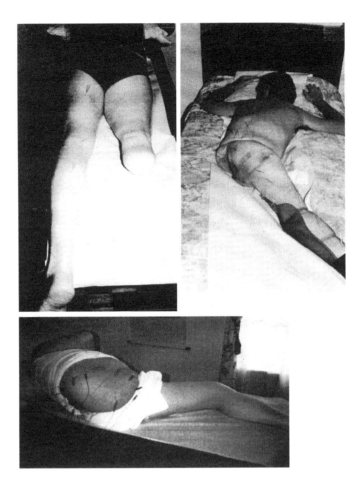

**FIGURE 15.9** Three patients with lower limb amputations. Acupuncture didn't help to stop their phantom limb pains.

Another three patients with lower limb amputations are seen in Figure 15.9. We assume that giving their names will not serve any useful purpose. Of the three, one patient had electrodes connected to the needles inserted. At that time, electrical stimulation was popular in acupuncture practice. We had tried it on a number of our patients, including those with phantom limb pain. Our conclusion is that the stimulation provides nothing but vibration of different frequencies and intensities to the needles. There is nothing to convince us that it enhances the efficacy of acupuncture. After taking care of patients with phantom limb pain, we are convinced that there must be some connection between the objective pain that patients have before amputation and the development of phantom limb pain after the surgery. Such a connection should not be difficult to prove with adequate study and research.

## 15.7 SPONDYLITIC ABNORMALITIES

Many patients with lower back pain are found to have nothing wrong in their vertebral column. A few of them do have abnormalities, as seen from the x-rays they provided. Medical terms used to describe these abnormalities by the patients include words such as "spondylitic." We thought that it would be appropriate to use "spondylitic abnormalities" to describe subjective pain with organic problems involving bones, particularly the vertebrae. Spondylitic abnormalities can include spondylosis, spondylitis, spondylolisthesis, and their associated adjectives, such as ankylosing, stenotic, etc. There are many reports of lower back pain in the literature [13–15]. We have three of our own to offer. They were all difficult patients to treat with acupuncture, and their results were all poor.

*Case 1*: David H. was a 24-year-old student and construction worker. He described his main problem as "lower back-slippage." The report from his orthopedic consultation stated that he has had multiple episodes of back pain over the years and was diagnosed with spondylolysis. The report also stated his present backache had started 3 to 4 months ago and also involved the posterior aspect of his right leg. Valsalva maneuvers did not increase the pain. Bowel or bladder function had not been altered. Physical examination by the orthopedic physician revealed equivocal straight leg raising, normal deep tendon reflexes, and motor and sensory exam results. He could walk on his heels and toes and had no selective atrophy, sciatic, or peroneal nerve tenderness. He had some mild spasming on his left paraspinal area and, oddly enough, his pain occurred mostly in the morning. X-rays revealed spondylolysis of L4 and L5 with no slippage. David was placed on a "stretching program," and was told "to stay in sports for now and we'll see how you feel when you get the back stretched out good in a month."

One month later, his report indicated "the patient is not any better." He apparently was not doing the stretching exercises properly, so he was retaught the technique and was to return in a month. After another month, the patient had some improvement but reaggravated the pain playing basketball. The pain had a radicular component in the right buttock and leg. X-rays were again performed, which revealed no change, but because his pain continued he had a CAT scan. He then was placed on a stretching program again. The CAT scan revealed "a HNP (herniated disc) of L4–5 that may require surgical treatment." It was also believed that David had "transitional vertebra with sacralization of transverse process L5 bilaterally and spina bifida occulta L5 and S1." He was referred to a variety of consultants, which finally revealed "grade 2 to grade 3 central disc herniation at L4–5 with a possibility of an extruded fragment and advanced facet hypertrophy with no evidence of sagittal lateral recess, or foraminal stenosis." It was now stated that David had "symptoms compatible with right L5 nerve root compression syndrome secondary to a combination of disc protrusion and spondylolysis bilaterally." It was felt by the consultants that "disc space exploration and probable fusion would eventually be required." The sequence of events described thus far seemed to us as medically complicated. Yet, after only three acupuncture treatments, David said that his pain was gone from the lower back to the bottom of his foot. He brought us the x-rays taken by his doctors (Figure 15.10). We are sure a radiologist can determine whether they are normal or not. Our motivation to present this case is, once again, to point out that whatever spondylitic abnormality can be, if the objective pain of the patient is low, good to excellent results are still possible. The objective pain in David was measured to be only at the third degree.

*Case 2*: Roman F. was a 31-year-old repairman. His first visit to the clinic was in March 1985. His back had been injured in 1974, when he was 20 years old, by a heavy falling pole. Chiropractic adjustment helped to ease some of his pain, but was unable to eradicate it totally. His chiropractor told him that one of his legs was shorter than the other so that he would have pain for the rest of his life. He also used a heating pad and took medications, but none of them helped. Medical doctors had told him that nothing was wrong from looking at his x-rays. The objective pain in Roman was also measured at third degree, and it took three treatments to stop his lower back pain.

*Case 3*: Harry Y. was a 67-year-old salesman and a typical example of difficult patients having subjective pain due to spondylitic abnormalities with poor results after acupuncture treatments. His problems began as "cervical spine and lower back pain." His neck pain was due to whiplash from a head-on automobile collision 35 years ago. He came well-prepared with a long medical report, which he had written himself. Included in the report were visits to multiple doctors, even to the Mayo Clinic. He quoted diagnoses provided by his physicians. "[The conditions] are severe degenerative disease in the lumbosacral spine, and sclerotic changes of the apophyseal joints, particularly in the lower lumbosacral spine. There is also some narrowing of the disc space at the level of L2 and L3. Concave defects are also seen in the inferior aspect of L5, probably representing a

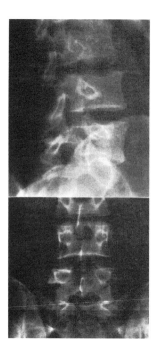

**FIGURE 15.10** Two photos printed from x-ray images brought to us by David on his visit to the clinic.

small Schmorl's node. There is also a break in the pars and interarticularis of L5 bilaterally with no evidence of spondylolisthesis." For the cervical spine, there was "extensive degenerative disease as evidenced by compromise of most of the neural foramina by bony lipins. There are also narrowed disc spaces, particularly most severe at the level of C5 and C6, C6 and C7. There is also an approximately 4 to 5 mm anterior displacement of C3 in relation to C4. Considering the previous history of trauma, this could be well related to a dislocation. Clinical correlation is suggested. The odontoid process is intact." Harry brought us many x-rays, from which we selected two for Figure 15.11. His objective pain was measured as seventh to eighth degree. After 15 treatments, he told us that his subjective pain had eased a little. After just a month or so, his pain returned, and he came back for a few more treatments. His repeated visits led us to conclude that his was a difficult case; his pain will stay with him for the foreseeable future.

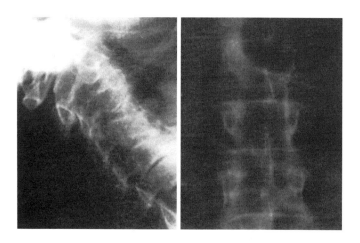

**FIGURE 15.11** X-ray images of Harry's cervical vertebrae.

## 15.8 REFLEX SYMPATHETIC DYSTROPHY

We learn that reflex sympathetic dystrophy (RSD) is also known as minor causalgia, posttraumatic pain syndrome, Sudeck atrophy, and sympathalgia. RSD can be caused by accidental injuries, surgical or other iatrogenic interventions, myocardial infarction, and neurological disorders. Clinical manifestations for RSD include causalgic pain, allodynia, hyperalgesia, hyperesthesia, skeletal muscle hypotonia, and vasomotor and sudomotor disturbances. The symptoms of RSA are graded at three different levels: grade 1 is severe, grade 2 is moderate, and grade 3 is mild. The disease can pass through three stages: the first stage is acute, the second stage is dystrophic, and the third stage is atrophic.

RSD is a rarely seen condition in our clinic. In general, acupuncture treatments will provide poor results, particularly if the disease is at grade 1 or 2, or at its second or third stage. Any single symptom of RSD alone is difficult enough to manage, not to mention a combination of them. To manage all of the symptoms described above for RSA is an impossibility. We can take allodynia as a case in point. Allodynia officially means pain in response to a normally nonpainful stimulus, but essentially, it appears to mean pain all over the entire body. We don't know if allodynia occurs before or after any particular injuries, accidents, or surgeries. Any RSD patient with allodynia must likely have had the pain before they had the disease. Of the few RSD patients we have seen, all were measured to have objective pain at seventh degree or higher. We believe difficult patients with objective pain at that level have allodynia. This fact is the reason that RSD often has poor results. In our opinion, RSD is an extension of old nociceptive disorders and not the beginning of new pain.

## 15.9 TAILBONE FRACTURE

Here, "tailbone" refers to the coccyx. The coccyx can be fractured when a person lands on the buttocks hard enough. The injury can cause pain at the lowest part of the back. This kind of pain is known as coccydynia. If the coccydynia is new and the patient has objective pain lower than fourth degree, acupuncture could produce good to excellent results after three or four treatments. However, if coccydynia is chronic and the patient becomes difficult to treat with a high degree of objective pain to manage, the results can be expected to be poor. The pain will become allodynic, spreading to the anal and genital areas. Inserting needles in any of these areas is not desirable for either the provider or the recipient. There are other factors that make pain in the tailbone difficult to handle, including discomfort in having sexual activities, as confessed by the victims. We have had three patients who suffered from coccydynia.

*Case 1*: Mildred C. was a 66-year-old housewife. She described her pain in the tailbone as "scar tissue from eight deliveries in life." She had been through 25 doctors and many pain pills. Her pain was so bad that she could not sit for any time without discomfort. She could only sleep on her side. Her objective pain was measured to be the 11th degree. After 26 treatments, she still had coccydynia. The benefits she received from acupuncture were that she didn't have to stand all the time and she slept better at nights.

*Case 2*: Joan M. was a 40-year-old psychotherapist. She described her suffering as "coccygeal pain, secondary to hips and pelvis" as the main problem. Her coccydynia began due to back surgery for disc degeneration in the lumbar vertebrae rather than a fall. Our opinion is that her coccydynia was not caused by the surgery, but because she already had seventh degree objective pain by the time of the operation. Her having allodynic pain in multiple locations was triggered by the surgery. Of course, we didn't have scientific evidence to make such a claim. Hopefully, other investigators will conduct clinical research at a future time to prove we are right. When she came for the first time, she was taking Vicodin, Clinoril, and Prednisone. She also had a sleep disorder and had to depend on medications to help her sleep. Other problems diagnosed by her physicians included the connective disease fibrocytis and collagen problems. She told us that she provides consultations to support groups of people with chronic illnesses and disabilities. She had never suggested acupuncture to any of them. Yet, she decided to try the treatment for herself. She had seventh degree objective pain. Her pain subsided for 10 days after six treatments. Of course, we didn't expect to cure her pain, and sure enough, she returned many times later on. We have not found Joan to be a difficult patient because she still had mixed and limited results.

*Case 3*: Kathy S. was a 34-year-old student/waitress/artist. Kathy described her problem as "lower back and tailbone pain." She was injured in a water-skiing accident in 1989, 7 years before seeing us. She went to a chiropractor, who fixed her back pain in one adjustment. In 1994, she fell from a lawn chair and landed on a concrete floor. Without medical consultation, she concluded that her "tailbone was broken." The pain was much more severe than after the skiing accident. The same chiropractor adjustments became useless. Her objective pain was measured as fourth degree. After eight treatments, she continued to have coccydynia but reported significant improvement in the lower back. After 6 months, she returned for her ninth treatment. Asked why she stopped coming, she replied that she had run out of money. We told her that treatments would be free thereafter, and she could visit as many times as necessary to get rid of her pain. She accepted the offer and came for three more treatments before her pain was resolved. Again, we use Kathy as an example to emphasize that similar pain to that of coccydynia can have good to excellent results, if the pain is cared for within a reasonable duration after the injury, and the patient has a low degree of objective pain. If the pain had been sustained for many years, and the patient had become difficult to treat because of a high degree of objective pain, the results of acupuncture treatment will be poor.

## 15.10　DIFFICULT PATIENTS WITH DIFFERENT RESULTS

There are many other kinds of pain that patients complain of when they come seeking help from acupuncture. Examples include multiple sclerosis, lupus erythematosus, itching skin, psoriatic arthritis, erythema multiforme, complications due to silicone breast implants, facial pain after plastic surgery, ulcerative colitis, and Crohn's disease. Some of the symptoms these patients have seem to benefit from acupuncture treatments, whereas some definitely do not. Results of managing their pain vary from excellent to mixed and limited to poor. It will take writing another entire book to describe them all meaningfully.

## 15.11　A FEW AFTERTHOUGHTS

We could write more about acupuncture. This book's basic purpose is to focus attention on pain management through acupuncture treatments. Our own clinical applications also validate that acupuncture is effective for treating allergic problems, nicotine addiction, tinnitus, and vertigo. Very little or nothing is said here about them for several reasons. One of these is unpredictability. Some patients with allergic problems such as rhinitis, sinusitis, asthma, nasal irritation, sneezing, rhinorrhea, nasal congestion, or blockage can be improved, whereas some cannot. We have no way to predict who will be which. Thus, we decided to avoid mentioning these problems. In addition, an overly lengthy book has the potential drawback of boring or wearing out readers. It will be more beneficial for us if readers peruse this book all the way through once they begin it. If they are willing to do so, then we expect a greater possibility for licensed physicians to learn acupuncture. That is the main goal for our spending time in writing this book. Finishing it up required substantial effort. Its purpose is not for financial gain, as a book of this nature is not profitable. Our wish is to see more medical doctors become more willing to perform acupuncture. There are many people suffering from chronic pain in this world, not to mention this country. We are certain acupuncture will be useful to help relieve their pain. From personal experiences and observations, we know for sure that there are many medical professionals who have a desire to learn to practice acupuncture. The question is, where would this opportunity be available?

The answer is: nowhere. As of this writing, no single medical school in the United States offers inculcation in acupuncture. We know there exists the opportunity to take a week's training course in California. One week may be sufficient time to attend many hours of didactic instruction in a classroom using a blackboard. However, ideal teaching and learning acupuncture requires that bedside training is available.

We believe that some review of anatomy will be needed, because in time, most medical school graduates will forget some of the basic sciences they learned in their freshmen year. After reading this book, it will become obvious that having a solid anatomical science background is certainly helpful in learning the acupuncture promulgated in this book. It is also useful to have experience using acupuncture to treat real patients with different kinds of pain. Through many years of offering anatomical acupuncture as an elective, I estimated that I had more than 200 students participate in the elective. None of them took the elective under the circumstances described above. Therefore, as far as I am concerned, their elective is incomplete. I always wonder if any of them had a chance to practice acupuncture after their medical school years. I have not received feedback from any of them. It would be very nice to be able to find out if the acupuncture they learned from me has been in use. My time is past, yet my dream to teach medical professionals to practice acupuncture is still alive. I hope there can be abundant opportunity for physicians to learn acupuncture because practitioners with proper medical training really are in great need in societies where so many people are suffering from the torture of pain.

We also ponder the potential for basic and clinical research in pain. Whether or not a given reader happens to have formal medical education, after reading through the book, it will not be difficult for her or him to realize that there is a great deal of potential to do research following the many phenomena we have observed and described. We believe the subjects of greater potential include:

First, are acupoints and trigger points the same? The difference is in their functional state. Determining whether this observation is accurate will not require elaborate experimental procedures. Anyone can test someone next to them to determine if there are any trigger points detectable.

Second, can trigger points be used for quantifying objective pain in all people? Doing so will certainly require some training and experience. Nevertheless, the testing can be done without question. It is our hope that some investigators are willing to study whether pain is, indeed, measurable.

Third, is it unreasonable to question the conventional way acute and chronic pain have been defined? What would be a reasonable way to distinguish them? We hope our way of differentiating acute from chronic pain will find some supporters in the near future.

Fourth, why is surgery to manage pain effective for some patients, but not for many others? We are sure many concerned surgeons will be curious to know the reasons behind this discrepancy. The answer could be in how much objective pain the patients have.

Fifth, the same speculation can be applied to patients who develop postherpetic neuralgia. Is it possible that patients with a high degree of objective pain will have their herpes infection become postherpetic neuralgia? We are sure that dermatologists will be interested in whether our hypothesis has any basis at all.

Sixth, does any scientist or medical expert really know if pain has memory? Pain is an unfortunate experience. We all want to forget the pain that we suffer. Yet, we feel that pain seems to have memory. Otherwise, why does it keep coming back to haunt the people who have had it before?

Seventh, does a pain grow? If not, why does chronic pain get worse in time, becoming harder to reduce or eradicate? If pain can grow, how can we tell? Could we detect this by an increase in the number of trigger points?

There are many more questions that can be asked in relation to pain and acupuncture. For the time being, those listed above are enough for curious people to ponder. Once we have the answer for any of these questions, we are sure other questions about pain and acupuncture will be asked.

Certainly, we know something about pain and acupuncture, although we do not know all we need to know. Yet, pain will doubtlessly stay with us for the foreseeable future. So will acupuncture, because it is a useful remedy to conquer pain.

One final piece of advice is that if you have pain, go to see your doctor first. If nothing serious is found, such as cancer or a tumor, try to manage your pain through acupuncture as quickly as your time permits. Acupuncture will do no harm; if it doesn't stop your pain, it cannot hurt you more, and you still have many other options to subdue the pain you have. Don't wait for pain to have the chance to grow on you. The longer your pain grows, the harder it will be for you to tackle it in the end.

## 15.12  EDITOR'S AFTERWORD

I have known Dr. Houchi Dung since 1986 or 1987, when I first became acquainted with his elder son and began visiting once a month or so to his home in San Antonio. I have seen his acupuncture clinic grow from a home-based office to its current location. When I initially moved to the city to work for the company his son cofounded, I saw him at his work almost daily.

I learned that after training himself and then his wife in acupuncture, Dr. Dung began growing his practice purely on a word-of-mouth basis; there was never any media advertising. And yet, any time I saw his clinic in operation, it was always busy. Business only continued to grow over the years, regardless of economic trends. He has since moved the clinic to a new, better location, and his younger son has taken over the practice, which still thrives, providing a solid income for his son and his family. The clinic has a phone book listing, but as far as I know, it has still never advertised in the media. Obviously, many people needed (and still need) the service Dr. Dung's acupuncture provides, enough that promoting his services by anything more than word of mouth is practically unnecessary.

For more than 20 years, through three editions of this book, I have seen Dr. Dung quietly crusade for the legitimization of his chosen practice as a proper medical treatment. He knows that acupuncture works to reduce or eliminate many kinds of pain, even if it isn't a miracle cure. His education in anatomical science has allowed him to analyze acupuncture to an extent I believe almost no one else has done. However, for acupuncture to become a proper medical modality, he knows it has to be researched and verified by people with medical science backgrounds. To that end, he has done his best to present to the world at large, and to interested people in the medical community in particular, his personal experiences, observations, and conclusions regarding acupuncture. I have found it worthwhile to aid him in this endeavor.

I speak here as someone with a college education but no medical or anatomical science background. In the course of editing this book (both the first and third editions), I have readily absorbed the basics of how acupuncture seems to work. I have at least some grasp of the principles of afferent and efferent nerves, myelinization, and neural signal transmission. I understand the ideas of primary, secondary, tertiary, and nonspecific acupoints, even if I don't have their locations memorized. I can see clearly from the examples presented that acupuncture works better in some situations than others, and that where it doesn't work, at least it has no ill aftereffects or lasting side effects. Sometimes, the medical terminology has left me a bit confused, but all in all, I believe I understand what this book is saying. If someone like me can understand that much, how much more could an actual doctor, medical school professor, or medical student draw from it? I dearly hope to find out within my lifetime.

## REFERENCES

1. Dung, H.C. Acupuncture for the treatment of postherpetic neuralgia. *American Journal of Acupuncture* 15:5, 1987.
2. Dyck, P.J. et al. *Peripheral Neuropathy,* 2nd edition, vol. I and II. W.B. Saunders Company, Philadelphia, 1984.

3. Eversmann, W.W. *Entrapment Neuropathies. Operative Hand Surgery,* vol. 2, edited by D.P. Green, Churchill Livingstone, New York, 1982.
4. Dawson, D.M. et al. *Entrapment Neuropathies.* Little Brown, Boston, 1984.
5. Sunderland, S. *Nerves and Nerve Injuries,* 2nd ed. Livingstone, Edinburgh, 1978.
6. Carlen, P.L. et al. Phantom limbs and related phenomena in recent traumatic amputations. *Neurology* 28:211, 1978.
7. Abramson, A.S. and A. Feibel. The phantom phenomenon: Its use and disuse. *Bulletin of the New York Academy of Medicine* 57:99, 1981.
8. Heusner, A.P. Phantom genitalia. *Transactions of the American Neurological Association* 75:128, 1950.
9. Bressler, B. et al. Bilateral breast phantom and breast phantom pain. *Journal of Nervous and Mental Disease* 122:315, 1955.
10. Hanowell, S.T. and S.F. Kennedy. Phantom tongue pain and causalgia: Case presentation and treatment. *Anesthesia and Analgesia* 58:436, 1979.
11. Bonica, J.J. *Management of Pain,* 1st ed. Lea & Febiger, Philadelphia, 1953.
12. Roberts, M.E.T. et al. Psoriatic arthritis. *Seminars in Arthritis and Rheumatism* 3:55, 1973.
13. Finneson, B.E. *Low Back Pain.* J.B. Lippincott Company, Philadelphia, 1973.
14. Gailliet, R. *Low Back Pain Syndrome,* 3rd ed. F.A. Davis Company, Philadelphia, 1981.
15. Kirdaldy-Willis, W.H. *Managing Low Back Pain.* Churchill Livingstone, New York, 1983.

# Index

Page numbers followed by f and t indicate figures and tables, respectively.

## A

Abducens nerve, 26
Achilles tendon, 80
    lateral, 80
    medial, 80
Action potential, 87–88
Active phase, acupoints, 91–92
Acupoints
    anatomical positions, 2
    body trunk, 55–67. *See also* Body trunk, acupoints of
    cranial nerves, 25–37. *See also* Cranial nerves
    dynamic nature of, 89–90
    formation, anatomical features contributing, 19–22
        bone foramina, passage through, 20
        concomitant blood vessels, 20–21, 21f
        deep fascia, penetration, 19–20
        depth, 19
        motor point, 20
        nerve fiber compositions, 21
        points of bifurcation, 21
        size, 19
        suture lines on skull, 22
        tendons and ligaments, points on, 21–22, 22f
    identification, 11–12, 22–23, 23f
    neck, 39–42
    phases of
        active phase, 91–92
        latent phase, 90
        passive phase, 90–91
    physical properties of, 92–94
        sensitivity, 92–93
        sequence, 93
        specificity, 93–94
    sensory nerves and, 12–16
    spinal nerve and. *See* Spinal nerve
    upper limb, 43–54
Acupoints in thigh, 76–79
    in lateral compartment, 77–79
        biceps femoris point, 79
        greater trochanter point, 78
        iliotibial tract point, 78
    in posterior compartment, 76–77
        gluteal fold point, 76–77
        inferior gluteal, 77
        posterior femoral cutaneous, 77
Acupoints of anterior compartment of leg, 81–82, 81f
Acupoints of lateral compartment of leg, 80–81
    peroneus brevis, 81
    peroneus longus, 80–81
    peroneus tertius, 81
Acupoints of lumbar plexus, 71–76
    cutaneous branches, 71–75
        anterior femoral cutaneous, 74
        cutaneous of obturator, 73–74
        genitofemoral, 73
        iliohypogastric, 71–72
        ilioinguinal, 70f, 72–73
        lateral femoral cutaneous, 74
        parapatellar, 75
        saphenous, 75
    muscular branches, 75–76
        femoral, 76
        obturator, 75
        rectus femoris, 75
        sartorius, 76
        vastus lateralis, 75–76
        vastus medialis, 76
Acupoints of popliteal fossa, 79
    lateral popliteal point, 79
    medial popliteal point, 79
    sciatic point, 79
Acupoints of posterior compartment of leg and ankle, 79–80
    lateral Achilles, 80
    medial Achilles, 80
    medial sural nerve, 80
    sural point, 80
Acupoints of sacral plexus, 76
Acupoints on foot, 82–85
    dorsal surface of foot, 82–84
        cuboid, 84
        cuneiforms, 83
        deep peroneal, 83
        dorsal digital, 83
        lateral calcaneous, 83
        lateroanterior malleolar, 83
        lateroinferior malleolar, 83
        metatarsal, 83
        superficial peroneal, 83
        talus, 83
    plantar surface of foot, 84–85
        calcaneus, 85
        first metatarsal point, 85
        flexor digitorum longus, 85
        lateral plantar point, 85
        medial calcaneous, 84
        medial plantar point, 85
        medioanterior malleolar, 84
        medioinferior malleolar, 84
        medioposterior malleolar, 84
        navicular point, 85
        plantar point, 85
        tibial point, 84
Acupuncture anesthesia, 7–8
Acupuncture Institute of the Academy of Traditional Chinese Medicine, 2

Acute vs. chronic pain, 146–147. *See also* Pain
Adenosine, 101
Afferent fibers, 16–18. *See also* Efferent fibers
   cranial nerves without acupoints, 25
   for general senses, 17–18, 18f, 58–59
   for special senses, 17
*AfroCubaWeb*, 4
Agonist, 95
*American Journal of Chinese Medicine*, 89
Amino acids as neurotransmitters, 100–101
Amputation, pain after, 213–214, 213f, 214f
Anatomy in acupuncture. *See also* Physiology in acupuncture
   acupoints
      formation, anatomical features contributing, 19–22
      identification, 11–12
   afferent fibers, 16–18
      for general senses, 17–18, 18f
      for special senses, 17
   confusion in presentation, 1–2, 2f
   cutaneous nerve branches, 19
   efferent fibers, 16
      autonomic nervous system, 16
      to skeletal muscles, 16
   general consideration, 11
   muscular nerve branches, 18–19
   overview, 1–9
   sensory nerves, 12–16
      divisions, 16
      histology, 14–16, 14f–15f
      neuron, 13–14, 13f, 14f
      peripheral nervous system, 13
Anesthesia, acupuncture, 7–8
Antagonist, 95
Anterior auricular point, 29f, 30f, 31f, 34
Anterior cutaneous points, 57f, 65–66
Anterior ramus, spinal nerve, 55
Anterior root, spinal nerve, 55
Applications, acupuncture
   body trunk, pain in, 159–163, 160f, 162f, 163f
   face and head, pain in, 152–155
   general guidelines, 149–150, 150t
   lower limb, pain in, 163–166
   with mixed and limited results. *See* Mixed and limited results, applications with
   neck and shoulders, pain in, 155–157, 156f, 157f
   pain for demonstration, 150–151, 151t, 152t
   results, 152
   upper limbs, pain in, 158–159
Arm, acupoints in, 47–52, 48f, 49f
Arthritic neck, 183
Arthritis, inside shoulder joint, 207, 207f
Atopic erythroid skin change, 102, 102f
Auriculotemporal point, 29–30, 29f, 30f
Autonomic nervous system, 16, 57–58
   parasympathetic nerves, 58
   sympathetic nerves, 57–58
Axillary point, 46f, 47–48

**B**

Back pain
   lower, 190–193, 191f, 192f
      after surgery, 210–211, 210f, 211f

Baker's cyst, 166
Bell's palsy, 34, 180, 181f
Bernhardt's disease, 74, 77, 164
Biceps brachii, 47, 48f
Biceps femoris point, 79
Biceps tendinitis, 185–186, 185f
Biochemistry in acupuncture
   agonist, 95
   antagonist, 95
   endorphin, importance of, 97–98
   granules, 96
   immediate acupuncture reactions, 101–103
      atopic erythroid skin change, 102, 102f
      sweating, 102–103
      syncope, 103
   neuromuscular junction, 96
   neuroreceptor, 95
   neurotransmitters. *See* Neurotransmitters
   overview, 95
   reactions after acupuncture
      drowsiness and sleeplessness, 104–105
      flare-up of pain, 104, 105f
      parasympathetic enhancement, 105
   synapse, 96
Blood circulation, poor
   endogenous origins, 109
Body trunk
   acupoints of, 55–67
   back of, distributions of acupoints, 59
   pain in, 159–163, 160f, 162f, 163f, 188–193
Bone foramina, 20
Brachial plexus, organization of, 43–44, 44f
Bregma point, 30f, 32
Bunions, 83, 85

**C**

Calcaneus fasciatis, 85
Cannon, Walter B., 121
Carpal tunnel syndrome, 186–188, 207–208
Catecholamines, 98–99
Chest
   dorsal surface of, acupoints on, 61–63, 62f
      posterior cutaneous points, 61, 62f
      thoracic spinal process, 62f, 63
Chest cage, lateral side of
   intercostobrachial point, 67, 67f
   lateral cutaneous nerve, 56f, 66–67
Chest cage point, angle of, 57f, 66
Chronic vs. acute pain, 146–147. *See also* Pain
Concomitant blood vessels, 20–21, 21f
Conductivity, 88
Connective tissue, acupoints of, 30–33, 31f, 32f
   Bregma point, 30f, 32
   coronal suture point, 32
   nasion point, 32
   pterion point, 30f, 32
   temporomandibular point, 29f, 32–33
Coronal suture point, 32
Cranial nerves
   acupoints of, 25–37
      facial nerve, 34–35
      glossopharyngeal nerve, 35
      spinal accessory nerve, 36–37

# Index

trigeminal nerve, 26–34. *See also* Trigeminal nerve, acupoints of
vagus nerve, 29f, 35–36, 36f
without acupoints, 25–26
  abducens nerve, 26
  hypoglossal nerve, 26
  oculomotor nerve, 26
  olfactory nerve, 25
  optic nerve, 25
  statoacoustic nerve, 25
  trochlear nerve, 26
Cupoints on foot, 85
Cutaneous branches of lumbar plexus, acupoints of, 71–75
  anterior femoral cutaneous, 74
  cutaneous of obturator, 73–74
  genitofemoral, 73
  iliohypogastric, 71–72
  ilioinguinal, 70f, 72–73
  lateral femoral cutaneous, 74
  parapatellar, 75
  saphenous, 75
Cutaneous branches of trigeminal nerve, acupoints of, 28–30, 28f
  arm and forearm, 50–51
  auriculotemporal point, 29–30, 29f, 30f
  infraorbital point, 29, 30f
  infratrochlear point, 28, 30f
  lacrimal point, 29, 30f
  mental point, 29, 30f
  neck, 40–42, 41f
  paranasal point, 30, 30f, 31f
  supraorbital point, 28, 30f
  supratrochlear point, 28, 30f
  wrist and hand, 54
  zygomaticofacial point, 29, 30f
  zygomaticotemporal point, 29, 30f
Cutaneous nerve branches, 19
  spinal nerve, 55–56, 56f, 57f

## D

Deep fascia, penetration, 19–20
Deep radial nerve, acupoint for, 49f, 50
Deformities, pain and, 208–209, 209f
Degeneration, endogenous origins, 109–110
Deltoid, acupoint for, 46f, 49
Deltoid ligament, 84
Diabetic peripheral neuropathy, 84
Difficult patients
  face and neck, pain in, 203–206, 204t, 205f
  pain after surgery, 209–213, 210f, 211f, 212f
  phantom limb pain, 213–214, 213f, 214f
  with poor results, 201–220
  profiles of, 201–203, 202t
  RSD, 217
  spondylitic abnormalities, 214–216, 216f
  tailbone fracture, 217–218
Dorsal root, spinal nerve, 55
Dorsal scapular nerve, 45–46, 46f
Dorsal surface of foot, 82–84
  cuboid, 84
  cuneiforms, 83
  deep peroneal, 83
  dorsal digital, 83

lateral calcaneous, 83
lateroanterior malleolar, 83
lateroinferior malleolar, 83
metatarsal, 83
superficial peroneal, 83
talus, 83
Drowsiness after acupuncture, 104–105

## E

Efferent fibers, 16. *See also* Afferent fibers
  autonomic nervous system, 16. *See also* Autonomic nervous system
  cranial nerves without acupoints, 26
  to skeletal muscles, 16, 57
Electrical activity in acupoints, 88–89
Electrical phenomena of body, 87–88
  action potential, 87–88
  conductivity, 88
  excitability, 87
  fatigue, 88
  polarization, 87–88
  threshold, 88
Endogenous origins, pathology in acupuncture, 107–110. *See also* Exogenous origins, pathology in acupuncture
  degeneration, 109–110
  hormonal imbalances, 108–109
  infections, 110
  poor blood circulation, 109
Endorphin, importance of, 97–98
*Essentials of Chinese Acupuncture*, 2
Excitability, 87
Exogenous origins, pathology in acupuncture, 110–111. *See also* Endogenous origins, pathology in acupuncture

## F

Face
  pain in, 152–155, 174–181, 203–206, 204t, 205f
  postherpetic neuralgia in, 179–180, 180f, 181f
Facial nerve, 34–35. *See also* Cranial nerves
Fascia lata, 74
Fatigue, 88
Femoral cutaneous, posterior, 77
Flare-up of pain, after acupuncture, 104, 105f
Foot, acupoints on, 82–85
  dorsal surface of foot, 82–84
    cuboid, 84
    cuneiforms, 83
    deep peroneal, 83
    dorsal digital, 83
    lateral calcaneous, 83
    lateroanterior malleolar, 83
    lateroinferior malleolar, 83
    metatarsal, 83
    superficial peroneal, 83
    talus, 83
  plantar surface of foot, 84–85
    calcaneus, 85
    first metatarsal point, 85
    flexor digitorum longus, 85
    lateral plantar point, 85

medial calcaneous, 84
medial plantar point, 85
medioanterior malleolar, 84
medioinferior malleolar, 84
medioposterior malleolar, 84
navicular point, 85
plantar point, 85
tibial point, 84
Foot, pain in, 197–198, 197f
Foramina, bone, 20
Forearm, acupoints in, 47–52, 48f, 49f
Fracture, tailbone, 217–218
Front of body, distributions of acupoints, 59

## G

Glossopharyngeal nerve, 35. *See also* Cranial nerves, acupoints of
Gluteal fold point, 76–77
Granules, 96
Greater auricular point, 40, 41f
Greater occipital nerve, 60–61, 60f
Greater trochanter point, 78

## H

Hammer toe, 83
Hand, acupoints, 52–54, 53f
Head
    pain in, 152–155, 174–181
    postherpetic neuralgia in, 179–180, 180f, 181f
*Heku*, 4
Hip replacement, pain after, 212–213, 212f
Histamine, 99–100
Histology, of nerves, 14–16, 14f–15f. *See also* Sensory nerves
Hormonal imbalances, endogenous origins, 108–109
Hunter's canal, 75, 76
Hypoglossal nerve, 26

## I

Iliotibial tract point, 74, 78
Ilitibial tract, acupoints along, 78f
Infections, endogenous origins, 110
Inferior gluteal, 77
Infertile pregnancy, 170–172, 170f, 171f
Infraorbital foramina, 20
Infraorbital point, 29, 30f
Infratrochlear point, 28, 30f
Intercostobrachial point, 23, 23f, 67, 67f
Interphalangeal joints, 83
Interphalangeal points, 54

## K

Knee pain, 164–166, 196–197, 196f

## L

Lacrimal point, 29, 30f
Lane, Kamala, 6
Latent phase, acupoints, 90

Lateral antebrachial cutaneous nerve, 49f, 51
Lateral brachial cutaneous nerve, 49f, 50–51
Lateral cutaneous nerve of chest cage, 56f, 66–67
Lateral popliteal point, 79
Lateral side, body
    distributions of acupoints, 59, 59f
Leg, acupoints of anterior compartment of, 81–82, 81f
Leg, acupoints of lateral compartment of, 80–81
    peroneus brevis, 81
    peroneus longus, 80–81
    peroneus tertius, 81
Leg and ankle, acupoints of posterior compartment of, 79–80
    lateral Achilles, 80
    medial Achilles, 80
    medial sural nerve, 80
    sural point, 80
Lesser occipital point, 40–41, 41f
Ligaments, acupoints, 21–22, 22f, 51–52. *See also* Acupoints
Lower back pain, 190–193, 191f, 192f
    after surgery, 210–211, 210f, 211f
Lower limb, pain in, 163–166, 193–198, 193f, 194f, 195f
    Bernhardt disease, 164
    region of knee joint, 164–166
Lumbar and sacral regions, acupoints on, 63–65, 63f, 64f
    lumbar spinous processes, 62f, 65
    posterior cutaneous of lumbar spinal nerves, 64, 64f
    posterior cutaneous of sacral spinal nerves, 63f, 65
    superior cluneal, 63f, 65
Lumbar plexus, 69, 70f
Lumbar plexus, acupoints of, 71–76
    cutaneous branches, 71–75
        anterior femoral cutaneous, 74
        cutaneous of obturator, 73–74
        genitofemoral, 73
        iliohypogastric, 71–72
        ilioinguinal, 72–73
        lateral femoral cutaneous, 74
        parapatellar, 75
        saphenous, 75
    muscular branches, 75–76
        femoral, 76
        obturator, 75
        rectus femoris, 75
        sartorius, 76
        vastus lateralis, 75–76
        vastus medialis, 76
Lumbar spinal nerves, posterior cutaneous of, 64, 64f
Lumbar spinous processes, acupoints on, 62f, 65

## M

Mandibular division, trigeminal nerve, 27, 27f
Masseter point, 33, 33f
Mathew, Roy J., 122
Maxillary division, trigeminal nerve, 27, 27f
Medial antebrachial cutaneous nerve, 49f, 51
Medial brachial cutaneous nerve, 49f, 51
Medial popliteal point, 79
Medial sural nerve, 80

# Index

Median point, 47, 48f
Menstrual cramping, 76
Mental foramina, 20
Mental point, 29, 30f
Meralgia paraesthetica, 164
Migraine, 174–177, 203. *See also* Head, pain in
Mixed and limited results, applications with
    body trunk, pain in, 188–193
    diffuse pain, 198–199
    face and head, pain in, 174–181
    irrelevant to pain, 168–172
        infertile pregnancy, 170–172, 170f, 171f
        weight reduction, 168–170, 169f
    lower limb, pain in, 193–198
    neck and shoulder, pain in, 182–183
    subjective pain perceived, 172–174
    in terms of number of treatments, 168
    in terms of pain relief and relapse, 168
    in terms of patient profiles, 167
    upper limb, pain in, 184–188
Morton's neuroma, 83, 85, 166
Motor nerves, 18. *See also* Muscular nerve
Motor point, 20
Muscular branches, 75–76
    acupoints of
        anterior auricular point, 29f, 30f, 31f, 34
        arm and forearm, 47–50
        Masseter point, 33, 33f
        superior auricular point, 30f, 31f, 34
        temporalis point, 30f, 33f, 34
        wrist and hand, 53–54
    acupoints of, neck, 42
    femoral, 76
    obturator, 75
    rectus femoris, 75
    sartorius, 76
    spinal nerve, 55
    vastus lateralis, 75–76
    vastus medialis, 76
Muscular nerve branches, 18–19

## N

Nasion point, 32
National Commission of Acupuncture, 4
Neck
    acupoints, 39–42
        boundaries of neck, 39
        cervical plexus, formation of, 39, 40f
        cutaneous branches, 40–42
        muscular branches, 42
    back of, distributions of acupoints, 60–61
        greater occipital nerve, 60–61, 60f
        third occipital nerve, 60f, 61
    pain in, 155–157, 156f, 157f, 182–183, 203–206, 204t, 205f
Nerve fiber, compositions, 21
Nervous system, organization of, 12. *See also* Peripheral nervous system
Neuroactive peptides, 100
Neuromuscular junction, 96
Neuron, 1, 13–14, 13f, 14f. *See also* Sensory nerves
Neuroreceptor, 95

Neurotransmitters
    adenosine, 101
    amino acids as, 100–101
    catecholamines, 98–99
    histamine, 99–100
    neuroactive peptides, 100
    relevance of, 96–97
    serotonin, 99
    terminologies in, 95–96
Nonspecific trigger points, 136, 138t, 139f. *See also* Trigger points

## O

Objective pain, 107. *See also* Pain
    *vs.* subjective pain, 130–131
Oculomotor nerve, 26
Olfactory nerve, 25
Ophthalmic division, trigeminal nerve, 27, 27f
Optic nerve, 25

## P

Pain
    after surgery, 209–213, 210f, 211f, 212f
        hip replacement, 212–213, 212f
        lower back pain, 210–211, 210f, 211f
    body trunk, 159–163, 160f, 162f, 163f, 188–193
    deformities and, 208–209, 209f
    for demonstration, sample of, 150–151, 151t, 152t
    diffuse pain, 198–199
    face, 152–155, 174–181, 203–206, 204t, 205f
    flare-up, after acupuncture, 104, 105f
    foot, 197–198, 197f
    head, 152–155, 174–181
    knee joint region, 164–166
    lower limb, 163–166, 193–198
    measurement, 129–147. *See also* Trigger points
        acute *vs.* chronic pain, 146–147
        challenge, 129
        results of, 139–146, 141t, 143t, 144f, 145f
        subjective pain *vs.* objective pain, 130–131
    mental attitude toward, 125–126, 126f
    neck, 155–157, 156f, 157f, 182–183, 203–206, 204t, 205f
    perception, historical prospect of, 124, 125f
    phantom limb pain, 213–214, 213f, 214f
    postamputation, 213–214, 213f, 214f
    psychology of, 121–124
    shoulder, 155–157, 156f, 157f, 182–183
    subjective pain perceived, 172–174
    upper limb, 158–159, 184–188
    vicious cycle of, 127–128, 127f
Paranasal point, 30, 30f, 31f
Parapatellar points, 75
Parasympathetic enhancement, after acupuncture, 105
Parasympathetic nerves, 58. *See also* Autonomic nervous system
Park, Alice, 123
Passive phase, acupoints, 90–91
Pathology in acupuncture
    endogenous origins, 107–110

degeneration, 109–110
hormonal imbalances, 108–109
infections, 110
poor blood circulation, 109
exogenous origins, 110–111
overview, 107
pathological origins, 107
trigger points appearance, modes for, 111–115
combination of systemic and regional appearances, 115, 116f–117f
regional appearance, 114–115
systemic appearance, 112–114
Pectoral region, acupoints on, 44, 45f
Peripheral nervous system, 13. *See also* Sensory nerves
Peroneus brevis, 81
Peroneus longus, 80–81
Peroneus tertius, 81
Phantom limb pain, 213–214, 213f, 214f
Phases, acupoints, 90–92
Physiology in acupuncture. *See also* Anatomy in acupuncture
dynamic nature of acupoints, 89–90
electrical activity in acupoints, 88–89
electrical phenomena of body, 87–88
action potential, 87–88
conductivity, 88
excitability, 87
fatigue, 88
polarization, 87–88
threshold, 88
phases of acupoints, 90–92
physical properties of acupoints, 92–94
Piriformis syndrome, 77
Plantar surface of foot, 84–85
calcaneus, 85
first metatarsal point, 85
flexor digitorum longus, 85
lateral plantar point, 85
medial calcaneous, 84
medial plantar point, 85
medioanterior malleolar, 84
medioinferior malleolar, 84
medioposterior malleolar, 84
navicular point, 85
plantar point, 85
tibial point, 84
Polarization, 87–88
Popliteal fossa, acupoints of, 79
lateral popliteal point, 79
medial popliteal point, 79
sciatic point, 79
Postamputation pain, 213–214, 213f, 214f
Posterior antebrachial cutaneous nerve, 49f, 51
Posterior brachial cutaneous nerve, 49f, 50
Posterior cutaneous nerve, 55, 56f
Posterior cutaneous points, 61, 62f
Posterior femoral cutaneous point, 77
Posterior interosseus nerve, 49f, 50
Posterior ramus, spinal nerve, 55
Posterior root, spinal nerve, 55
Postganglionic sympathetic nerves, 19
Postherpetic neuralgia, 188–190, 188t, 189f, 190f, 203–206, 204t, 205f
in face and head, 179–180, 180f, 181f

Primary rami, spinal nerve, 55
Primary trigger points, 132t, 133, 133f. *See also* Trigger points
Psychology in acupuncture, 121–128. *See also* Pain
acupuncture as placebo, 128
pain, 121–123
mental attitude toward, 125–126, 126f
perception, historical prospect of, 124, 125f
vicious cycle of pain, 127–128, 127f
Pterion point, 30f, 32
Pudendal nerve, 77

## R

Radial nerve, acupoint for, 49–50, 49f
Radiocarpal joint, 186
Reactions
acupuncture, immediate
atopic erythroid skin change, 102, 102f
sweating, 102–103
syncope, 103
after acupuncture
drowsiness and sleeplessness, 104–105
flare-up of pain, 104, 105f
parasympathetic enhancement, 105
Recurrent of median, 53
Reflex sympathetic dystrophy (RSD), 217
Regional anatomy, 69
Regional appearance, trigger points, 114–115
RSD. *See* Reflex sympathetic dystrophy (RSD)

## S

Sacral plexus, acupoints of, 71f, 76
Sacral spinal nerve plexus, 69–71
Sacral spinal nerves, posterior cutaneous of, 63f, 65
*San Antonio Express/News*, 6
Scapular region, acupoints over, 45–47, 46f
dorsal scapular nerve, 45–46, 46f
infraspinatus or suprascapular I nerve, 46–47, 46f
supraspinatus or suprascapular II nerve, 46, 46f
Sciatic point, 79
Secondary trigger points, 133–134, 134t, 135f. *See also* Trigger points
Sensitivity, acupoints, 92–93
Sensory nerves, 12–16
divisions, 16
histology, 14–16, 14f–15f
nervous system, organization of, 12
neuron, 13–14, 13f, 14f
peripheral nervous system, 13
Sequence, acupoints, 93
Serotonin, 99
Sheon, Robert P., 122
Shoulders, pain in, 155–157, 156f, 157f, 182–183
*Sibai*, 4
Simons, David G., 121
Skeletal muscles, efferent fibers to, 16, 57
Skull, suture lines on, 22
Sleeplessness after acupuncture, 104–105
Specificity, acupoints, 93–94
Spinal accessory nerve, 36–37. *See also* Cranial nerves, acupoints of

# Index

Spinal nerve, 56f
  composition of fibers, 57–59
    afferent fibers for general senses, 58–59
    autonomic nervous system, 57–58. *See also* Autonomic nervous system
    efferent fibers to skeletal muscles, 57
  cutaneous nerves with terminal branches, 55–56, 56f, 57f
  distributions of acupoints, 59
    back of body trunk, 59
    back of neck, 60–61
    dorsal surface of chest, 61–63, 62f
    front of body trunk, 59
    lateral side, 59, 59f
    lumbar and sacral regions, 63–65, 63f, 64f
  muscular branches, 55
  primary rami, 55
  roots, 55
Spinous processes, trigger points on, 136–139, 140f, 141f, 141t
Spondylitic abnormalities, 214–216, 216f
Statoacoustic nerve, 25
*Stedman's Medical Dictionary*, 182
Subjective pain. *See also* Pain
  perceived, 172–174
  *vs.* objective pain, 130–131
Superficial radial nerve, 54
Superior auricular point, 30f, 31f, 34
Superior cluneal point, 63f, 65
Supraclavicular point, 41f, 42
Supraorbital foramina, 20
Supraorbital point, 28, 30f
Suprascapular II nerve, 46, 46f
Suprascapular I nerve, 46–47, 46f
Supratrochlear point, 28, 30f
Sural nerve, medial, 80
Sural point, 80
Suture lines on skull, 22
Sweating, acupuncture reactions and, 102–103
Sympathetic nerves, 57–58. *See also* Autonomic nervous system
Synapse, 96
Syncope, acupuncture reactions and, 103
Systemic appearance, trigger points, 112–114

## T

Tailbone fracture, 217–218
Tarsal tunnel syndrome, 85
Teaching and learning, acupuncture
  obstacles in, 4
Temporalis point, 30f, 33f, 34
Temporomandibular point, 29f, 32–33
Tendons, acupoints, 21–22, 22f, 51–52, 52f, 53f. *See also* Acupoints
Teres minor, 46f, 48
Tertiary trigger points, 135, 136t, 137f. *See also* Trigger points
Theory of *qi*, 8
Thigh, acupoints in, 76–79
  in lateral compartment, 77–79
    biceps femoris point, 79
    greater trochanter point, 78
    iliotibial tract point, 78
  in posterior compartment, 76–77
    gluteal fold point, 76–77
    inferior gluteal, 77
    posterior femoral cutaneous, 77
Third occipital nerve, 60f, 61
Thoracic spinal process, acupoints of, 62f, 63
Threshold, 88
Tic douloureux. *See* Trigeminal neuralgia
Torticollis in perpetual motion, 206–207, 206f
Transverse cervical point, 41, 41f
Travell, Janet G., 121
Trigeminal nerve, acupoints of, 26–34. *See also* Cranial nerves, acupoints of
  connective tissue, 30–33, 31f, 32f
  cutaneous branches, 28–30, 28f, 29f, 30f, 31f
  cutaneous nerve supply, 27, 27f
  mandibular division, 27, 27f
  maxillary division, 27, 27f
  muscular branches, 30f, 31f, 33–34, 33f
  ophthalmic division, 27, 27f
Trigeminal neuralgia, 177–179, 178t
Trigger points, 107. *See also* Acupoints
  appearance, modes for
    combination of systemic and regional appearances, 115, 116f–117f
    regional appearance, 114–115
    systemic appearance, 112–114
  in four groups, 132–136
    nonspecific points, 136, 138t, 139f
    primary points, 132t, 133, 133f
    secondary points, 133–134, 134t, 135f
    tertiary points, 135, 136t, 137f
  ranking, 131–132, 131t, 132t
  on spinous processes, 136–139, 140f, 141f, 141t
Trochlear nerve, 26
*Tsusanli*, 89

## U

Ulnar nerve, 54
Umbilical point, 57f, 66
Upper limb
  acupoints, 43–54
    arm and forearm, 47–52, 48f, 49f
    over scapular region, 45–47, 46f
    on pectoral region, 44, 45f
    wrist and hand, 52–54, 53f
  brachial plexus, organization of, 43–44, 44f
  pain in, 158–159, 184–188, 184f
  topography of, 43

## V

Vagus nerve, 29f, 35–36, 36f. *See also* Cranial nerves
Ventral root, spinal nerve, 55

## W

Wallis, Claudia, 122–123
*Wall Street Journal*, 8
Weight reduction, 168–170, 169f
Whiplash, 182–183
Wrist, acupoints, 52–54, 53f

## X

Xiphoid point, 57f, 66

## Y

*Yang*, 8
*Yifeng*, 4
*Yin*, 8

## Z

*Zanzhu*, 4
Zygomaticofacial foramina, 20
Zygomaticofacial point, 29, 30f
Zygomaticotemporal foramina, 20
Zygomaticotemporal point, 29, 30f